D1430738

THE GREAT DOCTORS

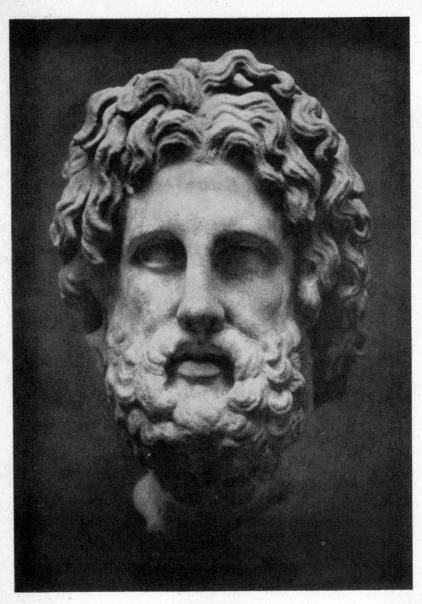

AESCULAPIUS

DR·HENRY·E·SIGERIST

PROFESSOR OF THE HISTORY OF MEDICINE
THE JOHNS HOPKINS UNIVERSITY

THE GREAT
DOCTORS

A BIOGRAPHICAL HISTORY
OF MEDICINE

Translated by Eden and Cedar Paul

DOVER PUBLICATIONS, INC.
NEW YORK

Published in Canada by General Publishing
Company, Ltd., 30 Lesmill Road, Don Mills,
Toronto, Ontario.

Published in the United Kingdom by Constable
and Company, Ltd., 10 Orange Street, London WC 2.

This Dover edition, first published in 1971, is an
unabridged republication of the English translation
originally published by W. W. Norton & Company,
Inc. in 1933.

International Standard Book Number: 0-486-22696-4
Library of Congress Catalog Card Number: 78-143674

Manufactured in the United States of America
Dover Publications, Inc.
180 Varick Street
New York, N. Y. 10014

*To the Unknown Doctor
who in unselfish and inconspicuous activities
fulfils the teachings of the Great Doctors
I dedicate this book*

CONTENTS

CONTENTS

ILLUSTRATIONS

ILLUSTRATIONS

PREFACE TO THE FIRST EDITION

DOUBTS assail me as I begin this book. I propose to write of great doctors, their lives and their work. But there has been such a multitude of great doctors, who were great doctors because, animated by the sacred fire of their mission, self-sacrificing in their daily doings, they helped numberless suffering fellow-creatures in bitter need. They dried many tears, brought much happiness, rendered bountiful achievements possible, by breaking the chains of illness.

When we look back into the past, we see an endless train of doctors on the march. Their dress, their language, their social position varies; their outlooks and their methods change from age to age. Some have a urine-glass in their hands, others a stethoscope. Yet one and all, from the shamans of primitive tribes down to the scientific physicians of our own day, are inspired by the same will. They seek the same goal and are guided by the same idea. Many of them have been veritably great.

But history has forgotten them. They lived their allotted span, and then they died. For a space the remembrance of them survived in the minds of those to whom they had brought help and healing. Then these too passed away, and a new generation grew. A name in the records of a university or a learned society, a date or two—what else is left of most to-day? They have suffered the same fate as the actor, the musician, who for many successive evenings were able to delight an audience, to make spectators forget their troubles—only to sink back into the waters of oblivion.

Posterity weaves garlands for those alone whose work has been creative. No doctors live on in the memory save the exceptional beings who enriched the healing art with new outlooks, who forged new weapons for the fight against disease. We remember those choice spirits who, becoming aware of divine thoughts that were still inchoate, were able, by strenuous labour, to make them generally known and practically applicable. It is only of such great doctors that I can write. Even of these there is no scarcity. Many hands have collaborated in upbuilding the edifice of medicine. Multiform energies have been requisite to make the leading principles of our science available for general use. I have, therefore, to concentrate; and have been compelled, in each epoch, to restrict my attention to a small number of doctors—to those whose activities were vital to the development of medicine; to those who incorporated a trend, founded a school, represented an era. The reader will miss name after name he might have expected me to mention. He must remember that the plan of my work excluded anything more than a passing allusion to the names of the living, and that for this reason an account of a number of momentous discoveries and important movements had to be omitted. Recent developments in psychological medicine, for instance. Besides, I did not aim at encyclopaedic completeness. I am content to bring into the limelight certain basic evolutionary tendencies in the science and art of medicine.

Is there anything uncongenial about a record in which no reference is made to any other than supreme achievements? Must we not feel that there is a great gulf fixed between ourselves and the pathfinders of medicine? No; for, throughout the centuries, we and they are linked by our common physicianship. One and all, in their several places, at the bedside or in the laboratory or at the writing-desk, were doctors. They were advancing towards the same goal as ourselves, pioneers on the road along which we of to-day still travel. We are about to study the life of each one of them, with its peaks and its valleys; to learn that, like us, they fought and suffered and erred, that, like us, they experienced joy and sorrow. To a large extent we shall recognise our own images in them. The fact that they were privileged to reach supreme heights makes them our masters and exemplars, the thought of whom can encourage and invigorate us when the trivialities of the daily round are tending to dim our faith in the splendour of our calling.

Bach and Mozart would be dead for ever, were it not for the living artists who are perpetually reviving their melodies. Pasteur and Koch would have lived in vain but for the everyday practitioners through whose activities their teachings are made effective. It is not so much the great theoreticians upon whom the health of the community depends, as the huge army of family doctors who succour the ailing from hour to hour.

That is why, at the outset of this book which is devoted to the creative masters of the healing art, I have in mind, above all, the practising physician and his labours. It is chiefly for him that these pages are written. To the "unknown doctor," *Great Doctors* is dedicated.

HENRY E. SIGERIST

LEIPZIG
   January 1931

PREFACE TO THE SECOND EDITION

IN this edition, called for within a year, and appearing simultaneously with the English translation, few changes have been made. These mainly consist in trifling emendations, but a new chapter has been added concerning William Osler. The author has been greatly encouraged by the cordial welcome given to his book.

HENRY E. SIGERIST

BALTIMORE
January 1933

GREAT DOCTORS

CHAPTER ONE

IMHOTEP AND AESCULAPIUS

ONCE upon a time (the story begins like a fairy tale) there was a wise minister of State, Imhotep by name, faithful servant of Zoser, the pharaoh who ruled the land of Egypt in the opening of the third millennium before Christ. He was a man of great learning, and skilled in all the arts of his day. For seven years in succession the annual inundation of the Nile failed to occur, and famine was widespread throughout the land. Imhotep, however, knew where to seek counsel. Studying the sacred books, he learned which were the gods that had charge of the sources of the Nile. The needful sacrifices were made, and, that night, the ram-headed god Chnum, the god of cataracts, appearing to Pharaoh in a dream, promised that thenceforward the Nile should fertilise Egypt as of old. It was with a light heart that the king awakened in the morning, and with the next harvest prosperity returned.

Son of an architect, Imhotep was an expert in that craft, and it was probably he who designed for his master's tomb the Step Pyramid at Sakkara which still stands after all these years and is believed to be the oldest pyramid in Egypt. It was also in accordance with Imhotep's designs that a temple dedicated to the god Horus was erected at Edfu.

In addition Imhotep was the priest who acted as reader to the king, was conductor of the sacred ritual, was an astronomer, and, last not least, a physician.

When he died, Imhotep was buried not far from his royal master in the mausoleum at Memphis. Though dead, he lived on in men's memories as one who had been a sage, kind of heart, and always ready to succour his fellows. The words of wisdom he had uttered became traditional. Every scribe made an oblation to Imhotep before beginning his work. In death as in life, Imhotep was sought by the sick in need of help, for his tomb became a place of pilgrimage where wonderful cures were wrought.

Thus his fame grew from century to century. Temples were dedicated to him. To these, patients in search of health flocked in ever-increasing numbers. From being a mortal, thought almost worthy of divine honours, Imhotep came at length to be regarded as a god, as the Egyptian god of healing. Now he was honoured as the first-born son of Ptah and Sekhmet, being regarded as able, not only to cure the sick, but also to make barren women bear children and to bring happiness to the unfortunate. Memphis remained the chief centre of his worship. In his temple, doctors were trained for the practice of their profession. The Ptolemies, the Greek kings of Egypt, consecrated a new shrine to Imhotep upon the island of Philae, a shrine which is in part still extant. Six times a year, festivals were held in commemoration of important incidents in his life.

Thus did the sage of those early days become transformed into a god of healing, so that it was natural for the Hellenes who visited Egypt to identify him with their own god of healing Aesculapius. Imhotep and Aesculapius were fused into the joint personality of "Imuthes-Asklepios." The temple at Memphis was styled the Asklepion. Nevertheless, though alike in function, the two gods of healing are markedly contrasted. Imhotep was a mortal who had been deified, whereas Aesculapius was a purely mythical deity whom human fancy had brought down to earth.

Or, rather, I should say that Aesculapius was a deity who had been brought forth from the depths of the earth. Originating in Thessaly, he had there been a subterranean elemental, his companion a serpent which likewise dwelt in a deep cleft. He was also accompanied by a hound.

Earth is the prime mother of all living creatures, nourishing them and healing them. He who has been wounded in the battles of life, who has been wearied by its struggles, lies on the earth for refreshment. He sleeps, and Aesculapius or the serpent of the god of healing appears to him in a dream. Thus he is made whole.

With the Thessalians the god migrated to the south and to the east, to the Peloponnesus and to Cos.

In Homer, Aesculapius appears as a Thessalian prince, whose sons Podalirius and Machaon are skilled in the medical art—as, indeed, though to a less extent, are all the Homeric heroes.

It is in Hesiod, however, that we find the old Thessalian saga. Apollo, one day, surprised Coronis—a virgin of the Lapithae—bathing in Lake Boebeis. He conceived a passion for her and possessed her. She became with child, but her father had chosen a husband for her, her cousin Ischus. What could she do but obey her father's will? The raven, Apollo's spy, brought news of the marriage. The wrathful god's first thought was to punish the bearer of evil tidings, and the bird which had hitherto been white bore thenceforward the hue of mourning. Ischus was slain by the arrows of Apollo, while the darts of Artemis laid Coronis and her innocent playmates low. Then, as Apollo contemplated the dead body of Coronis on the funeral pyre, he was struck with compassion for his unborn son, liberated the infant from the mother's womb, and took the babe to Mount Pelion, to the cave of Chiron the Centaur. There Aesculapius grew to manhood, learning from his wise tutor (half man, half horse) which plants had healing virtues, and many a charm that could cure illness. Thus he became a physician, greatly sought after. In the pride of his power, he ventured to transgress the laws of nature and to bring the dead back to life. Pluto, Lord of the underworld, complained that Hades was being depopulated, and thereupon Zeus slew Aesculapius with a thunderbolt.

This legend gives fine expression to the view that the healing art is essentially presumptuous, that the physician errs by interfering with the course of nature. To the men of old it always seemed necessary to find some peculiar justification for the work of the physician.

The first altars established in honour of Aesculapius were simple, under the open sky, or in caves; but, as the centuries passed, temples were built in his honour all over Greece, and especially in Epidaurus. There was a good reason why this town should have become the chief centre of the cult of Aesculapius, since, according to local legends, Coronis, when with child, had visited the place with her father. It was here that she had secretly given birth to Aesculapius, and she had abandoned the fruit of her womb, leaving the infant in a grove of myrtles. A goat had suckled the babe, and consequently the myrtle-crowned hill bears to this day the name of Titthion, the Hill of Teats. A hound kept watch over the infant. When Aresthanas the herdsman counted his flock, he found that one was missing, and also that his hound had vanished. Searching, he discovered the she-goat and the hound, together with the little boy. He stooped to lift the child, whereupon lightning flashed. Then he knew that this new-born baby must be of divine origin. Swiftly, the news spread over land and seas that Aesculapius could cure all illnesses and could even bring the dead back to life.

One who to-day walks along the road leading inland through vineyards from the seaport of Nauplia enters a valley in which he sees mighty ruins. They are the remains of the temple of Epidaurus, the most noted shrine of Aesculapius. Near by are the vestiges of a theatre, one of the finest of those which have survived from antiquity. So splendid, indeed, are these ruins that even Romans, familiar with an abundance of such relics, are amazed at them. For hours the traveller can wander among

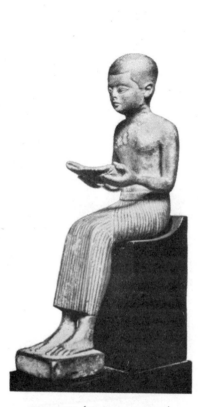 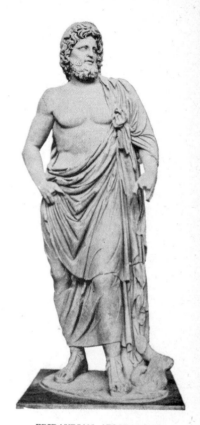

IMHOTEP (BERLIN MUSEUM) EPIDAURIAN AESCULAPIUS
(NATIONAL MUSEUM AT ATHENS)

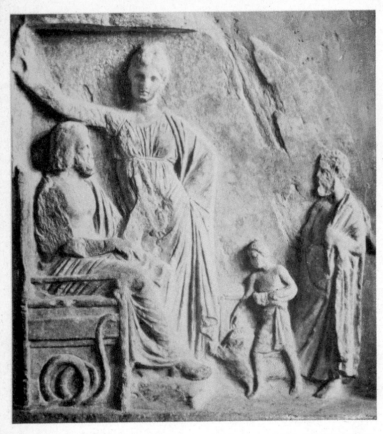

AESCULAPIUS, HYGIEIA, AND WORSHIPPERS, A VOTIVE TABLET FROM
THE ATHENIAN ASCLEPION (NATIONAL MUSEUM AT ATHENS)

the pediments where once statues stood, and among the marble baths. The pavement of the consecrated roadway is still discernible, and the lineaments of the ancient place of worship begin to rebuild themselves before the eyes of the imagination. As of old the sun smites pitilessly, Apollo sending his shafts upon the shrine where his son was worshipped. In fancy we see the great building resplendent as of yore. The sick and the cripples flock hither in crowds, on foot, on horseback, in litters, riding donkeys. The central shrine is fenced off, since only men and women pure of heart can enter. For women with child, for the dying, for the impure that is to say, a Roman senator, Antoninus by name, has built a house outside the precincts, where life and death join hands. A huge inn, with four courtyards, provides for the accommodation of pilgrims. There are swimming pools, an exercise ground, a large theatre and a small, a race-course for the amusement of visitors. They have to stay a good while before they are admitted to treatment, purifying themselves meanwhile by ablutions, prayers, sacrifices, and fasts. Daily they scan the votive tablets on which the god's miraculous healings are recorded. They read that Ambrosia, a woman from Athens, was blind of one eye, that Aesculapius slit the eye open, rubbed in balsam, and that thereafter the patient could see perfectly with both eyes. They read how Agestratus was cured of headaches which had been so severe that he was never able to sleep; how Gorgias, having a suppurating wound made by an arrow that had pierced his chest, slept beside the altar and awakened with a sound skin holding the arrow point in his hand. Who could doubt these wonders? Who among the pilgrims in search of health failed to expect that a like wonder would be worked in his own case?

When, by these preliminaries, the requisite tension had been induced, the sufferers were conducted, one evening, into the holy of holies. They made sacrifice before the gold and ivory statue of the god. Thereafter the patient would lie down to sleep within the courts of the temple. In his dream there would appear to him the god, Aesculapius, attended by the goddess Hygieia his daughter, and by the serpent who followed him wherever he went. Passing from patient to patient, he would lay his hands upon one, speak to another, slit open the belly of a third, give medicaments to all. Or, sometimes, the serpent would lick the open wound. When the glow of morning appeared on the hills, the blind would open their eyes and see. The deaf would hear the singing of the birds. Those who had been lame would find themselves able to walk without a limp. Pain had vanished, sores were healed. Thanks were offered up, and offerings representing the cured organs were made.

The renown of Aesculapius spread far and wide. In the fifth century before Christ, probably in the days of the great plague, a temple to Aesculapius was built upon the southern slope of the Acropolis. As at Epidaurus, there were altars for sacrifice, halls in which the patients could sleep, and wonder-working springs. The main walls of the structure exist to this day, and prayers are still said at one of the springs, though the light which burns there unceasingly is dedicated, no longer to Aesculapius, but to the Virgin Mary.

Even among the rationalist Athenians, prone to mockery, the cult of Aesculapius must have found numerous devotees, for after a time a second shrine, with all the proper appurtenances, was built in his honour. Reliefs depicting the god and his worshippers, and belonging to the best period of Greek art, are to be seen in the National Museum at Athens.

In the year 293 B.C. when a pestilence broke out in Rome and the native deities proved impotent, an embassy was sent to Epidaurus. Aesculapius took pity upon the travellers from afar and gave them his serpent. Hopefully, with a fair wind, the Romans made all possible speed homeward, and sailed up the Tiber. As soon as they reached the city, the serpent escaped their care, crawled on to the island in the Tiber, and announced that, in accordance with Aesculapius' will, it would take up its dwelling there. The sickness was stayed. A sanctuary was established. In commemoration of the successful voyage, the island was given the form of a ship, that of the trireme which had brought the god from Epidaurus. The holy serpent still coils round the bow.

What is the meaning of these old stories? They mean that at all times there have been persons who sought healing, even bodily healing, not from the physician but from the priest; who looked to religion for a cure. The old gods paled. Was Aesculapius the true healer, the saviour, or was Jesus Christ? Two learned writers, Celsus (the Platonist philosopher of that name, not the physician) and Origen disputed upon this question. Christ, declared Origen, was the true healer. He had wrought more cures; his personality was more in touch with ours; and, this being of supreme importance, he had devoted himself to the whole human race. All could turn to him for help; the poor, the unclean, and even sinners. The world decided in favour of Jesus. The old gods died. The Dioscuri, Castor and Pollux, passed out of men's minds, their places being taken by Cosmas and Damian, martyred under Diocletian, who, themselves physicians and medical missionaries, became the patrons of those who practised the healing art. Ended was the worship of Apollo, who, like his son Aesculapius, had of old come to Italy to drive away the plague. Benedict of Nursia had the sun-god's temple on Monte Cassino destroyed, and built a monastery for the Benedictines on its site. Whose help was now to be sought when pestilence came? That of Saint Sebastian! For Apollo's great temple on the Palatine had likewise been destroyed, and out of the same stones, in the same place, had been erected the first church consecrated to Sebastian the Christian martyr, revered as protector against the plague.

Down to the eighteenth century the sick continued to seek

healing at or would sleep within the precincts of the temple, though the temple had been renamed a church. Even in our own day, thousands upon thousands make pilgrimage to Lourdes, pious Catholics who hope for cures at the shrine of Bernadette. In the Protestant world, too, there are hundreds of churches, whose number continually increases, at which healing by the power of the spirit is promised.

This book is devoted to the lives and teaching of great doctors. The reader must not forget, however, that only a minority of the sick seek the aid of a physician. Many sufferers treat their own ailments, or are treated by their relatives in accordance with various principles which have nothing to do with scientific medicine. At all times people have looked to faith for the cure of illness. As in the days when Imhotep and Aesculapius were worshipped, so now.

CHAPTER TWO

HIPPOCRATES

FIFTH AND FOURTH CENTURIES B.C.

WE pass from myth to the opening of history. Whereas the medical literature of the ancient East, like its art, is anonymous, in Hellas for the first time we come into contact with great doctors who really lived on earth.

Little is known about the origin of Greek medicine. In the early days it must have been primitive, as at the beginning of every civilisation—a mish-mash of religion, magic, and empirically acquired ideas and practices. Not until the sixth century B.C. did the impulse to study nature begin to take shape. Growing self-conscious, people became puzzled about the world, and tried to discover a harmony in it. They formed notions about nature and about man who is himself a part of nature, made in nature's image. There were physicians among the pre-Socratic philosophers. The Pythagoreans, above all, were greatly interested in medical problems. They tried to discover a dietetics of the mind, but also of the body, which should safeguard human beings against noxious influences. In the sixth century there were doctors of note, and medical schools arose: at Croton, where Pythagoras dwelt; in Sicily; in Cyrene; also in Asia Minor and in the Archipelago—at Rhodes, but especially at Cnidus and Cos. It was on the island of Cos that Hippocrates was born, about the year 460 B.C. His name stands out among the physicians of antiquity. Down to our own time it is symbolical of the ideal doctor. To be spoken of as the Hippocrates of his day is the highest distinction that can befall a medical practitioner.

Who, then, was Hippocrates? Eagerly we examine the sources, only to be disillusioned! In truth we know little or nothing of Hippocrates. This much, at least, is certain, that he lived during the fifth century B.C.; that he was a famous practitioner of medicine and a teacher of the healing art; that, as aforesaid, he was born in Cos; and that he was an Asklepiad, this meaning that he was member of a guild supposed to have been founded by Aesculapius. So much is known thanks to certain passages in the dialogues of Plato, the only one of Hippocrates' contemporaries who mentioned his name. That is all. Unquestionably we know more of Hippocrates than of Homer, but we know very little.

Still, the Hippocratic writings are extant. Surely, even if his contemporaries were silent, his writings will tell us much about their author? Here, likewise, disappointment awaits us. The "Hippocratic writings" are a collection of heterogeneous works. They consist of monographs, textbooks, manuals, speeches, extracts, notes. They deal with all the provinces of medicine. Close study shows that they lack uniformity. The most contradictory views are expounded. Some of the utterances are expressly directed against others. It is impossible, therefore, to suppose that the "Hippocratic writings" were the works of one author. Which, among these various writers, was the true Hippocrates? Which of the scripts are genuine? We do not know. We have no data enabling us to decide. Why, then, do these writings bear the name of Hippocrates?

According to Ludwig Edelstein, the most recent authority, we must represent the matter to ourselves as follows. For Plato, and after him for Aristotle, Hippocrates was but one distinguished physician among many. Not until the Greeks had founded Alexandria and become the rulers of Egypt did Hippocrates begin to assume an outstanding position in men's minds. Yet to the early Alexandrians he ranked only with two other physicians, Praxagoras and Chrysippus, as one of the three leading authorities upon dietetics. From century to century, however, his fame grew. For the later Alexandrians he was the physician most worthy of remembrance, the first medical author, the doctor who reigned supreme over the whole domain of medicine. More and more the fifth century B.C. came to be regarded as the classical age of the healing art. In his particular field, Hippocrates ranked with Homer, with the tragedians, the philosophers, and the historians, of the age of Pericles. For Galen, finally, in the second century after Christ, Hippocrates became the ideal physician, and as such he has been regarded down to our own time.

Now let us turn back to the "Hippocratic writings." The more outstanding the position of Hippocrates seemed, the more important did his successors consider it to read his writings. In the great library at Alexandria the obtainable manuscripts of the past were being assembled. Unquestionably among them were medical books dating from the fifth and fourth centuries before Christ, anonymous compilations. Those who scanned these writings believed that in many of them they could recognise Hippocratic doctrines. Thus it was that, during the close of the third century before Christ, there came into existence a collection of medical scripts supposed to have been penned by Hippocrates. Still, even in those early days, there were many disputes as to the authenticity of this writing or of that. However, as time passed and readers grew less critical, the body of the works accepted as Hippocratic continually grew, until at last it came to include almost all the anonymous medical writings of the classical age.

As aforesaid, Hippocrates' contemporaries and immediate successors knew little about the details of his life. Now, when he had become the Father of Medicine, there was a demand for biographies. Legends arose, such as that recorded in the second century after Christ by Soranus of Ephesus, and others penned by subsequent authors. According to these tales he was the son of a doctor named Heraclides. His mother's name was Phenarete. He was born in 460. His first teacher had been his father; then he studied under Herodicus, Gorgias the sophist, and Democritus the philosopher. When his education was finished, he travelled widely. Under the promptings of a dream he went to Thessaly. Wandering from place to place, he traversed the whole of Greece, and his cures aroused general astonishment. The king of Macedon fell sick, and his doctors believed him to be consumptive. Hippocrates was called in consultation with Euryphon, the court physician, and recognised that the king's illness was not consumption but was what we should now call psychogenic—of mental causation. The philosopher Democritus had become insane, and the people of Abdera sent for Hippocrates to cure him, and also to free their city of the plague. In Athens, too, pestilence was raging. Hippocrates appeared upon the scene and noticed that the smiths were immune. Fire, then, must be a remedy, and Hippocrates had huge bonfires kept burning until the epidemic abated. The grateful Athenians erected an iron statue of the physician, bearing the inscription: "To our rescuer and benefactor Hippocrates." He was made a citizen of Athens, and a citizen of Argos, and was also initiated into the Eleusinian mysteries. His fame spread to Persia, and Artaxerxes, King of Kings, wanted to make him physician-in-ordinary. But Hippocrates, being a patriotic Hellene, refused the invitation. At length, advanced in years (the age of 104 is given) he died in Thessaly and was buried somewhere between Larissa and Gyrton. There was a beehive over his grave, and the honey made by these bees would cure children of thrush. He had two sons, Thessalus and Dracon, and numerous pupils.

These are but fables and anecdotes designed to show how great a physician was Hippocrates. No importance can be attached to them. In actual fact we know nothing whatever about his life. Only in one respect is tradition probably conformable with the facts, namely that Hippocrates was a great traveller. We know that the doctors of the fifth century before Christ were, as a rule, migratory practitioners. There were few doctors, and only the greatest cities of the day had settled physicians, salaried by the community. The others, like handi-

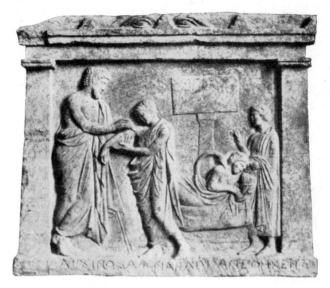

A CURATIVE DREAM, VOTIVE TABLET FROM THE AMPHIARAUS
NEAR OROPUS (NATIONAL MUSEUM AT ATHENS)

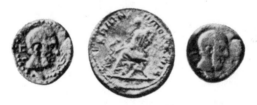

HIPPOCRATES, ON COINS FROM COS DURING
THE DAYS OF THE ROMAN EMPIRE

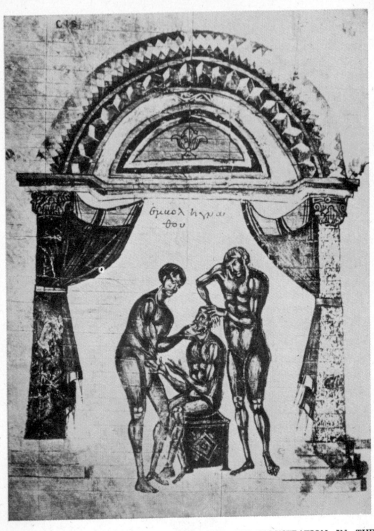

REDUCTION OF A DISLOCATED LOWER JAW. AN ILLUSTRATION IN THE
COMMENTARY ON AESCULAPIUS' WORK ON THE ARTICULATIONS,
BY APOLLONIUS OF CITIUM

craftsmen, moved from place to place, offering their services wherever they went. When a doctor was famous, as Hippocrates certainly was, his reputation preceded him. He would be received with much ceremony, and all the sick of the neighbourhood would flock to get the benefit of his ministrations.

Since the ancients knew nothing about the life of Hippocrates, we can readily understand why no authentic statues have come down to us. There are, plate facing p. 32, coins extant, minted at Cos, professing to show the physiognomy of Hippocrates, but, since they date from the days of the Roman empire, it is unlikely that they were based on portraits.[1]

Even though the "Hippocratic writings" are not homogeneous, and perhaps do not contain a single line penned by Hippocrates, they are still of incalculable value. They give us a clear notion of Hellenic medicine during the fifth and at the beginning of the fourth century before Christ, and enable us to picture the mentality of the doctors who were Hippocrates' contemporaries.

When, guided by these writings, we ask ourselves how medicine was practised in those days, we perceive that it was a highly developed healing art which had succeeded in ridding itself of the magical and religious elements that still clung to ancient oriental medicine, and that it was guided by observation and experiment. Many of the symptoms of disease had been recognised and accurately described. Clinical histories were recorded, enabling doctors to note how symptoms changed from time to time, and what these changes signified to the patient. It had become plain that certain symptoms are habitually linked, producing what we now call "symptom-complexes", and the study of these symptom-complexes in case after case enabled images of diseases to be formed. But these images of diseases were not rigidly conceived. The diseases were not

[1] A bust found at Albano, and now in the British Museum, which was for a long time described as that of Hippocrates, is now believed to be a representation of Chrysippus the stoic.

looked upon as entities which could be divorced from the sufferer and studied per se. What mattered was the sick man, the nature of the individual.

What is illness, and how does it originate? Various answers are given to this question. Health depends upon a condition of equilibrium. Disturbance of this equilibrium is known as illness. The contributors to the "Hippocratic writings" are agreed upon this matter. But what determines the equilibrium? The forces, or the qualities, which are at work in human beings; acidity, sweetness, bitterness. Or, perhaps, the juices, the "humours," of the body are the determinants. Man arises out of the seminal fluid, and for this reason the juices, the humours, are the essential constituents of the body. Some declare that there are many humours. Others insist that there are but two cardinal humours, bile and mucus. Others, again, speak of four humours, of two pairs of humours with opposed qualities, blood and black bile, yellow bile and mucus; these are the ideal sustainers of equilibrium. Should one of these humours be present in excess, or should it be corrupted in any way, the organism endeavours, by means of its natural healing forces, to restore the balance. The peccant humour undergoes a process which may be compared with boiling, and, when this process is finished, when the humour has "ripened," the peccant material is eliminated in the urine or in the stools, in the vomit or in pus. In one of the later Hippocratic writings this doctrine of the four humours makes its appearance. Subsequently systematised by Galen, it dominated medical science for centuries.

The human body maintains itself by continually taking in two substances from the environment, namely air and nutriment. Other Hippocratic physicians, therefore, held that these two substances must play a decisive part in the origination and in the mechanism of illnesses. Their opinions formed the starting-point of other far-reaching theories.

Men need a theory, for the phenomena that come under observation are so numerous that in default of a theory they would elude our grasp. Medicine must be guided by a theory, for otherwise medical doctrine could not be handed on from teacher to pupil. So long as theory and practice, science and practice, harmonise, so long as theory derives from practice and, in its turn, guides practice, medical science and practice will be fruitful. Every theory is philosophical in its nature. It works with the thoughts, with the concepts, available at any particular epoch, thus moulding the culture of the time. Thus, in the Hippocratic theories, there recur all the elements of the natural philosophy of pre-Socratic days. An attempt is made to solve the problem of health and disease conceptually and speculatively, setting out from observation. No other methods were then available, and it was not possible by this route to arrive at views which were of much help in practice.

The Hippocratic physician, called in to see a patient, examined him, tried to recognise as many symptoms as possible, and then made a prognosis. That is to say, he told the sick man what was likely to happen. The future course of the illness was, it need hardly be said, the patient's primary interest, and the prognosis gave the doctor a chance of manifesting his knowledge and of winning the sick man's confidence. Such a diagnosis as is the modern physician's first concern, a recognition of the disease, implies a conception of illness which was alien to the healing art of Hippocratic times. With us, diagnosis guides treatment. But our modern diagnosis presupposes numberless observations, a wealth of experience, the gathering of statistical evidence, etc.—matters which were not available to the physicians of antiquity.

Nature cures. The doctor's business, therefore, must be to increase the healing force of nature, to guide that force, to avoid counteracting it. The best mode of treatment is dietetic, a regulation of the manner of life, of the nutriment. The juices, the humours, are regenerated by food. We can

35

influence them most easily through the diet. The Hippocratic physician, guided by these ideas, achieved a mastery of dietetics which still deserves our admiration.

From dietetic methods to drug treatment, the transition was gradual. The effect of dietetic treatment can be intensified by that of drugs. A purgative effect can sometimes be achieved by a mere regulation of the diet. If this fails, the doctor must have recourse to medicaments. That was the line on which the Hippocratic doctors worked. The materia medica was still extremely restricted, consisting mainly of vegetable drugs collected by skilled herbalists.

When diet and drugs failed, recourse was had to the knife or the cautery. It also seemed reasonable to suppose that cure could be accelerated if the peccant humours were artificially discharged from the body, through artificial openings. By opening a vein, the physician gave outlet to the disordered blood. By lancing an abscess or by cutting into the thorax in a case of empyema, a channel was opened which the pent-up pus might never have found for itself, or would have found slowly. Furthermore, the doctors of classical times, like ourselves, had to deal with the multifarious results of mechanical injury, with fractures and dislocations, and with wounds, needing surgical intervention. There can be no doubt that accidents during sport must have been common, and that is why the surgery of fractures and dislocations was well developed in Hippocratic times, with the result that many a page of these early surgical treatises has a modern ring. Even major operations were performed, although with considerable hesitation. Scrupulous cleanliness was impressed upon the surgeon, and this provided, in some measure, for asepsis.

There is no space, in the present work, for more than the foregoing general indications concerning Hippocratic medicine.

All that we certainly know of Hippocrates is that he lived, and yet no doctor ever exerted a more far-reaching influence than he. Why bother about who he really was! The important thing is what he became in the imagination of his successors. To the ancients he was the ideal physician, the perfect embodiment of a specific conception of medical behaviour, the doctor who (as the "Hippocratic oath" declares) "lived his life and practised his art serenely and sacredly." Each successive epoch formed a new picture of Hippocrates. Each incorporated its own yearnings in his ideal figure. What people found wanting in the doctors of their own day, they thought of as having existed in Hippocrates, who thus became a perpetual exhortation, a prick to conscience, a leader on the road to true physicianship. Along these lines he will continue to manifest his power. Just as Caesar goes on training military commanders, just as Brutus stimulates tyrannicides, so will Hippocrates lastingly educate good doctors.

CHAPTER THREE

DIOCLES OF CARYSTUS
FOURTH CENTURY B.C.

THE Hippocratic tradition persisted. The fourth century before
Christ produced notable doctors. The school we have hitherto
been considering flourished in the Greek colonies, in Southern
Italy, and in Asia Minor; but in the second half of the fourth
century B.C. there arose a great doctor in Athens. Diocles by
name, he was born in Carystus, on the island of Euboea. The
son of a doctor named Archidamus, he did honour to his
father's memory by calling one of his books *Archidamus*. The
fragments of Diocles' writings which have come down to us
make it plain that he followed the custom of his day and
travelled widely. The Athenians esteemed him greatly, and
are said to have spoken of him as a second Hippocrates. To
subsequent ages, he seemed the chief of Hippocrates' successors, and Pliny wrote of him "secundus aetate famaque."
He was loved for his humankindliness, and was admired for
his oratorical gifts.

The Hippocratic writings were penned in the Ionic dialect,
Diocles having been the first medical author to write in Attic.
We know the titles of sixteen of his works. Not one of them
has come down to us entire, but we have fragments which
enable us to form some idea of his views. What did Diocles
write about? About prognosis, about the causes and the treatment of diseases, about fevers, about the evacuations, about
the diseases of women, and about surgery. These are the
themes to which the Hippocratic writings, likewise, are devoted.
It is true, moreover, that Diocles' views are closely akin to
those of the various Hippocratic authors. We find, however,
that he was most strongly influenced by the doctors of the
Sicilian school, in which matter he shows affinity to Plato,

38

whose medical views were likewise influenced by the Sicilians.

Among Diocles' writings, there are some whose titles instantly rivet our attention. For instance, he wrote an *Anatomy*. Now, although the Hippocratic writings include some short anatomical treatises, they are of trifling importance. Of course every doctor must be interested in the human body, must be eager to know what it is like inside and how it works. Still the Hippocratic healing art did not move along anatomical lines. To the Hippocratists, every illness was primarily a general disorder, even when its local manifestations were conspicuous. The school of Cnidus, indeed, conceived of diseases as localised, but their anatomy was crude. It was only the surgeon who demanded precise anatomical knowledge, and such knowledge as the surgeons of those days possessed did not go very deep. It consisted mainly of what we now call "topographical anatomy."

In the fourth century before Christ, the age of Aristotle, the study of nature took on a new impetus. Physicians were chiefly instrumental in promoting this development, and it was natural, therefore, that earnest attempts should be made to learn the structure of the animal organism. The human body was still taboo, so all sorts of lower animals were dissected, and from the data thus acquired the structure of the human body was inferred. Religious, moral, and aesthetic obstacles opposed the dissection of human beings. These barriers were accepted. No one seemed to feel it was necessary for them to be broken down. Even if Diocles was not the first anatomical author, he was one of the first. Moreover, if it be true, as Galen says, that he knew little of the human body, still his writings show that there was an awakening interest in anatomical study.

Plants were dissected as well as animals. Anticipating Theophrastus' famous work *On Plants*, Diocles wrote a *Rhizotomikon*, the earliest Greek treatise on botany we know of, a book which is said to have exercised a wide influence.

The author gives the various names of the plants, their habitat, the way of collecting them, and (of course) their medical use. A second book by Diocles described plants used for food; and a third, poisonous plants. We see, then, that pharmacological and toxicological studies were beginning.

Furthermore, Diocles wrote a great work on hygiene, of which a number of extremely interesting fragments have escaped destruction. Hygiene formulates an ideal of the healthy human being. In the Hellenic view, the ideal man was the harmonious man, the man who was equably made, who was well balanced both bodily and mentally. Such a man was esteemed as noble and handsome; he was also healthy. Hygiene discloses to us the path leading to this ideal.

We learn from Diocles how to spend the days hygienically. You should get up before sunrise, wash your face and hair, clean your teeth, massage your gums with powdered peppermint, and rub down the whole body with oil. Then you should take a short walk before beginning the daily work. In the course of the morning, you should pay a visit to the gymnasium, for bodily exercises. These exercises should be followed by a douche and by massage. Breakfast [you really "broke your fast" some hours after rising] should be a light meal, consisting of bread with a thin soup, some vegetables, cucumber, or what not, varying with the season, and simply prepared. Thirst should be quenched with water before eating. After the meal, drink a little white wine diluted with water and sweetened with honey. As usual in southern lands, breakfast [taken at a time corresponding to our luncheon or mid-day dinner, though it was the first meal] was to be followed, during the hot hours, by a siesta in a cool, shady, and retired spot. This rest should be succeeded by a further spell at the day's occupations, after which the gymnasium should again be visited. The chief meal of the day should be in the evening, which in summer would be just before sunset. It was to consist of fruit, vegetables, bread, and fish or meat. Then a

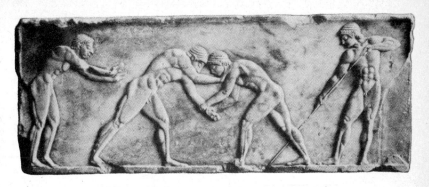

WRESTLING (NATIONAL MUSEUM AT ATHENS)

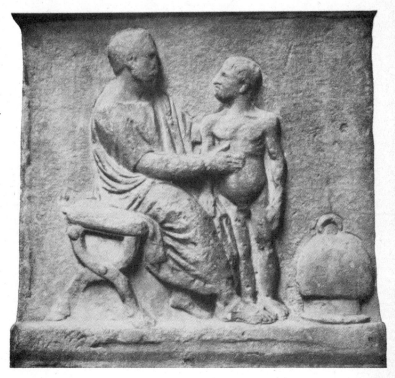

MORTUARY MONUMENT OF THE PHYSICIAN JASON (BRITISH MUSEUM)

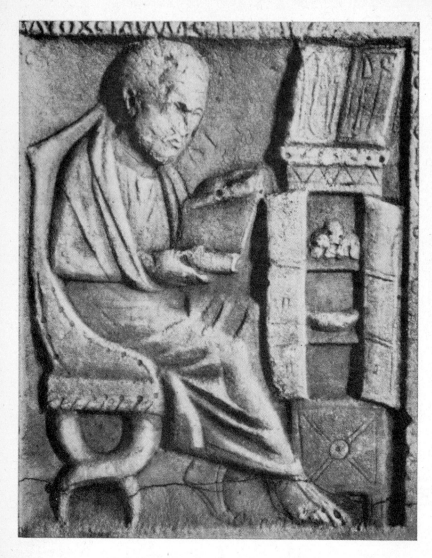

PORTRAIT OF AN UNKNOWN PHYSICIAN

short walk should be taken, followed by an early turn-in to bed.

We may suppose that the daily routine of the well-to-do Hellenes, of those belonging to the master class, may have been of the sort above described. Obviously the great mass of the population—the peasants, the handicraftsmen, and the slaves—can have lived in no such fashion. Still, we owe our thanks to Diocles and his Greek congeners for having formulated a regimen based upon the conception of the human being as a unity of body and mind, and at the same time one which, with few modifications, remains the hygienist's ideal for all time.

CHAPTER FOUR

HEROPHILUS AND ERASISTRATUS
ABOUT 300 B.C.   ABOUT 260 B.C.

ALEXANDER THE GREAT had conquered the world as known to the West. The Persians' realm had been shattered into fragments. Babylonian and Egyptian dominion were things of the past. The armies of "Iskander" had crossed the Indus and had overrun the Punjab. Wherever he wandered, he spread the Greek language, Greek art, Greek culture, far and wide. But the Greeks took, besides giving. Rival civilisations clashed and replaced one another. Hellenism was tinctured, fertilised, and disturbed by oriental knowledge, achievements, and views.

Alexander died prematurely in the year 323, when he was no more than thirty-two years of age. Though his realm was partitioned, the spiritual conquest remained intact. The viceroys became independent, but they continued the work of Hellenisation, each in his own sphere; in Macedonia, Bithynia, Pergamus, Syria; above all, in Egypt.

When, ten years before his death, Alexander had invaded Egypt, he had been welcomed as a liberator. A new city was founded on the Mediterranean coast at the western end of the delta of the Nile and was named after the conqueror. For many centuries thereafter, this town of Alexandria was to remain the acropolis of classical knowledge. It was the capital of the Ptolemies, the Greek kings of Egypt. An astronomical observatory was built; a library was founded; all the literature of the Hellenes was to be assembled within its walls. For millenniums Egypt had been famous as the source of papyrus, the best ancient variety of paper. Now, therefore, Alexandria became the centre of book-making and the book-trade. Intellectuals and artists were summoned to the new Egyptian court from various parts of the world. The Ptolemies, who were free-handed, enabled them to pursue their calling without material anxiety.

Among the learned men who answered the summons to Alexandria were two physicians, Herophilus and Erasistratus, whose writings were of considerable note. Mainly thanks to their influence, the science of medicine underwent a transformation, becoming, in fact, a true science, the incorporation of expert knowledge, whereas hitherto it had been mainly a handicraft. In a word, medical theory grew to much greater importance. The Hippocratic writings could be understood by any well-educated reader, but henceforward medical literature became a specialty for the understanding of which ordinary culture did not suffice. The body of medical knowledge increased from century to century. Through contact with the East, new morbid phenomena and new methods of cure became known to the West.

We know little more of the life of Herophilus than that he was born in the last third of the fourth century before Christ, at Chalcedon in Bithynia; that he learned the science and practice of medicine under a notable teacher, Praxagoras of Cos; and that he rose to fame in Alexandria both as a physician and as a teacher. His name has lived on in the modern anatomical nomenclature, the depression in the occipital bone at the confluence of a number of venous sinuses being known as the torcular Herophili. He was, in fact, a remarkably able anatomist for his day, having written a treatise on anatomy in at least three books which were greatly prized in antiquity. Whereas earlier anatomists had been mainly content to describe the anatomy of the lower animals, Herophilus gave detailed accounts of the organs of human beings, comparing them from time to time with those of other animals. We do not know for certain whether he systematically dissected human bodies; and we may reject as presumably fabulous an assertion which was current many centuries later that the Alexandrian physician vivisected criminals. But in Egypt, where the practice of embalming persisted, and where, as a preliminary, the viscera were removed, there must have been considerable opportunity of becoming acquainted with the anatomy of the internal organs.

The fragments of Herophilus' anatomical writings which have been preserved show that he was a careful observer. His description of the eye, the membranes of the brain, and the genital organs are excellent. It was he who gave the duodenum its name. His greatest discovery, however, was that he recognised the true nature of the nerves. Whereas Aristotle had failed to distinguish nerves from tendons, the Greek word "neuron" applying indifferently to both, Herophilus knew that the brain was the central organ of the nervous system, and that the peripheral nerves were the organs of sensation.

As far as medical theory and practice were concerned, Herophilus did not advance beyond the tradition of his day. He accepted the dominant humoral pathology, and wrote commentaries on some of the Hippocratic writings. According to him life was regulated by four energies; that of nutrition, that of warmth, that of sensation, and that of thought.

He held, however, that the traditional teaching must be further developed. Prognosis must be based upon the symptoms. For this reason, symptoms must be studied as carefully as possible and must be clearly defined. The manifestations of the pulse were among the most important symptoms, and, taking this view, Herophilus elaborated a far-reaching doctrine of the pulse. What is the essential phenomenon in the pulse? Rhythm, as in music. To understand the pulse, then, we must study the theory of music. Such was the course taken by Herophilus, who was guided, in this matter, chiefly by the musical theories of Aristoxenus of Tarentum, a Peripatetic philosopher and a musician, a pupil of Aristotle. By following this route, the doctrine of the pulse became so complicated that no one but a skilled musician could possibly understand it. Necessarily, therefore, the theory was stillborn, its chief outcome being that posterity was inclined to charge Herophilus with sophistry and hair-splitting.

Health, he declared, is a precious possession. In his treatise on dietetics he wrote: "Wisdom and art, strength and wealth, are of no avail if health be lacking." The physician must, therefore, strive to maintain or to restore his patient's health. Experience is of the utmost value here, but limits are imposed upon medical skill. "The best physician is he who can distinguish the possible from the impossible."

What are the chief implements of therapeutics? Dietetics come first, then drugs. If the physician prescribes a drug it is as if the deity were interfering with the course of an illness. Herophilus, in fact, termed medicaments "the hands of the gods," and he prescribed them in all diseases.

Medicine was not yet sufficiently advanced for surgery and midwifery to have become separate branches. Such knowledge as was available was at the command of a single individual, and therefore Herophilus was interested in surgery and midwifery as well as in medicine pure and simple. Indeed he wrote a treatise on midwifery which was widely circulated and greatly esteemed. Practical aid in childbirth was given chiefly by women, the services of the physician being called upon in grave cases; and it was of great importance that trustworthy instructions should be at the disposal of the midwife. There is an anecdote which shows Herophilus' decisive importance as regards the art of midwifery. In ancient Athens, we are told, there were as yet no midwives, since women were forbidden by law to practise any sort of healing activity. However, a noble-hearted woman, Agnodice by name, eager to help her sisters in the pangs of childbirth, dressed herself up as a man and, in this disguise, studied under Herophilus. Having thus acquired an extensive knowledge of the art of midwifery, she was of the utmost help to many women in labour. Thereupon the physicians became jealous of her, and laid an accusation against her before the Areopagus. Her women patients, however, most of whom were Athenians, came to bear witness in her behalf. She was acquitted, and the foolish law was repealed.

It need hardly be said that, as a matter of fact, midwives had practised in Athens long before the days of Herophilus. The only importance of the tale is to show that this man, whose name has come down to us above all as a skilled anatomist, was likewise a distinguished accoucheur.

Well on into the Christian era, many doctors looked back to Herophilus as the supreme master of their art.

Erasistratus, the second great Alexandrian physician, flourished about a generation later than Herophilus. They are commonly spoken of in the same breath, since their lives overlapped, they practised in the same city, and were both founders of schools. They differed greatly, however, in their medical theories.

Erasistratus sprang from a family of doctors. His mother was sister of a doctor; his father, Cleombrotus, was probably physician-in-ordinary to Seleucus I Nicator, King of Syria. Born at Iulis on the island of Ceos towards the close of the fourth century B.C., Erasistratus grew to manhood in Antioch. Having made up his mind to be a doctor he went, as the custom then was, to Athens as a student. His teacher was Metrodorus, who had married a daughter of Aristotle; and he is also said to have studied under Theophrastus, Aristotle's favourite pupil. In this way Erasistratus entered into close contact with the Peripatetic school, and also became acquainted with the philosophy of Democritus, which exercised a considerable influence upon his mind. From Athens he went to Cos, to study in the school of Praxagoras. But his most important impressions in medical matters were derived from the younger Chrysippus, a physician who had come from Cnidus to settle in Alexandria.

Whereas Herophilus, accepting the Hippocratic tradition,

had gone no farther than to attempt to develop it a little more fully, Erasistratus, who (as we have seen) had studied medicine in a number of different schools, soon took a line of his own.

Like Herophilus, however, Erasistratus was a student of nature. "Nature is the great artist who, in her care for living beings, has perfected all parts of the body and has organised them purposively." The ways of nature must, therefore, be explored. Erasistratus dissected animals, and some of the organs of human beings. He wrote two anatomical works. The fragments that are known to us contain excellent descriptions of the heart with its valves, of the upper air-passages with the epiglottis, of the liver and the bile-ducts, and of the brain. The nerves, he taught, do not only subserve the purposes of sensation; they likewise conduct voluntary impulses and arouse movement. He recognised, therefore, that there were two kinds of nerves, sensory and motor.

What more did he teach? That three sorts of conduit, veins, arteries, and nerves, traversed the whole body. They were intertwined to form organs as yarn is twisted into a rope. The ultimate parts of the organism, however, were the atoms. They were inalterable, and were animated by warmth from without. They were surrounded by empty space, which had an attractive force. This force drew the blood, the nutriment, out of the veins; the pneuma (air) out of the arteries; and the spiritual pneuma out of the nerves. The arteries did not contain blood, but only conveyed air, which was renovated by the breathing. If, none the less, a severed artery bled, it was because the pneuma (air) which issued from it drew with it blood by connecting channels with the veins.

Making post-mortem examinations, Erasistratus found organs which had manifestly been changed by disease. For instance, in a man who had died of dropsy he found the liver as hard as a stone. On the other hand, in the body of a patient who had died of snake-bite, the liver, the large intestine, and the bladder were softened. It was obvious, then, that illness exhibited local manifestations, in the form of changes in the organs. We could learn about it from a study of these diseased organs. Illness was not a vague "corruption of the humours." How, then, did it arise? To what mechanisms was it due?

Erasistratus wrote a book upon the causes of disease. The organism, he reiterated, was built up out of an interweaving of three sorts of tubes. The proper condition of these passages and their normal functioning were indispensable to health. The most important morbid process was plethora, a distension of the vessels with blood and nutritive materials. Thereby the veins were stretched and torn. Blood made its way into the arteries and blocked their passages, with the result that the pneuma could no longer move through them unhindered. Stagnation of the pneuma gave rise to inflammation. The arteries began to beat too vigorously, and fever ensued.

As regards particular diseases, they were determined by the particular regions or organs in which plethora occurred. According as the site varied, we had to do with pneumonia, pleurisy, epilepsy, disease of the stomach or the liver or the spleen, and so on.

Whilst plethora was the immediate cause of the symptoms of disease, it was incumbent upon the physician to look for the remoter causes which had given rise to the plethora, inasmuch as successful treatment depended upon the removal of these original causes. For the rest, treatment must be adapted to the individual case; and, in especial, Erasistratus was opposed to violent methods. There was no sense, he declared, in bleeding all the sick without distinction. The best way of counteracting the plethora was to see to it that only a small quantity of nutritive material should be ingested—in a word, fasting was useful. If blood were withdrawn from a fasting man or woman, this caused too much weakness, and thereby the cure was delayed. Dietetic treatment must take the first place. It was assisted by physical therapeutics: vapour baths, bodily exercises, poultices, frictions, etc. Drugs were also of use, although Erasistratus did not administer them so liberally as Herophilus. In many instances it was necessary to have recourse to the knife.

Prophylaxis, preventive treatment, however, was more important than remedial methods. Prevention was better than cure. If he could, a wise steersman would circumvent a storm, instead of exposing his ship to its fury. A shrewd physician would adopt a like measure. Erasistratus, therefore, wrote two books upon hygiene.

Let me repeat that Erasistratus was an innovator. He forsook the humoral pathology. Being a materialist, he considered disease from a mechanical standpoint. Not only did he dissect the human body, but he applied the data of his anatomical observations to pathology. Advancing along the lines already laid down by his teachers in Cnidus, he was on the way towards a pathology based upon a localised, an anatomical conception of disease. Nay more, he was on the way towards an ontological conception of illness. Naturally, therefore, a considerable proportion of his writings were monographs upon particular diseases or groups of diseases. For instance, he wrote books on fever, upon abdominal diseases, upon paralysis, gout, and dropsy. Still, as we have already noted, Greek medical science was predestined to follow another course. Erasistratus' teaching was thrust aside, and Galen, to whom the victory of Hippocratic theories was largely due, could not find invectives sufficiently strong for the expression of his contempt for the great Alexandrian physician.

There are many interesting anecdotes concerning Erasistratus. One of the best of these relates to the keenness of his medical insight. Antiochus, son of Seleucus I Nicator, King of Syria, was dangerously ill, and, when other physicians had failed to help him, Erasistratus was called in. While he was examining the patient, Stratonice, a young woman, one of the elderly king's wives, entered the room. From the quickening of the sick man's pulse and from the flush which spread over his cheeks, the doctor recognised that the illness was mental rather than bodily—that a passion for his inaccessible step-mother was at the root of the trouble. The cause having been discovered, the road to a cure had been opened. Seleucus, in order to save the life of his deeply enamoured son, divorced Stratonice, and gave her in marriage to young Antiochus, whereupon the prince recovered.

If there is any truth in the story, for chronological reasons we must infer that the physician who worked this cure cannot have been Erasistratus, but must have been (as Pliny maintains) his father Cleombrotus. The anecdote was transferred from the comparatively unknown father to the much more celebrated son. Presumably, however, the story is mythical, being a fable which turns up again and again in many parts of the East, and which in the West likewise has not infrequently secured pictorial expression.

According to another ancient tradition, Erasistratus presented the temple of the Pythian Apollo at Delphi with a pair of dental forceps made out of lead—as a hint that doctors would do well to extract only such teeth as were loose in their sockets.

At an advanced age he is supposed to have retired to Samos, and, having been attacked by an incurable disease, to have died a voluntary death, saying: "I die happy in that I have served my country." He had founded a school of medicine which was to endure for five hundred years.

CHAPTER FIVE

HERACLIDES OF TARENTUM
ABOUT 75 B.C.

WHICH was right, Herophilus or Erasistratus? Their disciples were incessantly disputing about the matter, hurling arguments at one another, quoting the words of their respective masters, splitting hairs. The rival doctrines were advocated with every weapon of dialectic.

But was not the controversy unmeaning? What is the doctor's business? To heal the sick. Are all these theories requisite for that purpose? No. Nature is unfathomable. This is already plain from the fact that no unity exists among philosophers and physicians. Why should one rather believe Hippocrates than Herophilus? Why give credence to one man more than to another? Good ground can be adduced for accepting the arguments of every one of them. Each wrought cures. Indeed, the philosophers would have been the greatest of physicians if philosophy sufficed to equip the doctor. But although the philosophers uttered wise words, they did not understand the art of healing. Besides, the art of medicine varies from place to place. It was necessary to practise according to one set of rules in Rome, according to another in Egypt, and according to yet another in Gaul. If diseases were produced everywhere by the same influences, then the same remedies could everywhere be used. If, moreover, the direct cause of an illness were known, a knowledge of how to cure it would come soon enough. But the causes are so often obscure! We should do best, therefore, to be guided by the results of accurate research. In this matter, as in others, experience is what teaches us. It is practice which makes perfect a peasant or a steersman —practice, not theory. However much the physiological and pathological ideas of different doctors may have varied, the doctors were successful, in many instances, in curing their patients. Why? Because their treatment was guided by experience, and not by theoretical considerations. The art of medicine was born out of experience.

Herophilus and Erasistratus were great anatomists, but of what use to a doctor is a knowledge of the structure of the human body? First of all, we do not even know whether the organs in the living body are really like those which we dissect in the dead. Even if this be so, a knowledge of the organs is needless for the curative art. What doctors are concerned with is practice, is experience, not theory. Illnesses are cured by remedies, and not by eloquence.

The physicians whose thoughts ran along these lines, and whose most notable representative was Heraclides of Tarentum, spoke of themselves as empirics. Their doctrine had been founded about the year 250 B.C. by Philinus of Cos, a pupil of Herophilus. In the first century B.C., Heraclides, who also belonged to the school of Herophilus, elaborated the ideas of the empirics. Philosophical scepticism was playing its part in the field of medicine. Therapeutics was on the way to become a pure science. Investigations were being made into the nature of man and the nature of illness. Discussions and speculations were rife. But since the firm foundations of an experimental and quantitative natural science had not yet been established, since people had not yet learned to concentrate but wished to embrace all knowledge simultaneously, their thoughts were apt to wander off into the void. The rise of the empirics was the outcome of a jejune reaction—of a reaction thanks to which (as happens often in the case of such movements) the child was emptied out with the bath-water, and every kind of explanation by the laws of nature was rejected. Practice was setting itself up against science, was demanding its rights as opposed to theory, and was imperiously reminding the doctor of his task. The dispute was one which was to recur again and again. Is medicine a science or an art; is it, in the last analysis, nothing more than a handicraft? The Hippocratists were handicraftsmen; but, nevertheless, a physician who was a philosopher as well, seemed to them quasi-divine. For them, art and science, theory and practice, were harmoniously combined, this being their great merit. On the other hand, in the case of Herophilus and Erasistratus, the trend towards theory, and in the case of the empirics, the trend towards practice, became one-sided.

The empirics did not constitute a school. They had no authoritative doctrine by which empirical practitioners were to be guided. They represented, rather, a trend of medicine. Their teaching was a method. Heraclides, like many doctors who had preceded him, wrote a great work upon the empirical method. Medicine, he said, was grounded upon experience; and, for each doctor, it was mainly grounded upon his own experience. Still, human life was short, and the experience that can be gathered by an individual is scanty. For this reason, doctors have to avail themselves of the experience of other doctors, handed down to them by tradition. Practising physicians, no matter to which school they belong, make observations for themselves, gather experience. Accept good things, whatever their source. The empirics, therefore, made a thorough study of the literature of the past, and Heraclides wrote a commentary upon the Hippocratic writings.

The practising physician, however, will often have to deal with cases of an unfamiliar type, cases concerning which there is no recorded experience to guide him. He will have to help himself out as best he may by analogies. When he has to treat a hitherto unknown illness, he will use remedies which have proved effective in illnesses more or less similar. Maybe, again, resemblances between the affected parts of the body, or a kinship between various remedies, will be of use to him and will determine his action. A clear indication is thus given of the best way for gathering new experience. That was the line along which the empirics moved; for, even though they

had a very different scientific ideal from that of their predecessors, they nevertheless made researches.

In view of the markedly practical attitude of the empirics,
their attention was, of course, mainly devoted to the practical
domain of medicine. Their work contributed to a knowledge of
symptomatology, and still more to a knowledge of therapeutics,
which at all times has had a strongly empirical tendency, and
upon which the empirics laid especial stress. Heraclides wrote
a treatise upon the treatment of internal disorders, and another
upon the treatment of external disorders. He also penned
a work on dietetics, in dialogue form, under the title of
Symposium; and he left behind him five books on pharmacology.
The fragments that have come down to us show him to have
been a sober-minded physician, a clear thinker, a man of wide
experience and extensive knowledge, able to make sound
criticisms upon his predecessors.

As regards the life of Heraclides we know practically nothing,
and are equally ignorant concerning the biographical details
relating to the other empirics. They must, for the most part,
have been ordinary sort of men, wholly devoted to medical
practice. It was part of their doctrine that the physician should
be a man of few words, that he should have no desire for
fame, that his personality should pass into the background
behind his work. From the little we know of them, we gather
that these doctors must have been characterised by extreme
sobriety, and by an inclination to the matter-of-fact. One of
them bluntly declared that he practised medicine in order to
make a living by it. These men were sceptics. Their writings
were merely compilations of experiences, and throw little light
upon the character of the writers. Heraclides is an exception
in this respect, but that is because he transcended the limits
of empiricism.

There can be no question that the empirics did a great deal
to increase the medical knowledge of ancient times. During
the third century before Christ, pharmacology began to take

on a rapid development, and this was in great measure the fruit of the work of the empirics. The pharmacologists of the days of the Roman Empire, Galen not excepted, borrowed freely from empirical sources.

The members of this school paid considerable attention to surgery and midwifery as well as to medicine in the narrower sense of the term. In the first century before Christ one of the empirics, Apollonius of Citium, wrote a commentary upon the Hippocratic treatise on the articulations, enriching it with a number of illustrations which are still extant. In this graphic method, we likewise see at work the desire to be chary in the use of words.

CHAPTER SIX

ASCLEPIADES OF PRUSA
FIRST CENTURY B.C.

In our study of ancient medicine, we now enter a new theatre. The oldest of the schools, those of the Hippocratic physicians, had been upon the periphery of the Hellenic world; in southern Italy, Sicily, northern Africa, the Aegean Islands, Asia Minor. Then came Diocles, who lived in Athens; followed by Herophilus and Erasistratus whose work founded the medical reputation of Alexandria. It was from Alexandria, likewise, that the empirical trend took its rise.

Now Rome was the centre of the medical art. Henceforward the development of medicine is associated with the capital of the Roman republic and the Roman empire. Rome had become the chief city of the Western world, and was exercising its irresistible charm. Whoever felt talent budding within him, whoever wanted to make a career for himself, was irresistibly impelled to try his luck in Rome, which offered such multifarious possibilities in medicine no less than in other fields of study and practice. How had this come about?

To begin with, Roman medicine had been primitive medicine. As everywhere else, so there, it had been a mishmash of religious and magical ideas with empirical knowledge. One who was stricken with fever, prayed to the goddess of fever. A pregnant woman offered up sacrifices to Lucina or Carmenta. Even during the era of the republic, the art of medicine remained extremely primitive. There were domestic remedies for pains and coughs and diarrhoea. Cabbage was regarded as an extremely valuable drug. A certain amount of knowledge had been acquired concerning the treatment of wounds, and splints were applied to a broken bone. But in addition to such means, or when they proved ineffective, recourse was had to

56

spells and charms. You never could tell! Common, too, was the practice of wearing amulets to protect against the evil eye and other sinister powers. One who owned numerous slaves was certain to have among them a person regarded as skilled in medical matters. Such a slave was extremely valuable in the household, and commanded a high price.

Then, in the course of the years, Greece was conquered and Greeks came to Rome. The Romans began to learn the refinements of Greek civilisation. Even though there was an inclination to regard Hellenic culture as softening in its effects and as unworthy of a Roman, by degrees those who dwelt in the City of the Seven Hills succumbed to its charm. Greek physicians settled there. According to the records, the first of these, Archagathos by name, from the Peloponnesus, arrived in the year 219 B.C. He was a freeman not a slave, and was much better informed than his Roman colleagues. Especially was he renowned as a surgeon, and was highly prized, being provided with rooms in which to practise his art, and, more important still, being made a Roman citizen, lest he should be tempted to return to Greece. A bold operator, he was successful for a time; but then, growing presumptuous, he became too ready with the knife, and his luck turned. Falling into evil odour, he was nicknamed Carnifex—the executioner! Archagathos, however, was but the first of innumerable Greek immigrant doctors. Nor was it only physicians and surgeons who arrived, for in their train followed midwives, masseurs, and charlatans. On the whole the newcomers were regarded with distrust, until at length one of them succeeded in establishing Greek medicine upon a firm footing in Rome. This was Asclepiades, a native of Bithynia.

He was a man of adventurous disposition who had studied philosophy and medicine in Greece and perhaps in Alexandria likewise, and had practised in various cities. Then, continuing his travels, he came to Rome at the opening of the first century before Christ. He established himself there at first, as an orator rather than as a physician. The foreign doctors were little loved, but there was need of rhetors. Any one who wanted to make a place for himself in the political world or as a lawyer had to be fluent of speech and must be able to persuade or to convince. Asclepiades was silver-tongued, and therefore began his career in Rome as a teacher of oratory.

Pupils flocked to his school of oratory, and as soon as he was well established he dropped the mask and disclosed himself as a physician. In this field, too, his oratorical gifts could be turned to good account. He knew how to blow his own trumpet. He promised "curare tuto, celeriter, et jucunde"—to cure safely, swiftly, and pleasantly. (This phrase originated with him.) A man, he said, would be a poor physician who had not two or three remedies ready for use in every case of illness; well-tried remedies. He himself had such remedies. Nor were these remedies the violent purgatives and vomitories of his colleagues. He cured by prescribing fasts, abstinence, massage, active and passive movements.

Then he had one of those strokes of luck which sometimes make a physician famous. A funeral train passed him. The "corpse" had been placed upon the pyre, and the torch-bearers were about to ignite it. But the man was not really dead! Asclepiades had him taken down from the pile and restored him to life.

Naturally patients thronged round this miracle-worker. He seemed a messenger from heaven rather than an ordinary physician. The houses of the great were opened to him. He was a welcome guest in those of Cicero, Croesus, Atticus, and Marcus Antonius. His reputation spread far beyond the walls of Rome. Mithridates, King of Pontus, wanted him as physician-in-ordinary, but Asclepiades declined the post with thanks, being content to send the king copies of his writings.

For Asclepiades was a voluminous writer. We know the titles of about twenty of his books. He was no charlatan, nor was he of the empiric school. He paid due honour to the teachings of experience; but he considered that medicine needed a theory to guide treatment. The workings of nature could be made comprehensible by research, and the characteristics of an illness disclosed the appropriate remedies. Beyond question much of what his predecessors had written was erroneous. Hippocrates? His treatment was positively murderous. Erasistratus had come nearest to the truth, but his doctrine, likewise, had been full of errors.

Asclepiades was a philosopher. He had studied to good purpose the atomist doctrines of Heraclides Ponticus, the epistemology of Epicurus, and the maxims of the Stoics. All the same, he constructed a system of his own.

The organism, he taught, was built up out of disconnected atoms, which attracted and repelled one another, and whose movements led to mutual clashes. Between them were pores. Health depended upon a proper size, form, and number of these primal corpuscles, and upon their having orderly movements. It was also essential that the pores should be of proper size. Illness arose through a standstill of the atoms and through a blocking of the pores. Of course there were juices or humours in the organism, and there existed a pneuma. Doubtless disturbances of the humours and of the pneuma gave rise to disease. But the atoms were the main determinants.

The essence of treatment lay in paying due regard to the principle of contraria contrariis. When there was an arrest of movement of the atoms, they must be brought into a proper motion. Since illness arises principally from mechanical causes, mechanical remedies are the most important. Asclepiades' therapeutics were principally physical. The forces he brought to bear upon the organism were heat and cold, also sunshine. He employed hydropathic treatment, giving water internally and applying it externally, using all kinds of baths, massage, active and passive movements. These methods were conjoined with a strictly regulated diet. He wrote a treatise upon the curative values of the different kinds of wine.

Indisputably, Asclepiades was a great physician and a man of strong character. A good many fragments of his writings have been preserved, and these suffice to show that he was determined to follow his own road, regardless of tradition. He paid special attention to mental disorders.

It is not difficult to understand why this man was so successful in Rome. His teachings appealed to the Romans. They were clear and simple. They expressed a philosophical trend congenial to the Romans and applied to the province of medicine. Thanks to the work of Asclepiades, the reputation of the Greek physicians rose to a higher level. They were efficient practitioners, and there was need of them. Competent physicians and surgeons! The latter were needed by the legions in the incessant wars. In the year 46 B.C., Julius Caesar bestowed the gift of Roman citizenship upon all Greek physicians that were freemen and were established upon Roman soil. This was a great boon, for in classical times foreigners had no rights. Augustus elevated his physician-in-ordinary Musa to the rank of eques (a knight). The physicians in Rome had begun to acquire a high social position.

If a doctor fell sick, laymen were wont to make fun of him, saying sarcastically "Medice cura te ipsum" (Physician, heal thyself). It is said that Asclepiades averred that he would no longer call himself a physician if he ever fell sick. The upshot was that, when well advanced in years, he did not die of illness but of an accident, through tumbling down a flight of stairs.

CHAPTER SEVEN

SORANUS OF EPHESUS

SECOND CENTURY A.D.

It was inevitable that a man with so strong a personality and such original views as Asclepiades should influence the development of medical science and should found a school. Asclepiades had a faithful pupil, Themison of Laodicea, who for many years followed strictly along the lines of his master's teaching. Not until after Asclepiades' death, when he himself was an old man, did Themison begin to strike out along a new route. It seemed to him that Asclepiades' teaching was not systematic, not precise enough. He therefore tried to consolidate it into a simplified method which would be more helpful to the practising physician.

What is or should be decisive in the treatment of a malady? Not its cause, but its fundamental type, which is recognisable by certain general manifestations. There are only three of these fundamental types: the status strictus, in which the pores are diminished; the status laxus, in which they are enlarged; and the status mixtus, in which the pores are diminished in certain parts of the body while they are enlarged in other parts.

If the skin is dry, if the excretions are scanty, if there is high fever, we have to do with a status strictus. If the symptoms are the opposite of the foregoing, we have to do with a status laxus. The aim of our treatment must be, in the former case to relax the pores, and in the latter case to constrict them. How is this to be achieved? Themison, like his teacher Asclepiades, put his trust in dietetics and in physical therapeutics generally. In applying these methods, however, two additional points had to be taken into consideration; first of all, the stage of the illness during which the intervention was being made; and, secondly, whether the illness was acute or chronic. Chronic maladies, said Themison, were not (as people had been accustomed to believe) invariably the result of acute conditions which had assumed a chronic course, for there were a great many diseases which were essentially chronic in their nature.

By these doctrines, medicine had been reduced to a simple formula. A principle had been laid down, a method had been established, which could be easily learned. The adherents of this school, which had a great vogue in Rome, called themselves "methodisers." Nevertheless, the excessive simplicity of their doctrine tended to promote charlatanism. One of these methodisers, Thessalus of Tralles, who lived during the reign of Nero, claimed that he was able to educate physicians in six months. He was the son of a Lydian weaver. Coming to Rome, he associated there chiefly with handicraftsmen, such as smiths, shoemakers, painters, etc., whom he took with him to visit his patients, and who, very soon, blossomed forth as doctors. Persons better instructed in the art of medicine, spoke of this gang of pseudo-physicians as "Thessalus' jackasses." Thessalus himself was preposterously vain. He declared that everything that had been written concerning the art of medicine before his own days was nonsense, and that Hippocrates had been no better than a liar. The true art of healing had begun with Thessalus of Tralles! He wrote various works, among others one on dietetics and one on surgery, which have not been preserved, but we know that they were dedicated to Nero. Wishing to persist in his role even after death, he had himself described on his tombstone as Iatronices—the Conqueror of Physicians.

Notwithstanding his foibles, this "know-all," as Galen termed him, must have been a shrewd fellow. Though he remained a methodiser, he amplified the system, especially as regards the treatment of chronic illnesses, which were to be dealt with in two stages. Thessalus perceived that in chronic disorders the tissues of the body had often undergone extensive changes. The aim of treatment, therefore, must be to

62

modify the organs in the direction of health once more. This, however, could not be instantly effected, for in many cases the patients had been so much weakened by protracted illness as to have become unable to bear vigorous treatment. They must be fortified before that could be begun. The first requisite was a circulus resumptivus, what we should nowadays call tonic or roborant measures, which were principally dietetic, but among which other physical methods were employed. As soon as, by these means, the patient's strength had been to some extent restored, a specific treatment began, the circulus metasyncriticus, an alterative or revulsive regimen, which was to whip up the organism. Various means could be used for this purpose. Some of them were dietetic, the nutriment being rhythmically varied. In other cases powerful purgatives were administered, followed by vigorous stimulation of one sort or another. In yet other instances, a change of air was prescribed, in the hope that thereby the nutritive processes of the body would be thoroughly transformed.

The reader will not fail to perceive that such ideas have a modern ring. We act in accordance with similar principles when we send a patient suffering from tuberculosis for a long stay at a health resort in the mountains.

This school of the "methodisers" would probably have decayed ere long in Rome had it not been that a man of genius, a man of wide medical experience, while adopting its principles, gave them a firmer scientific foundation, and at the same time adopted broader outlooks than those of his predecessors. This was Soranus of Ephesus, who ranks as the most notable representative of the methodisers. He was in many respects the antithesis of Thessalus, who had been an uncultured upstart. Soranus, on the other hand, having received an all-round education in Alexandria, was not a doctor merely, but also a philosopher and a grammarian, and author of a lengthy treatise upon the soul. Whereas Thessalus had regarded previous physicians with contempt, Soranus looked back to them with respect. No matter what trend they had represented, he studied their writings to learn by their experience. In his treatise comprising ten books he recorded what was known of the life and teachings of the great physicians of earlier days. Nothing remains of this beyond a fragment concerning Hippocrates. Soranus made extensive use of the medical knowledge handed down from the past. Thessalus apart, other medical authors of those days did the same. Soranus, however, was exceptional in this, that he was scrupulous in giving chapter and verse for whatever he quoted.

Very little is known about his life, beyond the fact that after his studies in Alexandria had been completed, he came to practise in Rome, during the reigns of Trajan and Hadrian, that is to say in the beginning of the second century after Christ. Nevertheless we know more about him than about most of the physicians of his day because so much of what he wrote has been preserved, either in the original Greek, or else in Latin translations. His writings are clear, simple, and impressive, being devoid of superfluous rhetoric.

As already said, Soranus was a convinced methodiser, some of his books being devoted to the exposition and elaboration of the doctrines of the school. His account of the "communities," that is to say the basic types of disease, was methodistic. He compiled extensive works upon special pathology and therapeutics, these, as was to be expected from a methodiser, treating separately of maladies as acute and chronic respectively. This great treatise was translated into Latin by Caelius Aurelanius, who flourished in the fifth or sixth century after Christ. The translation is extant, and is a rich mine to the student of the history of medicine, for it shows how the methodisers contemplated and treated particular maladies.

According to the methodistic view, anatomy, a knowledge of the structure of the normal body, was of no value whatever

64

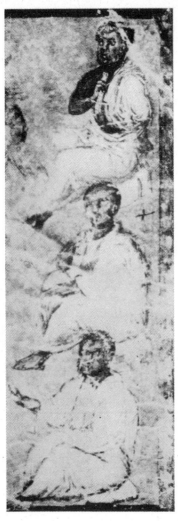

HERACLIDES OF TARENTUM (MIDDLE),
NIGRUS (ABOVE), AND MANTIAS (BELOW)

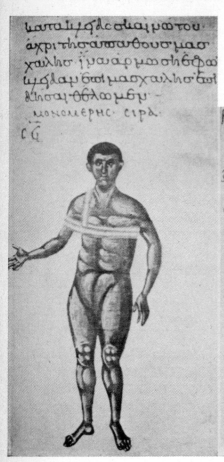

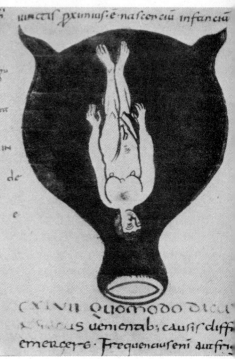

ONE OF THE ILLUSTRATIONS IN SORANUS'
TREATISE ON BANDAGING

ONE OF THE ILLUSTRATIONS IN SORANUS'
TREATISE ON MIDWIFERY

to the practitioner of the healing art. Soranus, no less than the others, held this opinion. Still, said Soranus, the doctor, who day by day inspects, palpates, and auscultates the human body, cannot but be interested in its structure and its functions. (His studies in Alexandria had left their mark upon Soranus!) Although anatomical knowledge may be useless, is in fact useless, it has an ornamental value for the scientific physician. Soranus himself, with remarkable industry, compiled a work giving the etymology and the definition of the anatomical and physiological terms in common use among experts. Not because such knowledge was necessary, but because it was interesting!

Such also was his attitude towards etiology. The doctor did not need to know anything about the causes of disease, but etiology was a remarkably stimulating province of inquiry, and etiological data rounded off our knowledge of disease. To supplement his writings upon special pathology and therapeutics, Soranus composed a work upon the causes of disease. It was in these respects that Soranus so greatly excelled the other methodisers, in that, departing from the rigid tenets of his school, animated by a spirit of scientific inquiry, he enlarged his studies far beyond the bounds of what he professed to regard as immediately necessary for medical practice.

In addition to the theoretical works already mentioned, Soranus wrote a number of books intended to guide practice: a treatise on hygiene; a work on pharmacology; a handbook on the practice of surgery; a manual on bandaging which was illustrated in ancient times, and whose illustrations have been preserved for us in a manuscript dating from the ninth century. These pictures show that the methods of bandaging in use to-day were known to the ancients; or, rather, that the modern practice of bandaging is the fruit of a tradition dating back a couple of thousands of years or more. The first requisite of a bandage is that it should stay in place. The simplest bandage that will do this is the best. In many instances the

65

surgeons of antiquity discovered these best and simplest methods of bandaging, as the illustrations to Soranus' book clearly show.

Above all, however, Soranus' fame rests upon his textbook of midwifery and gynecology. He is usually esteemed the ablest gynecologist of classical times. Unquestionably this textbook, the greater part of which remains in being, is excellent; but it is likely enough that there were better gynecologists than he, since he was not a specialist in the subject. We know him to have been skilled in internal medicine. He appears, moreover, to have practised extensively as a surgeon, though his surgical writings have not come down to us. As to gynecology, there must have been noted gynecologists in ancient days, both before and after Soranus, but unhappily their writings have vanished.

It would be extremely interesting, did space permit, to furnish a detailed account of Soranus' gynecological treatise, since this would give a picture of classical midwifery and gynecology in days when it had probably attained its climax. I must content myself, however, with a very brief outline of the work. First of all the author describes the skilled midwife. What bodily and mental qualities are requisite for success in this profession? She must be a person of high endowments, especially in regard to character. As for the remainder of the book, the greater part of it deals with the practical work of the midwife. This is considered in two sections: a physiologico-hygienic, and a pathologico-therapeutic. First an account is given of the structure of the female genital organs, from which the author passes on to their functions, to menstruation, conception, and pregnancy. Then the physiology of birth is described, with the aid that must be given by the midwife or the accoucheur; this being followed by an account of the care to be taken of the woman in childbed and of the new-born infant. That ends the physiological part of the work. Now comes the pathological section, an account of morbid

66

conditions; the treatment of these being considered in accordance respectively with dietetic, surgical, and pharmacological methods. The extent of the knowledge manifested in this treatise is amazing. A speculum was used for local examination. The practitioner was warned against meddlesomeness, but in difficult cases operative midwifery was essential. Version was practised, to induce, in some cases a head presentation, and in other cases a breech presentation. In the worst cases of difficult labour, embryotomy was requisite, to save the mother's life. Of course Soranus' book is not free from errors. To mention one of them, he believed (and it was still believed down to fairly recent times) that in the act of birth the pubic bones separate at the symphysis to give more room for the passing of the foetal head.

The book was illustrated, and copies of the illustrations have been preserved. Among them are diagrams of the uterus and the various positions of the child.

As a supplement to this treatise, Soranus wrote a small theoretical work concerning the nature of the semen and concerning the act of generation. He also made epitomised extracts from his treatise in the form of question and answer; a catechism for midwives, which, in Latin translation and illustrated, remained in use throughout the Middle Ages.

Soranus embodied the climax of the school of the methodisers, and this crowning figure of classical antiquity (in the days when the decline of the classical system had already begun) was to dominate medicine throughout the earlier part of the Middle Ages.

CHAPTER EIGHT

GALEN OF PERGAMUM

129 A.D. TO ABOUT 199

THERE are few great physicians whose value has been so variously esteemed as that of Galen. In his lifetime, though he had a large practice, he was but one distinguished physician among many. During the Middle Ages, his writings acquired a canonical status, so that he was regarded as authoritative to a degree in which he was only rivalled or excelled by Aristotle. Then came the Renaissance, when he fell into disrepute, and was even reviled. Down to our own day the campaign against him has continued, for many students of medical history describe him as a false prophet, and contrast with him the true prophet Hippocrates. Owing to this atmosphere of polemic, it is hard to form just views about his personality and his teaching.

If a teacher reads one of the Hippocratic writings with his students, he finds that the class is full of enthusiasm. If, on the other hand, he makes one of Galen's writings the subject of study, the very first sentences arouse fierce opposition. Involuntarily those who read become advocati diaboli—and yet they find it hard to persist in their incriminatory attitude. Now why is there such a difference between the outlook upon Hippocrates and that upon Galen? Let us ask, to begin with, who Galen was.

In Pergamum, the ancient capital of the Attalides, where such remarkable excavations have recently been made by German archaeologists, there lived in the second century after Christ an engineer named Nicon. He was a man of culture, well grounded in philosophy, mathematics, and natural science. He was "passionless, just, worthy, and amiable." He lived in easy circumstances, and would have been happy had it not been that he was unhappily married, his wife being "so ill-tempered that she sometimes bit her servant-maids, was continually screaming, was a scold, berating her husband more savagely than Xanthippe did Socrates." In the summer of the year 129 A.D. a son was born to this unequally matched pair, and the father named him Galen, thus giving expression to a deeply felt desire—for the Greek word "galenos" signifies "calm," denotes the condition of the sea when it is serene, waveless, unruffled by the winds.

He was a bright and lively youth, who was carefully trained by his father Nicon. At the school of philosophy in Pergamum, Galen became acquainted with the various philosophical systems. But he did not confine his studies to this field. When the lad was eighteen years old, Nicon had a dream which induced him to have his son trained as a physician. Dreams in those days were taken seriously. People were animated with a strong desire for expiation, for atonement, for deliverance from sin. They no longer made mock of Aesculapius, as of old had Aristophanes, the sceptical playwright. In Pergamum itself there was a famous sanctuary dedicated to the god of healing. Miraculous cures were matters of daily occurrence. Indeed, Galen was in later years cured at the shrine of Aesculapius.

But besides the priests at the temple of healing, there were in Pergamum ordinary practising physicians: Satyrus, who had written works on anatomy and was oné of the commentators upon Hippocrates; Straconicus; Aeschrion. Galen studied under these teachers, seeing and hearing much. The first cases of illness with which one makes close acquaintance as a student exert a powerful impression throughout life, and decades later Galen used to recount his early observations. He had made up his mind to become a great doctor. He studied all day and far on into the night, until his health suffered from overwork. Yet there is nothing from which a doctor learns more than from his own illnesses, and Galen observed his symptoms acutely.

69

When Galen was twenty, his father, with whom he had been linked by such close ties, passed away. There was nothing more to keep him in Pergamum. The time had come for him to follow the example of the illustrious doctors among his predecessors, to travel, to see other men and other cities, to study unfamiliar illnesses and fresh methods of treatment. He spent nine years upon his travels, from 148 to 157. His first remove was to Smyrna, close at hand, and there he studied under Pelops and other able physicians. Next he went to the Greek mainland, and was for a time in Corinth. But the goal of his wishes was Egypt, was Alexandria, where there was still a famous university, the best place in the ancient world for the study of anatomy, in which Galen had special interest. It was no longer, of course, the Alexandria of old days. Nearly five hundred years had passed since the time of Herophilus and Erastistratus. The organs of diseased human beings were no longer obtainable, and the would-be anatomist had to content himself with the study of the lower animals. However, Alexandria was a fine place in which to learn osteology. And Egypt was a wonderful country, too, in many other ways.

In the summer of 157, Galen returned to Pergamum. The gladiatorial shows held every summer in the capital of Pergamus were about to begin. Everything was ready, with one exception —the gladiators had no surgeon. The chief priest, who presided over the games, appointed young Galen to this important post. The gladiatorial shows took place. There were many wounded; Galen cared for them, and (an unusual thing) all the wounded recovered. Having thus made himself valued, he held the office of gladiatorial surgeon for three years in succession.

In his native city he now had a distinguished position, and plenty of work to do. The gladiators' doctor was not merely a surgeon, but had to guide the training of the fighters. This gave him ample opportunity to study the theory and practice of dietetics. He also had numerous private patients in the town, where people were glad that the son of Nicon had turned out so well. Persons of rank and fortune sought his advice. In the intervals of active professional work, he studied philosophy and he wrote.

In the year 161, the term of his appointment expired, and he was free from the trammels of office. Now the time had come for the great venture, for a transfer to the capital of the civilised world, to Rome. Taking ship at Troas, he sailed by way of Lemnos to Thessalonica, and then continued his journey until one day, in the opening of the year 162, he found himself at the gates of Rome. His heart beat fast as he entered the great city. How would he, a stranger from afar, be received? The place swarmed with doctors, some born there, and others immigrants like himself. There were specialists for each part of the body, for every kind of disease, representatives of all schools and trends, quacks, butchers, and assassins. They competed fiercely one with another, decrying one another, climbing on one another's shoulders. Any weapon that came to hand was acceptable in this struggle for professional success. Well, he would fight too, and would use whatever means came to his hands. It seemed to him of good omen that a philosopher, Marcus Aurelius Antoninus, had recently ascended the imperial throne. Such a man would at least be able to discern the difference between a philosopher and a humbug.

Galen was in Rome, but Rome did not seem to be aware of the fact. Asiatic Greeks, fine talkers, were there in plenty. One more made little difference. No use sitting idle in his lodgings; he must seek acquaintances. He called on various fellow-countrymen, upon those who had come from Pergamum to settle in Rome. Fortune favoured him. Among them there was a man of considerable distinction, Eudemus, an elderly man, an adherent of the Peripatetic school of philosophy, who moved in the best circles. Eudemus fell sick of a quartan fever, and called in, not young Galen, but the most famous doctor then practising in Rome. Under this distinguished physician's

71

treatment he grew worse and worse, until his life was despaired of. Then he bethought him of his fellow-townsman, Nicon's son, young Galen, with whom he had had some talks upon philosophy. Galen was summoned, and was thus given a great opportunity. He examined the patient, and made a prognosis. The illness ran the course he had predicted. He prescribed remedies, and the patient recovered. Visitors were calling in vast numbers to inquire after the health of the famous invalid. They made the acquaintance of the new doctor, about whose merits Eudemus was most enthusiastic, comparing Galen's prognosis with the utterances of the Delphic oracle. When he was fully restored to health, Eudemus could not find words strong enough in which to praise the doctor who had cured him.

Thus at one stride Galen had acquired a great reputation. It became the fashion to be treated by the newcomer, and, since Galen was really an able doctor, he knew how to maintain and consolidate his position. He was shrewd and cautious, displayed a great deal of psychological understanding, and was not above an occasional "bluff." Are we to blame him for this? Let us remember that the Rome in which he had begun to practise was not the Rome of five centuries B.C., but imperial Rome where there was a formidable competition among the doctors.

There is evidence enough that Galen's rise to eminence did not take place without resistance. The celebrated physicians who lost patients to him were green with envy, and did everything in their power to discredit him. Who was this Galen? To what school of medicine did he belong? To no school at all, rejoined Galen. How could a man of independent mind enrol himself in such a school? If he recognised any master, it was the founder of the healing art, the divine Hippocrates. Fierce polemics ensued. In lectures and in animated pamphlets, Galen took the field against his adversaries. His mother's passionate blood was stirring within him.

He made good. Patients of high rank sought his advice.

72

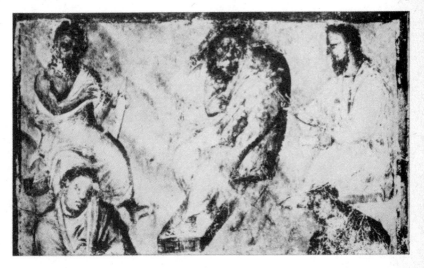

GALEN (IN THE MIDDLE). ON THE LEFT IS CRATUAS AND ON THE RIGHT IS DIOSCURIDES (FROM THE VIENNESE MANUSCRIPT BY JULIANA ANICIA, FIFTH CENTURY A.D.)

The wife of Flavius Boethus, the consul, was suffering from one of the diseases peculiar to women. Galen cured her. He received a fee of four hundred gold pieces and was appointed physician-in-ordinary to the family. Boethus was greatly interested in medical questions, and attended Galen's lectures. Above all he was fascinated by anatomy. In this field, Galen was an adept. A dissecting room was established where Galen demonstrated the anatomy of the lower animals. Boethus was delighted, and wanted to have his family doctor's demonstrations put on record. He engaged shorthand-writers who took down verbatim reports. In this way several of Galen's books on anatomy were compiled.

He had even more distinguished patrons. One of them was Marcus Civica Barbarus, an uncle of the Emperor Verus; and another was Claudius Severus, son-in-law of Marcus Aurelius. The road to the highest position attainable by a doctor was open to him, the road to the court. Once firmly established as physician to the emperor, his enemies would be able to do nothing against him. Boethus and Severus wanted to recommend Galen to Marcus Aurelius Antoninus.

Then a strange thing happened. Galen, the ambitious Galen, now thirty-seven years of age and on the threshold of his supreme triumph, requested his patrons to abstain from mentioning his name to the emperor. Hastily disposing of his household goods, he set out on foot through the Campagna, crossed the peninsula to Brundusium, took ship for Greece, and then travelled to Pergamum, returning to his native city in the year 166.

He had spent only four years in Rome. During this brief space of time, the stranger had risen in the ranks of his profession with unexampled speed. Then, when about to attain the highest pinnacle of a doctor's ambition, he had fled. Why?

It is unlikely that the precise reason will ever be learned. All we know is that that year a raging pestilence visited Italy from the east. As to whether it was bubonic plague, smallpox, or typhus, remains uncertain, for the descriptions lack precision. Beyond question it claimed innumerable victims. Did Galen run away from the malady? If so he ran only to meet it in Asia Minor. Can he really have been a coward? Perhaps he felt that when so desperate a disease was epidemic, the proper place for him was his native city. Other reasons may have been at work. We do not know.

Having returned to Pergamum, he took up his old practice in that city. Was his great career at an end? Had Rome been no more than an episode, a dream? Would he grow old in this provincial city as a respected general practitioner, wax fat, and die? That was not to be his fate? His name had bulked too largely in Rome. The court remembered him in his retirement. If ever good doctors were needed, it was now. One day there came an imperial missive to Pergamum, summoning Galen to Italy. Without undue haste, he followed the call. In the winter of 168–169, he joined the court at Aquileia. Hardly had he arrived when the pestilence broke out once more. The two emperors, Marcus Aurelius and his adoptive brother Verus, with their train, fled southward towards Rome. On the way Verus fell sick of the disease and died.

Galen had remained in Aquileia. But once more the emperor sent for him. The barbarians were threatening the boundaries of the empire in the north. Marcus Aurelius was arming against the Marcomanni. Galen was to accompany him. A campaign in the uncivilised north? Well, a doctor could gather fresh experience there, and would be able to dissect the bodies of slaughtered barbarians. On the other hand, the war might go on for ages. That would be a great interruption to his studies. Surely Commodus, the heir apparent, needed a physician-in-ordinary? Galen was able to persuade Marcus Aurelius that he could do better work in Rome.

There Galen stayed for another thirty years, until his death. Medical and surgical practice, literary labours, lectures, the teaching of the medical art, polemics—these filled his days. Marcus Aurelius died in 180, while still prosecuting the campaign against the Marcomanni. Commodus succeeded his father, but was murdered after a reign lasting twelve years. There ensued the brief reigns of Pertinax and Didius Julianus, and then Septimius Severus became emperor. Galen continued to hold his position at court. It was his duty to give the emperor the daily dose of theriac, the universal antidote which the rulers of the empire, who dreaded poison, were accustomed to take. Occasionally he was called in consultation.

He suffered a great distress when, in the year 192 (the year before the accession of Septimius Severus), his library was destroyed by fire. Copies existed of most of his writings, but a good many of them were unique. He rewrote some of these; the others were lost for ever. Towards the year 199, at the age of seventy or thereabouts, he died.

Galen had been a voluminous writer. His works dealt with all the provinces of medicine and with numerous departments of philosophy. Although so many of them have been lost, those that have been preserved fill many volumes. The question, however, arises why Galen exerted so profound an influence upon his successors. Neither the quality nor the quantity of his writings can fully account for this influence.

We have already learned that he did not belong to any school. He was an eclectic. From the body of medical writings then available, he took whatever seemed good to him. He had no scruples about plagiarising from his forerunners, for this was the custom of his time. Still, he was no mere bookmaker, but chose his excerpts under the guidance of personal leanings. Like the empirics, he prized experience; like the dogmatists, he liked to have a sound theoretical basis for his views and his practice. But, above all, he was a Hippocratist. Hippocrates was the master to whom he continually referred. Hippocrates had begun the good work. Galen's mission was to build upon Hippocratic foundations. Six hundred years had elapsed since

Hippocrates had flourished. Much had been learned during these centuries. Galen thought it incumbent upon him to systematise the huge body of new knowledge that had come into being. He aspired to establish formulas which would free medical practitioners from perpetual uncertainty, would give them sound guidance to suit every occasion.

In the Hippocratic writings, the most diversified theoretical views had been propounded. Galen made an amalgam of them all; the doctrine of qualities, the doctrine of the four humours, the doctrine of the pneuma, the doctrine of the physis. The most important innovation since Hippocrates had been the growth of a precise knowledge of the bodily organs. This must be built into the system. Continually Galen was endeavouring to erect such a composite system, all through his life, and in each of his writings from a different standpoint. He never succeeded in completing the unique system he desiderated. In not a single one of his writings did he formulate any system consistently throughout. Yet his books are so full of systematic or systematised statements that it was easy during the Middle Ages to compound elements from the Galenic writings into a Galenic system which was predominantly founded upon the doctrine of the four humours and the doctrine of qualities.

In Galen, the ideas of the Hippocratic writers were maintained, but were given a peculiar, a Galenic stamp.

In old age he wrote: "I have continued my practice on until old age, and never as yet have I gone far astray whether in treatment or in prognosis, as have so many other doctors of great reputation. If any one wishes to gain fame through these, and not through clever talk, all that he needs is, without more ado, to accept what I have been able to establish by zealous research." Prophetic words! Galen's successors showed themselves only too willing to renounce the trouble of making their own investigations, only too willing to regard Galen as an unchallengeable authority.

Troublous times were at hand. Science was at a standstill. The historians of the healing art will look vainly in the four or five centuries that followed the death of Galen for physicians who manifested originality, for investigators who had ideas of their own. There were still efficient practitioners in the Roman world. Books were still written, but those who wrote medical books were no more than copyists, and they copied by preference from Galen. Religious problems rather than medical were the main interest of those days. The new faith, Christianity, had surged up mightily from the depths; it was fought with words, with steel, and with fire; then it proved victorious, and became the religion of the State. What this signified for the healing art we shall learn in a later chapter.

Meanwhile the Teutons were a gathering storm upon the north-western frontiers of the Empire. Towards the close of the fourth century the storm burst. The world changed its countenance. The period of the folk migrations had begun. Then, when the Roman world had been overrun by the barbarians, in the East Mohammed was born.

CHAPTER NINE

RHAZES AND AVICENNA
865–925   ABOUT 980–1037

MOHAMMED was born at Mecca in the year 570. He was not only the Prophet of the One God, but worked something akin to a miracle upon his people, disciplining and uniting the savage and sundered Arabian tribes. He imposed upon them strict cleanliness. At the appointed hours they said the appointed prayers. Mecca drove forth the Prophet, but he returned to it as a conqueror. He became lord of Araby.

Then, under his successors, under the first caliphs, the Arab armies began to cross the frontier. The Semitic kettle was boiling over once again. Arabia was a desert, an impoverished land. East, west, and north was the lure of splendid booty. Inspired by the new faith, the Arabs raided in all directions, conquered, and settled down. Provinces and kingdoms fell before their onslaught; Syria, Palestine, and the Neo-Persian realm, Damascus, Jerusalem, Ctesiphon were theirs. They overran Egypt, and, degrading Alexandria to the level of a provincial town, founded Cairo as the capital of a tributary kingdom. Streaming westward across the desert lands of northern Africa, they destroyed the new Carthage which had arisen to replace the one wiped out near a thousand years before by the Romans. Still moving westward, the Moslem armies at length reached the Atlantic Ocean. Looking northward across the straits they saw a mountainous rock, and one of their captains, Tarik, transported a force to this eminence, which was called, after him, Gibraltar. The Visigoth army was defeated. The raiders moved northward, ever northward through Spain, crossed the Pyrenees, and thrust into the very heart of the Frankish empire. At length their progress was stayed by Charles Martel, in the great battle which raged between Tours and Poitiers. The armies of the East and the armies of the West, which were to contend for centuries in the crusades, had measured strength against one another.

This was in the year 732 of the Christian era, and no more than one hundred and ten years since the Hegira, when Mohammed had fled from Mecca to Medina. Thus in little over a century the Arabs or "Saracens" had become rulers of an empire which stretched from the Pyrenees to the Indus, a realm containing the most diversified nations and races, held together by the bonds of the faith. All their looks turned towards a centre, towards the sacred city of Mecca. They were united, likewise, by the bond of a common speech, for the translation of the Koran had been forbidden, and Arabic soon became the tongue of letters throughout the realm of the caliphs.

In the middle of the seventh century, when the rule of the Ommiade caliphs began, Damascus was the capital of the Mohammedan world. The Ommiade dynasty was followed by that of the Abbaside caliphs, who removed their seat of government farther south, to Bagdad. There, a contemporary of Charlemagne, reigned Haroun al-Rashid, the man round whose figure so many quasi-fabulous stories have accreted.

Most of the lands conquered by the Arabs or Saracens were regions of ancient civilisation. Wherever they went, the conquerors took over the relics of Greco-Roman culture. Damascus was a flourishing city, with magnificent buildings. Alexandria was still a busy centre of scientific life. In Alexandria dwelt Paulus Aegineta, the last of the noteworthy Greek physicians. Classical technique (aqueducts, bridges, and the like) could not fail to arouse the admiration of the invaders. At first, of course, they had little time and probably little inclination to attend to cultural questions. By degrees, however, when peace was established within their borders, there awakened in them a passion to turn these alien technical and artistic abilities to account. They had castles and palaces built by foreign architects. They welcomed foreign technicians, foreign chemists, and also foreign physicians. Nor were they slow to perceive that Greek prescriptions were more effective than Arabic amulets. They learned, moreover, that the wisdom of ancient Greece and Rome had been embodied in written words. A demand for the manuscripts arose, and, conquest apart, many of them were acquired by diplomatic channels. When treaties of peace were signed, one of the stipulations was that scientific books should be handed over to the Arabs. The Greek imaginative writers did not interest them. The works they wanted were philosophical, mathematical, astronomical, and, above all, medical. These books could not, however, be turned to good account until they had been translated into Arabic. Translation was facilitated by the fact that many of them had already been rendered into another Semitic tongue, Syriac. At Gondeshapur, on the northern shore of the Persian Gulf, there had long existed a Syriac medical school. Thence doctors and translators were summoned. In this matter, during the ninth century, a Christian named Hunain ibn Ishaq was a most efficient go-between.

Libraries were established, schools arose, hospitals were built. Education was extended to all classes. Doctors were trained. Most of these were Persians, who excelled in the science of that day, but they wrote in Arabic instead of in their native tongue. The great doctors who flourished in the East during those times were numerous. Two of them need especial mention, not only because they were probably the ablest, but also because they exercised so marked an influence upon western medical science.

One of these is known to us as Rhazes [pronounced in two syllables, rah-zees], a Latinized form of a name that became attached to him because he was born at Raj in Khorassan, north-eastern Persia. The full name by which he is known in

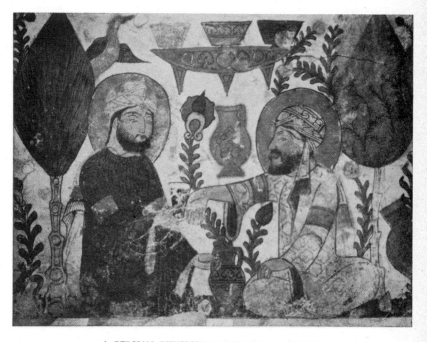

A PERSIAN PHYSICIAN OFFERING A POTION

the East is Abu Bekr Mohammed ibn Zakkariya, Ar-Razi. In his earlier days as a student he devoted himself, not to medicine, but to philosophy and to music. He was an accomplished lute-player. One of his most intimate friends was an elderly apothecary at the hospital, discussions with whom aroused Rhazes' interest in medicine. He was long past his first youth when he made up his mind to devote himself exclusively to the healing art. Having made rapid progress in his medical studies, he soon became famous. His first promotion was to be chief of the hospital in his native town, whither numerous scholars flocked to learn from him. After a while he was summoned to Bagdad, where a new and large hospital was to be built, and the first task imposed upon him in the capital was to choose the most suitable site. The story runs that he had uncooked joints hung in various places which were in most respects favourable. The site in which the meat took longest to become putrid was, he declared, obviously the place where the air must be most healthy, and this was therefore chosen for the hospital.

In old age he is said to have gone blind. Since we know very little about the details of his life, the chroniclers have let their fancy run upon such matters. They inform us that when it was proposed to operate upon the blind old man, he rejected the proposal on the ground that he had seen enough of this world. Another anecdote endeavours to give an explanation of his blindness. Rhazes, who had devoted much attention to chemistry, had dedicated a work on alchemy to a man of high rank, and had been given a great reward. But the patron wished proof of the efficacy of the method by which, according to Rhazes, baser metals could be transmuted into gold. When Rhazes tried to evade the test, he was given a violent blow upon the head which blinded him. In another version of the tale, the physician and alchemist was strangled because of his failure. But these fables are scarcely worth considering.

Rhazes was a prolific writer, composing more than a

hundred, some say more than two hundred, works. Very few of them have been printed, so that it is difficult for western physicians to appraise the quality of his writings. Nor did he write medical books alone, many of his treatises being concerned with philosophical, chemical, mathematical, astronomical, and physical questions.

During the Middle Ages, the West held in high esteem a book which Rhazes wrote for the ruler of Khorassan, *Mansur ibn Ishaq*, and which was therefore known as *Kidab el-Mansuri* (*Liber Almansoris*). It was a concise general account of medical science, and was of much value as a practical handbook.

To-day, however, we appreciate most highly, among the works of Rhazes, a treatise *On Smallpox and Measles*. It is valued especially for the reason that it was one of the first monographs on a disease. It is doubtless a defect that measles and smallpox are not sharply distinguished one from another. Still, the little book, one of the classics of medicine, contains excellent clinical descriptions, and a vigorous spirit of observation breathes through it. Rhazes also penned one of the first known monographs on the diseases of children.

Rhazes' fame among the Arabs was, however, mainly grounded upon a huge compilation, a sort of encyclopaedia of the medical knowledge of his day, so compendious that the Arabs spoke of it as *El-Hawi*—Latinised as *Continens*. This was a posthumous work, and not penned by the master himself, but put together after his death by his pupils. It recorded and elaborated all that had been known to Greek, Arabian, and Indian physicians, and was enriched by Rhazes' own observations. It is from a study of this book, above all, that we have come to regard Rhazes as the greatest clinician of the world of Islam. He was not concerned with systematisation, but with particular cases and their treatment. His chief method of demonstration was the clinical history, his writings being packed with such histories. He inveighed against theoretical hair-splitting, and especially against attempts at undue precision in prognosis—a method which among the physicians of old days was often improperly used by those grasping at a reputation, the more unworthy of them using the arts of the modern "confidence-man."

We know no more than a small part of Rhazes' works, and these are mainly handbooks. Now, to form an opinion concerning an investigator from handbooks is to form a caricature. Every handbook is necessarily, to some extent, a mere compilation. If, in due time, the numerous monographs penned by Rhazes become available, there can be no doubt that he will appear a more original thinker than he seems to us at present. We can infer as much from the monograph upon smallpox and measles.

Avicenna, likewise a Persian, was born about forty-five years after Rhazes' death. His life took a different trend and had a very different tempo. To give him his full name, Abu Ali Husain ibn Abdullah ibn Sina, the son of a highly placed official, was born in the neighbourhood of Bokhara, that is near the periphery of the Islam empire, about the year 980. He was an infant prodigy. At ten, he knew the Koran by heart, and was so well read in the classical authors that his knowledge seemed almost miraculous. After a while he turned to the study of philosophy, then to that of jurisprudence, and then to mathematics (Euclid). At sixteen he took up the study of medicine, which came easily to him. By the direct observation of sick persons he supplemented what he read, learning a great deal which was not to be found in the books.

He was dominated by an insatiable thirst for knowledge. "At home of nights," he relates, "by lamplight, I read and I wrote, and when I grew so sleepy that I felt my powers of work were failing me I drank a glass of wine to restore my energies and resumed my labours. When at length I fell asleep, I was still so full of my studies, that often on waking I found that problems which had perplexed me had been solved during slumber. Thus I continued my studies until I had attained to a complete knowledge of dialectics, physics, and mathematics. Then I turned to theology and metaphysics."

When no more than eighteen he had already acquired fame as a physician, and was then consulted by a prince who, grateful for renewed health, opened to the young doctor the treasure-house of his library. A few years later he wrote his first book, an encyclopaedia running to twenty volumes. At this time he was one-and-twenty years of age. Now his father died, and for a time he had difficulty in earning a livelihood. He entered the service of one ruler after another, but those were troublous days, and he was not always lucky in his choice of patrons. At length he reached Hamadan, at a time when the emir, Sham ud-Daula, was suffering from severe colic. Avicenna cured him. When the emir discovered the wide range of his faculties, he appointed him vizier. But there was a militarist party at Hamadan, and the new minister of State was by no means to their taste. Soldiers stormed his house, seized him, and demanded that he should be put to death. The emir stood out against this demand, but, yielding to pressure, agreed that his vizier should be banished. Then, at the right moment, the royal patron's colic returned. Again Avicenna cured him, and was reinstated as chief minister.

A time of unresting activity followed. The days were filled with cares of State, while at night Avicenna studied, gave lectures, and wrote. But it must not be imagined that he was a dryasdust. A man of the world, he loved wine, women, and song—more ardently, perhaps, than was good for his health.

His subsequent career was a further succession of ups and downs. At one time he would be high in princely favour, and at another time he would be in gaol. At length, settling in Ispahan, he devoted himself exclusively to science. On Fridays a number of learned men would assemble to learn more from his wisdom. But before he reached the age of fifty-eight his bodily powers were exhausted, and he died.

He left behind him a great number of works, many of them extremely comprehensive, and dealing with innumerable branches of science. He had done remarkable work in every field. His fame excelled that of all other scholars of his day. Himself an Aristotelian, he was regarded by posterity as a second Aristotle.

His most important medical work was a treatise entitled *The Canon of Medicine*. It was divided into five sections, devoted respectively to the theory of medicine, the simpler drugs, special pathology and therapeutics, general diseases, and the pharmacopoeia. Each section was further subdivided into subsections, and these were split up into smaller divisions. Avicenna's method was that of the Aristotelian dialectic, and his work was a product of Arabian scholasticism.

It would hardly be possible to conceive of a greater contrast than that between Rhazes and Avicenna. Rhazes was a musician and an imaginative man, whereas Avicenna was a purely logical thinker. Rhazes was a clinician, but Avicenna was the systematist of Arabian medicine. Rhazes was fond of clinical history, of individual cases. Avicenna, too, was a good observer, he, too, studied particular patients; but what interested him in them was that which was general to the type. Just as Aristotle was his master in philosophical matters, so Galen was his medical teacher. Like Galen, Avicenna was continually endeavouring to construct a watertight system. In his hands, medicine became a huge, unified, circumscribed, logical edifice, embracing the whole of Greek and Arabian knowledge. He did his utmost to realise the ideal of making the healing art into a quasi-mathematical discipline.

Obviously such a "system," however much it might do violence to nature, could not fail to prove attractive. It was easy to learn and easy to apply; it freed the mind from doubt, and those who accepted it felt that they were no longer groping

85

in the dark. Naturally, then, it exercised a widespread influence, becoming, as its name portended, canonical; so that its dominance persisted, in the West from the time when it became known in the thirteenth century until well on into the seventeenth century, and in the East down to our own day.

The huge Arabian realm lasted no more than a few centuries. In the beginning of the thirteenth century, led by Genghis Khan, the Mongols began to overrun it from the north and from the east. In the year 1258 they took Bagdad, and the dynasty of the Abbaside caliphs fell. In the fourteenth century began the inroads of the Turks, who likewise destroyed what was left of the Roman empire when they took Constantinople in the year 1453. But Arabic civilisation persisted. The conquering invaders were assimilated, and adopted the creed of Islam. For them, too, the Koran became the guide of life; and their physicians were trained in the doctrines of the great Arabian masters.

Above all, Arabic medicine lived and developed in Spain, an Arabic province which carried on an independent life. When the Ommiades were overthrown by the Abbasides in the eighth century, one of the former, Abd-er-Rahman by name, surviving the massacre of his relatives, took refuge in Mauretania, and was invited by a party of the Arabs in Spain to come to them as their sovereign. Quickly establishing his power, he became emir of Cordova, and two centuries later his successors took the title of caliph. The sciences and the arts flourished at their courts. In due time minor Arab States became established in Sevilla and Granada, which, though small, could offer numerous advantages to men of learning. Moslem rule persisted over large parts of Spain down to the year 1492, the year in which Columbus discovered the New World. During the days of the Moorish dominion, there flourished many men who were eminent both as philosophers and physicians, such men as Averroes, Maimonides, and Avenzoar. There were also noted Arab surgeons in Spain, such as Abul-Kasim; and distinguished pharmacologists like Ibn el-Baitar. Toledo was the chief university of the western caliphate, a centre where the cultures of the East and of the West met to fertilise one another.

CHAPTER TEN

CONSTANTINE OF AFRICA, ABOUT 1010–1087, AND THE SCHOOL OF SALERNO

IT is to western civilisation that we must now return. The beginning of the folk migrations has already been described. Wave following wave, Celtic and Teutonic tribes had moved southward and westward, overrunning the outworn Roman empire, and (like the Mongols and the Turks in the East) adopting the civilisations and the creeds of those whom they conquered. It was Christianity which gave the new developments their stamp. The glad tidings had come to the sick as well as to the hale. Illness was freed from the odium of sin and inferiority which had clung to it from primitive times and throughout the days of classical culture. Suffering was a mark of God's grace and denoted transfiguration. The patient was a privileged person. Through compassion, the healthy could participate in his privileges. Indeed, it became a Christian duty to do all that could be done for the poor and the sick.

In due time the care of the sick was organised upon the grand scale. Great hospitals were built. Benedict of Nursia instructed the monks of the order he established to pay special attention to the care of the sick.

Although at the outset Christianity was fundamentally hostile to classical science, by degrees the new faith became reconciled to it, and even to pagan medicine. Obviously a Christian equipped with medical knowledge could be more helpful to the sick than could any ignoramus. Cassiodorus, who held high office under Theodoric, and who subsequently became a monk, declared that a study of classical literature was meritorious for a Christian. The library of the monastery in which he lived to a great age contained, among others, medical

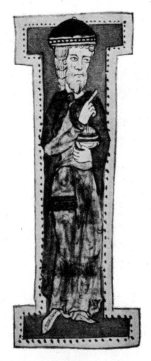

CONSTANTINE OF AFRICA,
1010–1087

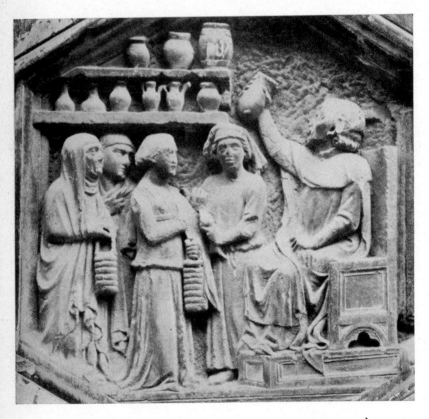

URINOSCOPY (A RELIEF FROM THE CAMPANILE IN FLORENCE)

books. The Benedictines gradually adopted Cassiodorus'
principles, with the result that wherever Benedictine monasteries were established, there were centres for the study and
practice of medicine, places to which the sick were welcomed
for Christ's sake, and where likewise the medical lore of the
ancient world was studied, in so far as it had been preserved
from destruction. Among such centres, Bobbio, St. Gall,
Reichenau, and Fulda, deserve special mention.

In the early Middle Ages, doctors were in holy orders.
Doubtless there were lay practitioners as well, but they formed
an infinitesimal minority. Priests and monks were mainly
responsible for keeping the literature of medicine alive, as well
as for being medical practitioners. We have, therefore, good
reason for speaking of this period as that of "monastic
medicine."

Whereas in the East the works of the great Greek physicians
were early translated into Arabic and their contents assimilated,
they long remained closed books to the Latin-speaking West.
No doubt some of the writings of Hippocrates, Soranus, and
other Greek doctors had been Latinised, but they were too
complicated, and secured little acceptance. Much more
successful were brief treatises, extracts and condensations
from the Greek masters, making certain essentials immediately
available for practice. The upshot was that the early medieval
literature of medicine consisted mainly of collections of recipes,
of brief dietetic hints, and of concise monographs upon the
pulse, fever, the urine, and blood-letting. These were sometimes couched as letters, sometimes in catechismal form, and
sometimes penned in macaronic verse, to be remembered the
more easily.

We shall look in vain in the medical literature of those
days for original ideas, but the medical teachings already
extant were sedulously preserved. Nor were they blindly
transcribed. The monastic medical authors made compilations,
indeed, but often did so understandingly, and incorporated

89

their knowledge of popular medicine into the text. The great service of the Church was, that it not only undertook the care of the sick, but furthermore in the Dark Ages kept the spark of medical science glowing, so that, when the time was ripe, new fires could be kindled. It was not, however, until the second half of the Middle Ages had begun that there came a man, Constantine of Africa, who was to give a decisive impetus to medieval medicine.

Yet I cannot but hesitate to describe Constantine as one of the "great doctors." We really know nothing whatever about his capacity as a physician. His importance to medical science did not lie in the field of practice, though none the less his works had great influence. Who, then, was this Constantine?

He was born at Carthage, somewhere about the year 1010. Legend clings to his personality. His biographer, Petrus Diaconus, informs us that he visited Babylon, to study there the medical and other sciences of the Chaldeans, the Arabs, the Persians, and the Saracens; that from Babylon he went farther afield to India, whence he returned by way of Ethiopia and Egypt, absorbing on his travels the wisdom of these lands. His journeyings lasted for nine-and-thirty years, and he was heavily burdened with knowledge when he returned to his native city. His compatriots, however, regarded him as a sinister figure, and they planned to put him to death. Having got wind of the intended assassination, he took refuge on board a ship sailing to Salerno. He remained there for a time in hiding, disguised as a beggar. Then it happened that the brother of the king of Babylon passed through Salerno, and recognised Constantine, who thereupon was treated with great honour at the court of Robert Guiscard. But he did not find court life congenial, so he retired to Monte Cassino. Securing a friendly reception from Abbot Desiderius, he became a monk. In the peace of the cloister he devoted himself to the translation of medical works from Arabic into Latin until, in the year 1087, the pen dropped from his hand. His fellow-monks remembered him as "magister orientis et occidentis," as a new Hippocrates.

This is all we know about Constantine of Africa; not very much, and yet it suffices. The account is, of course, legendary, but, like all legends, it contains a kernel of truth. There can be no question that Constantine came into close contact with the world of Islam, that he studied oriental science, and transmitted it to the West. We have also ample evidence that he was well informed in the western science of his day, and we know that he wrote in excellent Latin, differing greatly from the barbaric phrasing of the monastic medical writers of previous centuries.

Constantine's significance lies in this role of intermediary. As if with a magic key, he opened the world of the East to the West. Medical literature had become arid. The monastic medical writers had been chewing the same texts for half a millennium. Although these texts had sufficed for a time to guide medical practice, they were being superseded. Medicine was in the act of breaking away from the Church. Education was no longer exclusively a clerical affair; there were educated laymen as well. Centuries were still to elapse before independent productive work was once more to become possible, but intelligent men were thirsting for better instruction. Constantine had made it accessible to them. They were enabled, in his translations, to read the writings of Arabic physicians; though not those of Rhazes or Avicenna, which would have been beyond their comprehension. The works translated by Constantine were those of much less noted authors, tenth-century writers such as Isaac the Jew, Ali ibn el-Abbas, etc. By the same Arabic route, the practitioners of that day became acquainted with the writings of the old Greek physicians, with the *Aphorisms* of Hippocrates, his *Prognosis*, his *Dietetics*— books which many hundred years before had been translated into Latin, but had not been understood, and had therefore been forgotten. Now, returning to the West by way of the

East, they were eagerly read. With Hippocrates came Galen, Galen's commentary on the Hippocratic writings, his great work on therapeutics, and his little *Ars medicinae*. Galen, who already dominated oriental medicine, now began to achieve the conquest of the healing art in the western world.

What gave Constantine's translations so speedy an influence was that they became textbooks at the School of Salerno, where they appeared at an apt moment. Salerno was a flourishing seaport lying not far to the south of Naples. It was an archiepiscopal see, had a famous cathedral, and many monasteries. Of late it had become widely known for its medical school. As early as the beginning of the tenth century, Salernian physicians had acquired a fair measure of reputation beyond the boundaries of the principality—not merely as men of learning, but as competent practitioners. Very diversified influences were at work in the place. Classical learning had never completely died out there. Greek was still understood, forming a supplementary language to the local Italian dialect and the Latin of the learned. There was a brisk trade between the town and the Levant. Arabic knowledge found its way into the place from the adjoining island of Sicily. There is a legend relating to the foundation of the School, to the effect that one day four doctors, a Greek, a Roman, a Saracen, and a Jew, decided upon the joint composition of a book of recipes or prescriptions. This story gives a key to the characteristics of Salerno. It was a place where laymen and clerics could collaborate in friendly rivalry.

Now, in this little community of Salernian physicians, the translations of Constantine became known. The fertilising effect was amazing. Those who had been no more than family practitioners became men of learning. Salerno developed into a "civitas hippocratica," just as, at an earlier date, Gondeshapur had in the East. A medical faculty, the first medical faculty of the West, came into being. In the twelfth century the School gave birth to an extensive literature: prescription books; textbooks of special pathology and therapeutics; monographs upon fever, the urine, the pulse, diet; treatises on surgery and on gynecology. Anatomy was once more being studied. Animals, especially swine, were prepared for anatomical demonstrations, and brief handbooks on the subject were penned. Throughout these writings, in every line, we feel the influence of Constantine. The new knowledge which he had brought to the West was being elaborated; the teachings of the Greeks and of the Arabs were being harmonised with the experience of the Salernians. But the latter felt humble-minded in face of the achievements of the great masters.

We should err were we to suppose that the Salernians of the twelfth century did original scientific work, or that it would have been reasonable to expect such work from them. They wanted to learn. They learned in the practice of medicine, at the bedside. They learned also from the new literature. Working over and over what they had learned, they passed it on to others: by word of mouth to the pupils who came in increasing numbers to Salerno; and in their books, in the new medical literature they produced, which was enormously superior to the writings of monastic medicine. They saw no reason for formulating new theories. The Greco-Arabic science, whose wealth had so recently and surprisingly been disclosed to them, provided sufficient explanations, and fully gratified their scientific thirst.

We know the names of many of the Salernian physicians: Magistri Bartholomaeus, Platearius, and Copho; that of Magister Ferrarius; at a somewhat later date those of Magistri Maurus, Urso, etc. But it is hard to discern the human beings behind these names. We can glean very little concerning their individual lives; and their books seldom convey a personal note. The work of the School of Salerno resembles that done by a guild. That is why I have made no attempt to deal with any one of the Salernians as a great doctor, and have merely made brief reference to the School as a whole, the account being supplementary to the chapter upon Constantine of Africa.

Moreover, the School of Salerno had but a brief blossoming, that of an instructive, nay stimulating impetus in the history of medicine. It flourished most abundantly during and shortly after the days of Robert Guiscard. Then, in 1195, the town was sacked by Emperor Henry VI. Thirty years later, in 1225, the university of Naples, which was soon to become a formidable rival, was founded by Emperor Frederick II. However, even after this, Salerno maintained its repute for a time. According to ordinances issued by Roger II of Sicily and by Emperor Frederick II, no doctors were to be allowed to practise in their realms unless they had received the "approbatur" of the physicians at Salerno.

CHAPTER ELEVEN

PIETRO D'ABANO
1250–1315

CONSTANTINE had made an eloquent gesture towards the East. His translations had opened a new world of medical learning. It was only to be expected that others should pass along the road he had opened. In the year 1085 Toledo was conquered by Alfonso VI of Castile. The acropolis of western Mohammedan science was seized by the Christians. At Toledo there were large libraries, and many men who were good linguists. There, surely, if anywhere, it would be possible to discover the wisdom of which Christendom stood in need. During the latter half of the twelfth century an Italian, Girardo of Cremona, made his way to Toledo, learned Arabic there, and ransacked the libraries. He made discovery after discovery. The treasures were far more valuable than he had expected. He devoted himself ardently to their exploitation. Numerous pupils flocked round him. A school of translators came into being, and displayed a febrile activity. Within a few decades, dozens upon dozens of folios had been filled with these translations, the writings of philosophers, mathematicians, astronomers, and doctors being rendered into Latin from Arabic. It was in this way that the West first came into full possession of Aristotle, Euclid, Ptolemy the astronomer, and of hitherto unknown Galenic and Hippocratic writings. Thus, too, was diffused a knowledge of Rhazes, Avicenna, and many other Arabian physicians.

At various other places where East and West came into contact, similar translations from the Arabic were now being made. Sicily was one of these fruitful regions. Whereas during the eleventh century the influx of the new literature was scanty, the stream broadened throughout the twelfth century,

95

and in the thirteenth century an enormous mass of traditional knowledge was made available to the Christian world. The maintenance and the elaboration of this knowledge became the task of the universities that were springing up throughout Europe. In the twelfth century the medical school of Montpellier began to come to the fore, and the universities of Oxford, Cambridge, and Bologna were founded. During the thirteenth century came the establishment of the universities of Paris and Naples, that of Messina, and above all that of Padua. The foundation of the universities of Prague, Vienna, Heidelberg, Cologne, and Erfurt occurred in the fourteenth century. Montpellier, a Spanish outpost in Provence, was the first of the before-mentioned places to be strongly influenced by the wave of translation, being fertilised by it as Salerno had been by the translations of Constantine. The new knowledge, however abundant, and perhaps because it was so abundant, was not readily comprehensible. Many of the translations, made with great speed, were badly done, and in so abominable a Latin that even to-day we can only read them (as Albrecht von Haller said) "superata nausea." Numbers of the Arabic technical terms, misunderstood or not understood at all, were simply transliterated without any attempt to translate them, with the result that a new jargon was created of which the world had great difficulty in ridding itself.

Those who study such texts to-day can do so as dispassionate historians, recognising them to be products of the time. But the attitude of the thirteenth century was altogether different. It took over the new literature as a living whole, and wanted to apply it forthwith in medical practice. Naturally great difficulties were encountered. Many of the descriptions of illnesses and many of the recipes were unintelligible. What had been applicable under Greek, Persian, or Egyptian conditions, could not be transferred without modification to the European world. Much work had therefore to be done in order to clarify these traditions, to explain apparent contra-

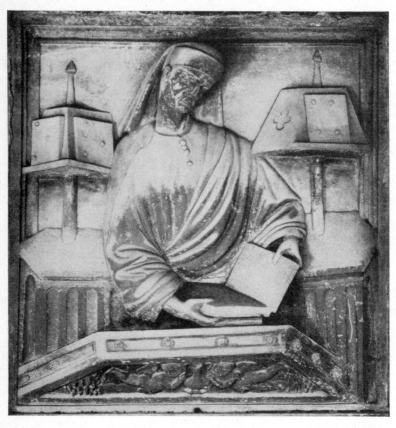

PIETRO D'ABANO, 1250–1315 (A RELIEF FROM THE PALAZZO DELLA
RAGIONE IN PADUA)

dictions, to make the new knowledge fruitful. Aristotle had taught the method, which was known as dialectics. The up-shot in the West was what it had been in the East, the growth of scholasticism. Galen and Avicenna, regarded as infallible authorities, dominated the medical mind. The business of these medieval universities was not merely to make a doctrine known but to guard it against infraction.

We shall find it easier to grasp the mental outlook of the medical scholastics if we study the writings of one of their notable representatives. For this purpose I have chosen the Italian, Pietro d'Abano.

Abano is a spa near Padua, famous for its sulphur springs, and Pietro d'Abano took his name from his birthplace. He was a typical polyhistor of the later Middle Ages. Born in 1250, he studied medicine and philosophy at Padua. One of his titles to fame was that he knew Greek, a rare acquirement in the days before the Renaissance. The writings of the Greek physicians had been studied in Latin translations by way of Arabic. Why not go direct to the original sources? Pietro went to Constantinople. We know practically nothing about his days in the imperial capital, but we are probably entitled to assume that a thirst for knowledge led him there; that he wanted to improve his command of Greek and to study Greek manuscripts. Anyhow it is certain that soon after this visit he translated a number of Galen's writings from Greek into Latin.

Next we hear of him in Paris, where he became an instructor at the university. There he wrote many of his great works, dealing not only with medicine and philosophy, but also with astronomy and physiognomy. The Church, however, regarded his doctrines with suspicion, and believed him to be engaged in the study of the occult. He was denounced to the Inquisition, the Dominicans bringing no less than fifty-five charges against him. "He practised sorcery and necromancy; he did not believe in miracles; he was lukewarm in religious matters." Happily he was successful in his defence, and was acquitted.

At the beginning of the fourteenth century, Pietro returned to Padua and became one of the shining lights of the university there. Dante was in Padua for a time at this period, and we may well suppose that the two men became acquainted. Once more Pietro was denounced to the Inquisition, and died while the trial was proceeding. Since the inquisitors could not burn him alive, they committed his corpse to the flames.

Pietro's opus magnum in the medical field is entitled *Conciliator differentiarum philosophorum et praecipue medicorum*. The medical science of the scholastics was a part of the universitas litterarum. It was a closed doctrine, resting upon the two pillars of "ratio" and "auctoritas." It formed part of the ecclesiastical picture of the universe and it was the handmaid of theology.

What did the scholastic physician write? Commentaries upon authoritative texts; dictionaries for the elucidation of difficult topics or concepts; concordances in which similar opinions were brought together. The object of Pietro's *Conciliator* was to dispel the contradictions which were so numerous in the field of medical tradition. The work was divided into three parts, the first dealing with general questions, the second with the theory of medicine, and the third with its practice. In matters of detail the work is rigidly systematic. A problem is enunciated, and then the authorities are adduced in a spate of quotations. This is followed by (the most important part for a scholastic) the argumentative section, in which the pros and the cons are sedulously balanced, in the hope that the truth will emerge and the contradictions be resolved.

In the end, the correct doctrine, purified, coordinated, could be transmitted as a circumscribed whole.

The foregoing indications must suffice to show along what

lines the healing art of those days moved. The scholastic physicians were only to a very minor degree interested in their own experience. Experience, of course, they had, and probably recorded it most freely in the "concilia"—opinions concerning particular cases, which were often written out at length. Primarily, however, the scholastic physicians were philosophers. The methods of thought had been prescribed for them by Aristotle and the learned men of Araby. They regarded logical thinking as the first requisite, endeavouring, with its aid, to achieve the systematisation of knowledge.

There were many noted doctors of this type besides Pietro d'Abano. For instance: Taddeo Alberotti, Arnold of Villanova, Giacomo dei Dondi, Bernard Gordon, and others. They all worked along kindred lines, and were apt to find themselves in conflict with the Church because they attempted to overstep the limits it imposed.

CHAPTER TWELVE

GIROLAMO FRACASTORO
1478–1553

DURING the first years of the sixteenth century there were sitting side by side on the benches of the university of Padua Gaspare Contarini, Andrea Navagero, Giambattista Ramusio, and Girolamo Fracastoro. A young Pole of German extraction, Nicolaus Koppernigk (usually known by the Latinised name of Copernicus) was one of their fellow-students. He was older than the rest, having studied law in Bologna, other subjects elsewhere, and having now, in the year 1501, enrolled himself at the medical faculty in Padua.

Padua was a sleepy old town, its streets well beset with trees. It was still famous as a seat of learning, a magnet attracting students from all parts of the world. But in these Renaissance days it was being renovated and beautified. In front of the church of St. Antony there now stood a fine equestrian statue, the work of the Florentine sculptor Donatello. The Loggia del Consiglio had just been finished. No building so fine as this had existed in Padua before. The general feeling of the place was that the glories of classical antiquity were being revived. The inhabitants of the city were enthusiasts for art. The ruins that abounded had become for them witnesses to a great past instead of mere cumberers of the ground. Fine statues were erected everywhere. There was a cult of the beauty of the human form. The moderns were endeavouring to rival or even to outdo the ancient artists.

Pietro d'Abano had taught at the university of Padua two centuries before. He had not been forgotten. His *Conciliator* was printed for the first time at Mantua in the year 1472, and there had been many subsequent editions. The art of printing with movable types had recently been discovered, so that books were rapidly becoming more numerous and cheaper than manuscripts. One who wrote a noteworthy book could count upon having the fruit of his thought speedily and widely diffused.

The most noted teachers at Padua in those days were Alessandro Achillini and Pietro Pomponazzi (Pomponatius). Both of them were Aristotelians like Pietro d'Abano, and Achillini (like Avicenna) was spoken of as "the second Aristotle." Achillini, too, was an admirer of Arabic learning, and especially esteemed the philosopher Averroes. But Achillini was something which Pietro d'Abano had never been —an anatomist. He dissected human bodies, and was a good observer. As early as the fourteenth century, not so very long after the death of Pietro, doctors began to realise the need for a thorough knowledge of the human body. Wishing to acquire a better understanding of the classical anatomical textbooks, they dissected the human body for themselves.

Pomponatius, as well, had close ties with Pietro. His brand of Aristotelianism was that of the famous commentator Alexander of Aphrodisias, an author whom Pietro had translated. But Pomponatius was an original thinker. He insisted upon the necessity of studying natural laws, so that the world might be made explicable through a knowledge of demonstrable successions. Being an investigator of physical science, he was in opposition to the Church and to the dominant religious outlook. Moreover, he was a pagan. In that age of the Church, before fanaticism had been tightened up anew by the Reformation, it was once more possible to be a pagan. Religious ties were being dissolved.

As of yore, classical philosophy was taught at the university of Padua. As of yore, the physicians of ancient days were being interpreted. There had, however, been in progress a gradual movement away from Arabic learning. Whereas until recently the Greek physicians had been known only through Arabic translators and commentators, doctors were now returning to the sources. In 1453, Constantinople had been taken by the Turks, and numbers of Greek intellectuals had fled to Italy. A knowledge of the Greek tongue was no longer markedly exceptional. Many learned men in Italy and the other countries of western Europe were able to read Greek medical textbooks. New Latin translations, direct translations, were made and printed, and revised Greek editions were also issued from the press. Previously unknown or insufficiently known authors came to light: Celsus, Aretaeus, Rufus, Paulus Aegineta. Purified texts of the Hippocratic writings were published. Antiquity was still dominant. Its reproduction still seemed the leading ideal. But what was wanted was no longer a systematised antiquity, no longer antiquity in a strait waist-coat. Classicism was being revived in its entirety. The Renaissance, for instance, had, above all, rediscovered the sculpture and the poesy of the ancient world.

This rediscovery brought about a profound modification in men's attitude towards their fellow-men and towards the universe in general. A new society had grown up. In the West the individual was awakening, was feeling the need for activity and self-expression. Humanism became the moral ideal of the Renaissance; the utmost possible development of the humanity in man, the supreme unfolding of personality. Entering imaginatively into the life of the most flourishing days of the ancient Greek and Roman commonwealths, people trained themselves in accordance with what they believed those commonwealths to have been.

Consequently the young fellows whom we have mentioned by name as studying in Padua were humanists. They were not content with learning philosophy and medicine. It was not their ambition to become experts, but human beings with a worldwide culture. One day, therefore, they would study Hippocrates; the next, Horace; and the day after, an astronomer or a geographer.

Let us contemplate them a number of years later and see

what had become of these sometime youths. Contarini, now a cardinal, is at the Diet of Ratisbon in the year 1541, trying to effect a reconciliation between the Protestants and the Catholics. Navagero has become a leading light upon classical literature, and is editing fine editions of Cicero, Quintilian, Terence, Vergil, and Ovid for the Aldine printing-house in Venice. The first edition of Pindar is dedicated to him. Ramusio has published in Venice a great work entitled *Viaggi e Navigazione*. In the field of travel and navigation, the first decade of the sixteenth century has been occupied in reaping the harvest of Columbus' discovery. A great world which was utterly unknown to the Greeks has been discovered—new continents, new kinds of human beings, new animals and new plants. This conquest of our planet is attracting universal attention. Copernicus has not abandoned medicine, but he gives most of his time to astronomy, and in his work *De revolutionibus orbium caelestium* he has reached out into the cosmos, creating a new picture of the universe, not speculative merely, but based upon precise calculations.

What about Fracastoro?

Near Verona there is a fine country mansion, with rooms looking to the south and others to the north, cool in summer but warm in winter, and far from noise and vexation. The owner of the place, a stumpy broad-shouldered man with a luxuriant growth of black hair, is Fracastoro. His nose is somewhat pinched, and it is a joke among his friends that this is because he spends so much time star-gazing.

Fracastoro prefers a country life. Here he has everything he wants: his library, which is a perpetual source of pleasure; his globes, upon which he follows the new voyages of discovery; his astrolabes. He also practises medicine, and when summoned to a patient he takes with him a volume of Plutarch to read on the way.

Here, at his country manor, with its comfortable rooms, he receives his friends. They make music, read one another the latest poems, discuss, laugh. Fracastoro is also a writer penning witty letters to friends in foreign parts, finely chiselled Latin verses, and scientific works. He writes about the art of poetry, about the soul, about sympathy and antipathy. He compiles a treatise on astronomy; and he is a contributor to geographical textbooks.

Above all, Fracastoro was the author of two medical works which have made his name immortal and have given him a firm footing in the history of medicine. He was greatly interested in epidemic diseases. In the fourteenth century there had been a terrible epidemic of bubonic plague, the Black Death, which had devastated the known world. Nearly one-fourth of the population of Europe had died of the plague which, since then, had never wholly ceased, flickering up here and there from time to time, so that its menace was continually felt. People had done their best to avert the evil, following the principles that had been tried and found useful in warding off another pestilence, leprosy—principles clearly enunciated in the Old Testament. Like the illness "zara'ath," leprosy, and now the plague or Black Death, were dealt with by notification, examination, isolation, and disinfection. People had come to recognise that there were certain illnesses which fell into an entirely different category from the rest; that they had peculiar characteristics, a physiognomy of their own; that their nature was to attack large numbers of persons in one place and at one time, to be transferable from person to person and from place to place, to be transmitted by some kind of infective material. Not only leprosy and oriental plague were thus infective, or contagious, but also anthrax, scabies, tuberculosis, and erysipelas.

These were the diseases to which Fracastoro devoted special attention. But since the close of the fifteenth century a new malady of the same class had been discovered, had undergone wide diffusion, attacking gentle and simple alike. At the outset the apparatus of quarantine, etc., had been set to work against it, until the authorities realised that it was in many respects

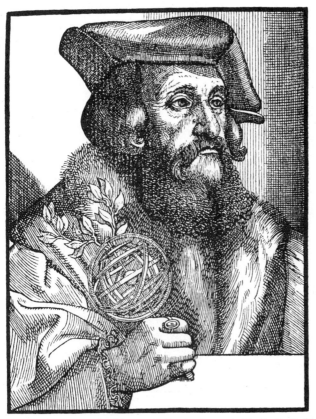

HIERONYMI FRACASTORII.

GIROLAMO FRACASTORO, 1478–1553

less dangerous than plague and leprosy. It was not almost invariably and speedily fatal like the plague; and, as contrasted with leprosy, it was curable. Nevertheless, it was a terrible scourge, for it poisoned love. After enjoying the intimate embraces of a woman, a man was always in danger of finding himself infected with this illness a few weeks later. He suffered from multifarious pains. Pustules broke out over the whole body, so that the sufferer became a horrible sight. This new disease was the "love-pestilence." It appeared to have spread with great rapidity as a sequel to King Charles VIII's campaign against Naples in the year 1495. But where had the disease originally come from? Naturally enough, its origin was ascribed to the New World.

Fracastoro studied this "love-pestilence." He was moved to describe it, its source, its manifestations, its treatment. In what way? As a dry dissertation? Of course, that was feasible. But there were poetic motifs attaching to the new malady. Many supposed that it had been sent by the gods to punish men for their sins? Classical reminiscences floated through his mind. Yes, this would be the way of it. Fracastoro wrote, and his words formed themselves into hexameters: "Qui casus varii, quae semina morbum. . . ." Was not Apollo, the god of healing, also the god of poesy? In the New World, the Spaniards had sacrilegiously killed the sacred birds, and had for this reason been chastised by infection with a previously unknown and loathsome malady, which had existed in those parts from ancient days. The natives had a legend as to the origin of the disease. A herdsman had committed sacrilege. Renouncing obedience to the sun-god, he erected altars to his mundane king, Alcithous by name. The whole population of the country followed him in his wickedness. The vengeance of the god was swift. His shafts filled the air, the earth, and the water with poisonous germs. The pestilence came into being, starting first with the herdsman, and soon affecting the whole population.

What had been the herdsman's name? In this part of his narration, Fracastoro sought inspiration from Ovid's story of the son of Niobe. Niobe's second son was named Sipylus. Niobe herself dwelt on Mt. Sipylus, and was turned into stone by Zeus, after the slaughter of her fourteen children by the arrows of Apollo and Artemis. A slight modification of the classical name sufficed (such modifications were in vogue among the writers of the humanist epoch), and Fracastoro named his hero Syphilus. The poem about Syphilus was the "Syphilid," just as the poem about Aeneas was the "Aeneid." Thanks to this, "syphilis" became the name of the "love-pestilence," which has retained this poetic name ever since the days of Fracastoro.

It was in the year 1530 that the three books entitled *Syphilidis sive de morbo gallico* were published, and they were received with unequalled approval. Every one knew the disease, and there were but too many who knew it through personal experience. Now there was a printed textbook containing valuable advice upon its treatment, and this in a form which charmed every person of culture.

As he grew older, Fracastoro continued to study the problem of syphilis, but no longer in isolation. He considered it in association with the other infectious or contagious diseases. In 1546 appeared the book which gave the most solid foundation to his fame, *De contagionibus*, likewise a work in three sections, a discussion of contagious maladies and their treatment. In the simplest and clearest fashion he explained how infectious disorders were transmitted by an infective material, in part transmitted directly from human being to human being, by contact, and in part indirectly, in cases where the contagion clung to intermediary transmitting objects (subsequently known as "fomites"). To some extent, however, contagion was also transmitted through the air. We know to-day that this contagion is a "contagium vivum"; that it is not a dead substance, but consists of extremely minute living organisms, for the most part bacteria and their congeners. In

106

his day, when the microscope had still to be invented, Fracastoro could know nothing of this. Nevertheless his theory was shrewdly formulated, and was competent to disseminate a general understanding of the nature of infectious disorders. It gave, moreover, valuable aid in the campaign against their spread.

Fracastoro did not confine himself to theory. He gave detailed descriptions of the various infective disorders, in so far as they were known in his day. Nay, he went farther, opening new ground. He showed that many fevers are not just "fevers" unqualified, but have a specific character. Distinguishing one kind of fever from another, he gave a clear account of their respective peculiarities. Thus he became the discoverer of the disease we now know as typhus. Furthermore, contemplating particular diseases as entities, he was a pioneer on the road to the establishment of that ontological conception of disease which Sydenham was to make widely acceptable a little more than a century later.

Fracastoro's literary activities attracted general attention, so that it was difficult for him to persist in leading a retired life in his Tusculum. Secular rulers and princes of the Church heaped honours upon him and tried to attract him to their courts. In general, however, he affably but persistently refused such invitations, being content to show his gratitude in the dedications of his works. He made only one exception, when Pope Paul III appointed him medicus ordinarius to the Council of Trent. Still he did not stay long at the Council, which lasted nearly twenty years; he speedily returned to his country mansion near Verona. He died there when seventy years of age, from a stroke of apoplexy which began while he was seated at the dinner-table.

The Veronese honoured his memory by erecting a monument to him two years after his death. One who to-day enters the Piazza dei Signori from the direction of the Piazza Erbe finds himself in front of the magnificent early Renaissance building of the Loggia, most impressive in its simplicity. The edifice is adorned with statues of famous Veronese of the days of classical antiquity: Cornelius Nepos, Catullus, Vitruvius, the younger Pliny, and Vergil's friend Aemilius Macer. Hard by, over an arched doorway, stands Fracastoro, the man who, filled with classical inspiration, described new things in ancient language and ancient metres—a modern through and through, notwithstanding his antique dress—a man of the Italian Renaissance.

Fracastoro was a typical representative of one of the specific mental outlooks of the Renaissance. He was one of those who lived through that animated and troubled period without becoming engaged in fierce or dangerous contentions. He was on good terms with the Church. He valued classical culture above all things, and he respected tradition. Yet the spirit of the ancient world, the spirit of research, was alive in him, and guided him incessantly in his activities. He was stirred by an impulse towards research. Following this impulse, he made discoveries without being thereby brought into conflict with tradition.

He and his fellows gave science a new tongue in which it was able to express itself clearly. They did much to initiate the discovery of the world in which we live. Conrad Gesner, Leonhard Fuchs, Brunfels, Bock, and others of their generation, the men who worked to enrich our knowledge of the animal and vegetable kingdom, were of the same calibre as Fracastoro. They helped greatly to fructify the healing art. Yet it was not they who were to bring about the decisively new trend that medicine required. For that, persons of a different calibre were requisite, persons less happy in that they lived lives of struggle. We must now turn to these fighters.

CHAPTER THIRTEEN

PARACELSUS
1493–1541

NORTH of the Alps, the revised lore of the ancient world had made its way. There, too, great enthusiasm was being shown for classical authors, and their works were being reprinted in splendid editions.

Not far from the monastery of Our Lady at Einsiedeln in Switzerland, where the Sihl roars along its deep channel amid the pine forests, a physician had settled down to practise. His name was Wilhelm Bombast von Hohenheim, and he was a man of Swabian lineage. He married a Swiss girl; the region pleased him, and was well suited for medical practice. Past his house ran the pilgrim's way which after crossing the St. Gothard led northward through Schwyz to the famous Benedictine monastery. Year after year thousands of the faithful came to worship at the shrine of the Black Mother of God in Einsiedeln, and not a few of them found it necessary to consult the doctor, seeking relief after the hardships of the journey. Two years after Hohenheim's marriage, a son was born to him. This was in the year 1493, when Columbus returned from his first voyage to the New World. The boy was christened Philipp Theophrastus, or, to give him his full Latinised appellation, Philippus Aureolus Theophrastus Bombastus von Hohenheim. Why "Theophrastus"? Was the name in the calendar? No, Theophrastus had been a disciple of Aristotle, and had succeeded that great philosopher as head of the Peripatetic school. He was the author of a *History of Plants* which had at length found its way into print, about ten years before.

In the forest of Einsiedeln, the youngster grew up among persons who were not clad in silk and who were accustomed to utter their thoughts without circumlocution in the rough and pithy patois of the district. His father took the boy with him on his rounds, where he was perpetually in contact with nature. Father Wilhelm taught young Theophrastus about plants and their wonderful healing qualities. From the neighbouring hills the lad could see the whole chain of the Alps, which looked extraordinarily close on warm days when the Föhn was blowing—alarming mountains, and yet mysteriously alluring. He shuddered as he looked, just as he shuddered in church when the clouds of incense were rising and the sacring-bell rang.

On the long winter evenings, when the countryside was wrapped in snow, no doubt his father would take a book from the library and would initiate his boy into the secrets of the written word.

Modern psychological research has taught us how decisive in our career is the influence of our early years. Thus we can understand the mental peculiarities of Theophrastus von Hohenheim much better when we know the environment of his childhood.

He was ten years old when his father removed from Switzerland to Carinthia to practise thenceforward at Villach. The mother was dead. Father and son were alone in the world. We can guess what had attracted the elder Hohenheim to Villach. There were mines in the neighbourhood, and there was a school of mining in which, according to tradition, Wilhelm von Hohenheim taught. Here, too, were Count Füger's smelting-works. A new world, a new side of nature, opened to young Theophrastus. He had occasion to learn the practical arts. He saw how the elements attracted and repelled one another, combining to form new substances. He learned the fundamentals of chemical analysis, and came to recognise its imminent practical importance.

The years ran their course, and it was time for the young man to go to a university where he could systematically study for the medical profession. To which one? To Prague? To Vienna? No, he would go to Italy. There the new science was in its prime.

Thus, one day, Hohenheim reached Ferrara. His master was Leoniceno, a grey-headed humanist who had translated the aphorisms of Hippocrates into elegant Latin, and who had been one of the first to read classical authors with a critical mind, discovering numberless errors in the writings of Pliny and others. He also had been one of the first to describe the new "love-pestilence"—decades before Fracastoro.

Hohenheim studied after the manner of other students of his day, studied in the way Fracastoro had studied. He took his doctor's degree, and, following the fashion of the humanists, Latinised his name to Paracelsus. Would he become a humanist like the rest, edit the works of classical authors, write Latin verses? There was something within him which revolted against a career of peaceful studies. As he walked through the trim gardens of Ferrara, with their carefully clipped yew-hedges, the forests of his birthplace rose before the eyes of his imagination. This was finished art; that had been nature, in communion with which he had lived, and where he had felt at home. Were not the doctrines of his professors likewise highly artificialised? Galen's theory of the four humours, the doctrine of qualities—they were logical, doubtless, and the intelligent could readily grasp them; but how would they stand the test of examination by one in tune with nature? They were sustained by the appeal to persons of great authority. But what did authorities matter if experience contradicted their teaching? Paracelsus had already had experiences of his own. He did not come from the nursery to the university. He had grown up in touch with nature, had learned how to observe, had from earliest childhood been in contact with the sick. The miners and the analysts side by side with whom he had worked, were they not much closer to nature, had they not learned far more of nature's secrets, than these dryasdust professors with their books?

A ferment was stirring in the young physician, just as at this same period a ferment was stirring in a certain Augustinian monk who was likewise beginning to doubt the infallibility of the authorities, and who, driven by his conscience, was arming for the struggle against the world in order to help on the victory of truth.

Away from the stuffy atmosphere of the class-room, into the free air, back to nature! There was true art to be found. It would not seek any one out, but must be eagerly pursued. He took a pilgrim's staff into his hand, realising that no one could become a geographical discoverer who remained seated beside the fire. "If a man wishes to become acquainted with many diseases, he must set forth on his travels. If he travels far, he will gather much experience, and will win much knowledge." On his travels, the young man learned, not only about illnesses, but also about remedies. Peasants, old wives, handicraftsmen, the barbers and the barber-surgeons—such people often had knowledge well worth acquiring, although the professors at the universities knew nothing of it.

Paracelsus set forth on his voyage of discovery through the world, upon a journey which, with trifling interruptions, was to last until death, and led him through all the lands of western Europe. He visited the mining districts, studied the healing springs, made long series of chemical experiments. He continued to practise as a physician, to help, to heal, where he could. He had thrown away his doctorial biretta and wore an ordinary slouch hat. Disciples joined their fortunes to his, apprentices of low degree often enough. Thus it was a motley company that moved from place to place.

As he travelled, it grew more and more plain to him that the traditional art of healing was on a false road. Its theories were false and its therapeutic methods were false. He began to keep a record of his own observations and ideas. He wrote, as he thought, in his mother-tongue. He had not yet become fluent in its use, and often found it difficult to express himself

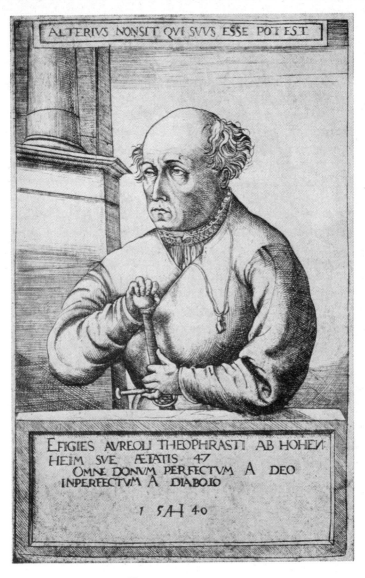

EFIGIES AVREOLI THEOPHRASTI AB HOHEN
HEIM SVE ÆTATIS 47
OMNE DONVM PERFECTVM A DEO
INPERFECTVM A DIABOIO

1 5A⌐ 40

PARACELSUS, 1493–1541

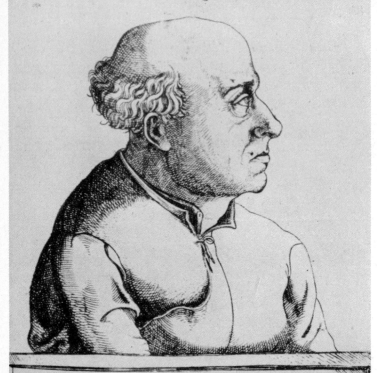

PARACELSUS, 1493–1541

clearly. Many concepts were still lacking to his verbal treasury. Many terms were hard to find. But he coined them, and by degrees fluency came. He penned observations concerning particular diseases. Especially was he interested in gout. He also wrote a little book upon disease and the healthy life which bore the strange title *Paramirum*. It was but a sketch, callow in many ways, and yet it was the draft of great things to come.

Five spheres, five entia, determine human life. The first is the "ens astrale." Every human being has his constellation. Every man is the child of his own time. The creation is a unified product, and human beings are linked in an orderly chain. Man and his environment are mutually hostile; yet man has need of the environment, and must draw nutriment or sustenance from it in order to keep himself alive. That is the second sphere, "ens veneni." The third sphere, "ens naturale," concerns the vital force of man, concerns the circulation he makes from birth to death, concerns the determination which each individual bears within him. Last of all, man is a spiritual being. He has not only consciousness, but self-consciousness. Through the spirit, through the working of the mind, the environment becomes the world in which he finds himself as a thinking and creative being. This sphere is the "ens spirituale." Out of these four spheres there rears itself against man the menace of disease. He is healthy when the fourfold ordering is fulfilled. Disturbances in that ordering lead to disease: to disease of the world, as manifested in pestilences; to disease resulting from disorders in the environment, such as occurs in consequence of nutritive disturbances. But man's course of life can also give rise to disease; and, finally, disease may arise from spiritual or mental causes.

Over-arching these four spheres is the fifth, "ens Dei," which concerns healing. In it, man returns from disorder to order. The task of the physician is to guide him to this road, to restore him to his place in the realm of order.

The *Paramirum* was a fragment, an introduction. A detailed

work on practical therapeutics was to follow. But even the sketch bears witness to the vigour of Paracelsus' mind, for it is a bold attempt to construct a medical anthropology which, undismayed, seeks to solve the basic problems that confront every practitioner of the healing art. We see that from the outset Paracelsus was following his own road, and we see whither that road was leading.

By the time he was thirty, Paracelsus was already a mature man. He had seen and learned much. He paid a visit to his father at Villach, went thence to Salzburg, and lived there for a time. Were his wanderings at an end? Perhaps they might have been, had it not been for the Peasants' War which now broke out. In such troublous times there could be no question of a tranquil practice, so Paracelsus set forth once more, to the Black Forest, to Freiburg, to Strasburg. He was weary of journeying, and longed for some fixed establishment, where, while practising his profession, he could continue his studies and elaborate his experiences; where he would have a laboratory and assistants, and where he could get his books printed. For by now he had written many books. He had studied the natural treasures of his homeland, its plants, its minerals, its healing springs. What need to buy foreign drugs at great expense, and adulterated for the most part, when such valuable sources existed close at hand? Strasburg, with its vigorous intellectual life, with its famous printing-presses, with its renowned surgical school, would be an ideal place to settle down in. On December 5, 1526, he was enrolled as a citizen of Strasburg.

Here, too, there was to be no abiding. At Basle, less than a hundred miles up the Rhine, the famous book-printer Frobenius was seriously ill. As the outcome of an accident five years before, he had horrible pains in the right foot. The doctors dreaded gangrene, and advised amputation. But the fame of the wandering physician who had recently come to Strasburg had reached Basle; and, before deciding to undergo this formidable operation, Frobenius wished to get his opinion.

Paracelsus came to Basle, took over the treatment of the case, and was able to cure the patient without the use of the knife, so that Frobenius was soon well enough to ride all the way to Frankfort.

Since Frobenius was a man of note, this cure naturally attracted much attention. In Frobenius' house lived Erasmus of Rotterdam. He too fell sick, and he too consulted Paracelsus, who thus acquired still greater fame in Basle. Since the office of town physician fell vacant at this time, it was natural that the municipal council should offer him the appointment, which carried with it the right to give lectures at the university.

Could it be true? Was he at length to have a settled establishment? More than that, was he to be professor at a university? It would give him the possibility of delivering his mind of its wealth of ideas. He would have many pupils, would be able to guide young men along the paths leading to true physicianship. No doubt the faculty—oh, well, what did it matter if the faculty were disgruntled?

He accepted the call, and in the spring of 1527 transferred to Basle. Now the moment had come for initiating the reforms in medicine of which he had dreamed for so long. He sketched a programme, which was printed as a pamphlet, and widely distributed. It had a revolutionary ring. The art of medicine, he said, had decayed. "But we shall free it from its worst errors. Not by following that which those of old taught, but by our own observation of nature, confirmed by extensive practice and long experience. Who does not know that most doctors to-day make terrible mistakes, greatly to the harm of their patients? Who does not know that this is because they cling too anxiously to the teachings of Hippocrates, Galen, Avicenna, and others?" What the doctor needed was a profound knowledge of nature and its secrets. "Day after day I publicly elucidate for two hours with great industry and to the great advantage of my hearers books on practical and theoretical medicine, internal medicine, and surgery, books written by myself. I did not, like other medical writers, compile these books out of extracts from Hippocrates or Galen, but in ceaseless toil I created them anew, upon the foundation of experience, the supreme teacher of all things. If I want to prove anything, I shall not try to do it by quoting authorities, but by experiment and by reasoning thereon. If therefore, my dear readers, one of you should feel the impulse to penetrate these divine mysteries, if within a brief space of time he should want to fathom the depths of medicine, let him come to me at Basle, and he will find much more than I can utter in a few words. To express myself more plainly, let me say, by way of example, that I do not believe in the ancient doctrine of the complexions and the humours, which have been falsely supposed to account for all diseases. It is because these doctrines prevail that so few physicians have a precise knowledge of illnesses, their causes, and their critical days. I forbid you, therefore, to pass a facile judgment upon Theophrastus until you have heard him for yourselves. Farewell, and come with a good will to study our attempt to reform medicine. Basle, June 5, 1527."

This was a declaration of war. The faculty was aghast. It had not been consulted as to the appointment of the new town physician. Besides, Paracelsus openly ignored it, and abstained from the customary formalities, from having himself entered upon the register, from presenting his diplomas, from the disputation which was prescribed for such cases. The riposte was speedy! The faculty forbade Paracelsus to use the lecture-theatre, and wanted even to forbid his practising in the town. Battle had been joined. Paracelsus applied to the town council, which had summoned him to Basle, and now insisted upon his right to use the lecture-theatre. As for graduation as a member of the university, and the right to officiate as one of the medical faculty of Basle, that he had never asked for.

Heedless of the storm of opposition he was arousing, he ardently began his teaching activities, lecturing during the summer term, lecturing in the vacation and the winter term of

1527–1528, upon special pathology and therapeutics, upon the preparation of medicines and the art of prescribing, upon the examination of the pulse and of the urine, upon purgation and venesection, upon injuries and surgical disorders. An unheard-of innovation, his surgical lectures were given in the vernacular, in the German tongue instead of in Latin! He had new things to say, and they needed a new language. Besides, medicine was not for him an esoteric art and science which must be hidden away behind Latin furbelows.

With increasing wrath the faculty watched the behaviour of this innovator who was disregarding the forms sanctified by use and wont, who was teaching unprecedented doctrines, and who seemed to regard his colleagues as little better than idiots. They would have to fight him tooth and nail if they wished to maintain their own positions.

Paracelsus had expected nothing else from the faculty. But what about the young folk, the future for which he lived and worked? Surely they would stand by him? No, they likewise disowned him. One morning there were posted on the doors of various churches and upon that of the new bourse copies of a vulgar versified lampoon upon Paracelsus, obviously written by a student. This poisoned shaft wounded him to the core. His patron Frobenius was dead. He had only the council left on his side. From the council he demanded protection—protection against his own students. They were to be questioned one by one, until the offender was discovered. A strange reformer this, who aspired after a following of youthful disciples and was now asking to be protected against these same youthful disciples by the town beadle.

At this juncture, moreover, Paracelsus quarrelled with the town council over the paltry question of a fee. He had cured a canon of the Church, and had demanded a good round sum for his services, considering that the rich ought to give of their superfluity so that the poor might be treated for nothing. The canon refused to pay, and the case came into court. The decision went against Paracelsus. In a fury, he railed against all and sundry, and he no longer had any friends in the town. The medical faculty was delighted, the students made fun of the affair, the whole place turned against him.

The upshot was that his stay in Basle lasted no more than ten months. One foggy night in February 1528 he left the city to renew a migratory existence. Prophets can find no abiding place, for they are citizens of the world. People were not yet ripe for his teaching, not even the younger generation. But his day would come.

Returning to Alsace, he settled for a time in Colmar. The MS. notes of his lectures at Basle were to be elaborated into books. He was eager to voice his views, to justify himself after his defeat at Basle, to announce the kernel of his teaching.

This was effected in *Paragranum*. "Herein I disclose the foundation upon which I write, the foundation without which no physician can become established." Paracelsus knew that now, if ever, he was in arms against the world. He assumed a challenging tone: "You must follow in my footsteps, I will not follow in yours. Not one of you will be able to find a corner so retired but that the dogs will come and lift their legs in order to defile you. I shall become monarch, mine will be the monarchy, over which I shall rule to make you gird up your loins. What think you of Cacophrastus? You will have to eat dirt."

The books treat of the four pillars upon which the healing art stands. The first pillar is philosophy. This philosophy, however, is not medieval scholasticism, but knowledge of nature. Disease is the outcome of nature, and so is healing. Who can be a better teacher in these matters than nature? . . . Just as the physician is an outgrowth from nature, what can nature be other than philosophy? What else is philosophy than invisible nature?

The second pillar is astronomy. Heaven's attitude toward the creature is that of the father to the son. Heaven works in us, and we shall not understand human beings unless we recognise their cosmic affiliations.

The third pillar of medicine is chemistry. Its object is not to transmute baser metals into gold and silver, but to provide effective drugs and to throw light upon biological processes. Nature is the ideal chemist. The chemist who does not follow nature's ways is like a bungler of a cook who does not understand his job.

Herein lay one of Paracelsus' greatest merits, that he enlisted chemistry in the service of therapeutics as never before. He taught the use of sulphur, lead, antimony, mercury, iron, copper, in their various combinations. He was fiercely opposed to the traditional polypharmacy, to the administration of vague mixtures of large numbers of vegetable products. He was reproached with giving his patients poisons, and he replied: "All things are poisons, for there is nothing without poisonous qualities. It is only the dose which makes a thing a poison." The essential drugs were active principles which must be extracted from the raw materials. "I separate that which is arcanum from that which is not arcanum, and I administer the arcanum in its proper dose." Specific, purposive treatment was the ideal of therapeutics.

It was his knowledge of chemistry which gave Paracelsus the key to the understanding of the processes in inorganic and organic nature. Everywhere he discovered three principles; the combustible (sulphur); the volatile (mercury); and the incombustible, which remained behind as ash (salts). What transformed the non-living into the living was a peculiar force to which he gave the name of "archeus."

The fourth pillar of medicine is virtue. Love is the foundation of the healing art. Only a sincere, God-fearing, unselfish man can be a good physician.

Confident in the soundness of his mission, he wrote: "Do not despise my writings, and do not allow yourselves to be estranged from me because I stand alone, because what I write is new, because I am German." Since he was forbidden opportunities for teaching by word of mouth, he would teach in writing.

But no one would print his books. It seemed to him that there must be a conspiracy against him. Then in Nuremberg he found a town council whose members were more liberal-minded than those in other cities, and were prepared to publish his works. In 1529 appeared two books on syphilis; but thereupon the medical faculty of Leipzig entered a protest, and he could get nothing more printed in Nuremberg.

He continued his travels, though no longer going very far afield. The region in which he had passed his childhood exercised an attraction upon him. In the year 1531 he was in St. Gall, where he got into touch with the humanist Vadian. The town was in a ferment because of the Reformation, and had no taste for the medical reforms of Paracelsus.

Besides, at this juncture Paracelsus himself was passing through a religious crisis concerning which we are very inadequately informed. While staying in the canton of Appenzell he wrote certain theological books about which little is known. Had he abandoned the theory and practice of medicine, had he given up the struggle?

No, for when in 1535 the plague broke out in the Inn valley, the doctor in him reawakened. He wrote a treatise on the disease for the town of Sterzing. At the same time he penned surgical treatises. Once more he justified himself and his doctrine in seven admirable defensive writings.

Hirschvogel's portrait, made in the year 1538, presents him to us when he was no more than forty-five years of age, but we are looking at an old man who has suffered greatly. Still, we note the tough Alemannic skull, made for butting against thick walls; we note the hard-bitten features of a man ready to defy the world.

He was in Carinthia when Prince Ernest of Bavaria, a patron of the natural sciences, summoned him to Salzburg. He followed the call, but died, prematurely worn out, on December 24, 1541.

When Paracelsus died, Fracastoro, fifteen years older than he, was living in the fine country-house near Verona, surrounded by a brilliant circle of friends. It was autumn, when the figs were ripe and the vintage had begun. Two different worlds, sundered for ever by the granite masses of the Alps! Fracastoro's home was in the south, with its warm air and its bright sunshine, which gave cheerful colours to the landscape. Paracelsus' lot was passed and his days drew to a close in the chill, misty, but vivifying north.

It was with Paracelsus that the northern world appeared upon the stage of medicine. Its entry was fierce, impetuous, characterised by a Faustian urge towards completion. Fracastoro wrote and was applauded. Paracelsus wrote and was laughed to scorn. Fracastoro made valuable contributions in respect of particular medical topics. In his day, he advanced medical science, fertilised it, but his influence was fleeting, so that to-day he is numbered wholly with the dead. Paracelsus broached the basic problems of the healing art, those which will for all time be part of the essentials of physicianship. He did not found a school. It was hard for his discoveries to secure incorporation into the general body of medical doctrine. Yet his work, originating at one of the turning-points of western medicine, is still very much alive to-day.

Paracelsus was thoroughly German in his mode of thought, and perhaps no one but a German can really understand him. But whenever a German doctor meditates upon his calling, he cannot fail to think of Paracelsus and to find in Paracelsus a leader.

CHAPTER FOURTEEN

ANDREAS VESALIUS
1514–1564

THE discovery of the world went on. People had again grown aware of the beauty of the human body. There was nothing sinful in this beauty. On the contrary, man's body and woman's body were the most perfected works of the Creator. It was artists, not physicians, who led the way in studying the human body, that they might be better able to depict it nude in all its splendour. They studied the classical statues, which were such magnificent representations of the nude; and they also studied nature. Trying to grasp the plastique of life, they followed the play of the muscles beneath the skin. What sort of a muscle is it which, shaped like a delta, forms the roundness of the shoulder? Or that muscle which, with teeth like those of a saw, grips the thorax from behind? Scientific curiosity awakened among artists as well as among men of science. Many of the Renaissance artists were not content with the study of outward form, but, getting access to the bodies of the dead, removed the skin in order to expose, to see, and to touch the various muscles.

The leader of these artistic anatomists was Leonardo da Vinci. He, too, was a man with multifarious, nay universal interests; artist, scientist, and technician; the painter who created for posterity the enigmatic and enthralling smile of Mona Lisa; who would next day, as an engineer, draft the plans for a canal; and who, the day after, would design a new cannon. He, likewise, was an innovator, sharply opposed to traditional science, and he wrote, not in Latin, but in the living vernacular. For him the essence of knowledge lay in measurement. Mathematics was at the focus of cognition, and proportion was its medium. He studied the whole of nature, the realm of perfect configuration, trying to fathom its determinisms by the instruments of experience and reason.

His interest was centred upon man. He wanted to learn everything he could about man's structure and functions, and about the laws that control human action. He dissected numerous bodies. With knife and crayon he penetrated the mysteries of the organism. Hundreds upon hundreds of sheets of paper were covered with his sketches and his notes. In conjunction with his friend the anatomist Marcantonio della Torre, he planned a great anatomical work which was to describe human beings from the moment of procreation. Unfortunately this was never completed, was never made ready for the press. Only a circle of intimate pupils knew of these studies. The manuscript and sketches fell into the hands of ignoramuses who scattered them or destroyed them, so that their fruit was lost to science. It was inevitable that Leonardo's work should remain a fragment, since his aim was to acquire and transmit a knowledge of the whole cosmos.

But what about the Renaissance physicians? They were busied on the same task. They, too, were driven to the study of anatomy as if possessed by a demon. From the beginning of the fourteenth century—first of all in Bologna, whence the movement gradually spread to other places—the dissection of corpses had been going on. The days of anatomical demonstrations were red-letter days in the academic calendar. The authorities would place the corpse of an executed criminal at the disposal of the university authorities. Doctors and students would be invited. The professor sat at his desk, reading aloud from a textbook of anatomy. Meanwhile a surgeon was dissecting, and a demonstrator was indicating with a wooden pointer the parts as they were successively mentioned. It was plain to all hearers that the human body must have greatly changed since the days of antiquity—for at this date no one dreamed of imagining that the ancient authors could have made any mistake.

When the Renaissance was in its bloom, corpses were more readily obtainable. The various schools were no longer obliged to restrict themselves to dissecting one body each year. The professor came down from his desk and himself wielded scalpel and forceps. There were doctors who could boast of having dissected in the course of their life several hundred bodies. They described what they saw or believed themselves to see, for they all of them looked through Galen's spectacles now that Galen's anatomical works printed from revised texts were in every one's hands.

The Giunta publishing house in Venice planned a monumental edition of the Galenic works in Latin translation. A staff of humanists was recruited for the work. Who was to undertake the anatomical writings? In Padua, near by, there had been established for two years as professor of anatomy and surgery a young man one of whose publications had attracted widespread attention. In the year 1538 he had issued an atlas of anatomy, containing six full-page plates; three of them pictures of the bones drawn from actual specimens by a pupil of Titian's, an artist from the Low Countries named Johann Stephan von Kalkar; and three of them plates of the vascular system, from the professor's own dissections. To these plates detailed descriptions were appended. The atlas had bumper sales, being better than anything of the kind hitherto attempted.

In other fields of medicine this young anatomist was already a writer of note. A few years before he had translated into good Latin the ninth book of Rhazes' *Liber Almansoris*; and he had subsequently issued a new edition of the *Anatomical Institutions* of Winter von Andernach, professor at Paris—as a text to his own anatomical atlas. Recently, too, he had given plain proof of the importance of anatomy in medical practice by a letter upon venesection, in which, moreover, he had given an excellent description of the azygos vein—and one which differed in many respects from that of Galen. Indubitably he was a man with a critical intelligence, the very man for the Giunta printing house. He was therefore commissioned to do the work.

This young professor at Padua had come from Brussels, and his name was Andreas Vesalius. How had he found his way to Italy? The son of the imperial court apothecary, he had been born on New Year's night 1514-1515. The family hailed from Wesel, of which the father's name Vesalius was a Latinised and adjectival form. From early youth, Andreas had manifested an uncontrollable impulse towards the study of nature, and especially towards anatomy. No animal was safe from him. Dogs and cats, mice, rats and moles, whatever he could get hold of, were meticulously dissected by him.

He went to school at Louvain, and then was sent to Paris for the study of medicine. No doubt at this famous university there must have already been possibilities of learning human anatomy, but Andreas Vesalius was bitterly disappointed. One of his teachers, Jacques Dubois, was content, at the anatomy class, to read Galenic texts over the organs of dogs, and while doing this he made a practice of skipping the most important passages as too difficult. As for the other professor, the already mentioned Winter von Andernach, he was a learned student of classical literature who "every day translated as much as a scribe could take down from his dictation," with the result that very often time was lacking in which to read over what he had dictated. He had been the first to translate Galen's chief anatomical treatise from Greek into Latin. But as for using the knife, Vesalius never saw him do that anywhere except at the dinner-table.

What, then, could the enthusiastic young anatomist do but dissect animals, and vary this by going from time to time to the cemetery or to the place of execution in search of bones, which he would study until he could identify them with closed eyes. But as at other universities, so in Paris, there were now and again dissections of human bodies. Vesalius had attracted notice by his zeal. At the third of these dissections, the professor asked him to undertake the job. At length his opportunity had come. For the first time, scalpel in hand, he stood beside a human corpse. He acquitted himself well, and was asked to act as dissector upon a subsequent occasion.

The outbreak of war made it necessary for Vesalius to quit Paris. He continued his studies at Louvain and Brussels, getting a chance at dissection from time to time. He was able to fulfil his ambition in another respect, becoming (at great risks) the possessor of a complete skeleton by stealing a body from the gallows. What next? Italy, the land of the new sciences, exerted its lure. He crossed the Alps, reached Venice, encountered there his fellow-countryman the painter Johann Stephan von Kalkar, and the two went on together to Padua. On December 5, 1537, he took his doctor's degree at the university of that town. Next day he was appointed professor of surgery and anatomy, although he was but three-and-twenty years of age.

Now began a period of unresting activity, so strenuous that one might almost imagine Vesalius knew his life was to be a short one. The before-mentioned atlas was published within a few months of his appointment as professor.

Then came the editorial work upon Galen's anatomical writings. He read them, compared the different editions, studied variorum readings, did his best to understand. There were so many statements that were obviously incorrect. The lower jaw was said to consist of two parts. The sternum was made up of seven distinct bones. The liver had several lobes. Now Vesalius, in his dissections, had never come across anything of the kind. Of course it is human to err, yet how could such a man as Galen make gross errors? Were they errors after all? Perhaps what Galen was describing was not human anatomy at all, but the anatomy of the lower animals. That explained it! Galen's anatomical writings concerned the anatomy of monkeys, swine, goats. Vesalius could have kicked himself for not having realised this before!

The recognition of the true facts of the case brought with it a sense of liberation. The fetters of tradition had been broken. Galen had never dissected a human body. He was not the unchallengeable authority he had been supposed. Doctors needed to know the structure of the human body, and since existing books on the subject were untrustworthy Vesalius must set out upon a voyage of discovery, must himself write an authoritative work upon the anatomy of man.

He worked at this self-imposed task with febrile energy, assisted by Kalkar as draughtsman. By August 1, 1542, he finished the manuscript of his great treatise on anatomy, *De humani corporis fabrica libri septem*. He was then seven-and-twenty years of age.

Now came the question of publication. Vesalius was fully aware of the historical importance of his book, and great care was therefore given to the type-setting. Although Venice was a famous centre of printing, he preferred to publish in Basle, the heart of Europe, at the printing house of Oporinus. The blocks for the illustrations were laden upon mules and sent over the Alps. Vesalius travelled with them, for he intended to keep watch upon the printing. The faculty of Basle gave him a friendly reception. In the Swiss university town he dissected a body whose skeleton is still preserved there as a relic in the Anatomical Institute.

In June 1543, the year in which Copernicus created for his contemporaries a new picture of the universe, Vesalius' great book was published, containing 663 folio pages and over 300 illustrations. Simultaneously there was published an epitome, for class-room use. This appeared not only in Latin, but also in a German translation which had been made by the rector of Basle university, Albanus Torinus.

Vesalius was now twenty-eight, and the course of his life had reached its apogee. He had, in fact, finished his work, although he lived for twenty-one years more. After his return to Italy he quarrelled with his colleagues, finding that they regarded him with envy and disfavour. Thereupon he followed his father's example by entering the court service, as physician-in-ordinary to Emperor Charles V and subsequently to King Philip II of Spain. He formulated various plans, taking up his pen from time to time, especially for the preparation of a second edition of his opus magnum. But he became involved in deplorable polemics. The defenders of Galen showered abuse upon the innovator. Some of these attacks came from Padua. He was reproached for making mistakes, though obviously no one who broke so vast an extent of new ground could avoid an error here and there. He did his best to defend himself, but his dissecting-room was in an imperial palace. Under such circumstances, what chance had he of effective reply, corroborated by sufficient references to physical facts?

One day therefore in the year 1564, a prey to dull disquiet, he left the court, recrossed the Alps, and found himself in Venice once more. Twenty-seven years had passed since he had first entered the City of the Lagoons. Then he was on his way to Padua. Whither now? He took ship for Palestine, intending to go to Jerusalem. During the voyage to the Holy Land he fell sick, and died on one of the Ionian Islands.

What had led the great anatomist to start upon this adventurous pilgrimage? There are various rumours. One story runs to the effect that he had opened the body of a presumably dead woman to find with horror that her heart was still beating. He was brought before the Inquisition, and the emperor rescued him with difficulty. Others declare that he was consumed with home-sickness, was weary of the court, and had made a vow to visit Jerusalem in search of health. Yet others tell us that he had merely made a pleasure voyage to Cyprus. On the return journey he fell sick and died, just when he was about to be recalled to Padua.

Gossip about the matter continued for a long time. We shall

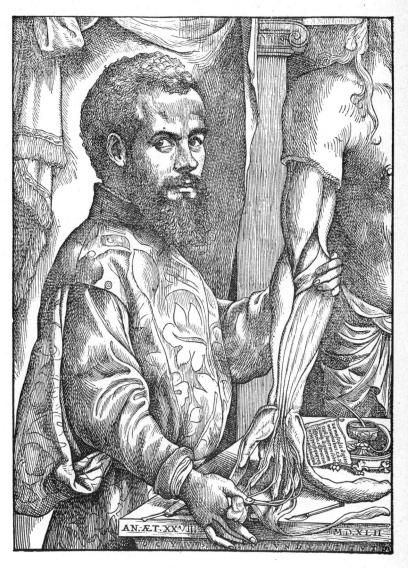

AN·ÆT·XXVIII

M·D·XLII

And. Vesalius

VESALIUS, 1514–1564

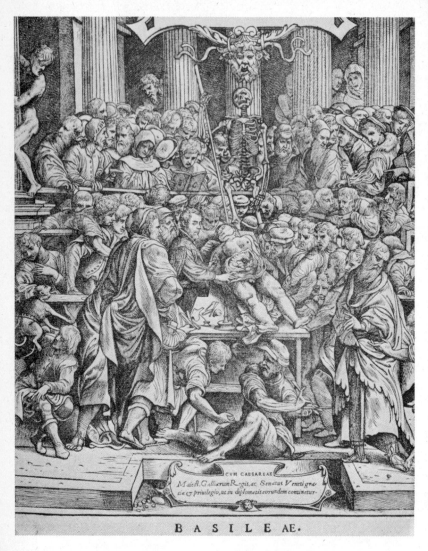

CVM CAESAREAE

Maiest. Galliarum Regis, ac Senatus Veneti gratia & priuilegio, ut in diplomatis eorundem continetur.

BASILEAE.

VESALIUS GIVING A DEMONSTRATION OF ANATOMY

never learn the truth. Vesalius took the secret with him to the grave.

Vesalius was dead, but there remained as monument his *De humani corporis fabrica*, the first complete text-book of human anatomy known to history. Thus the year 1543 stands out in the story of medicine no less than in the story of astronomy. Galen's authority was even more convincingly refuted by the sober factual demonstrations of Vesalius than it had been by the onslaught of Paracelsus. Nor was Vesalius content to be a destroyer; he was a creator as well. He fashioned the methods of modern descriptive anatomy, and, by his own use of them, achieved valuable results. To a greater extent than even he had anticipated, anatomy was to become the basis of medicine; nay more, was to become one of the "forms of thought" of the western healing art. We shall learn in the sequel how anatomical thought was henceforward to run like a red thread through all the developments of medical science.

Fracastoro, Paracelsus, Vesalius—the three of them passed through the Italian universities. The three of them were likewise products of the humanist culture of their day. Yet how greatly they differed! Fracastoro and Paracelsus were both of them polyhistors of the Renaissance, but one of them was cheerful and easy-going, whereas the other had the tortured spirit of a Faust. Vesalius, like Paracelsus, was from the colder regions that lay northward of the Alps, was equipped with the fighting vigour of the North. In five years he did enough work to last another man for a long lifetime. But he sounded a new note, being somewhat one-sided—a specialist instead of a universalist. He did not make all knowledge his province, nor even devote himself to the wide field of medicine as a whole. He concentrated his energies upon one topic, upon a topic whose fundamental importance he had recognised. It is perhaps still too early in the history of medicine to talk of "specialism," but in the case of Vesalius we are beginning to foresee the lines medical development was destined to take.

CHAPTER FIFTEEN

AMBROISE PARÉ
1510–1590

IN 1536 began the third war between Francis I and Charles V. It was on this account that Vesalius had quitted Paris. Paracelsus, who was living near Augsburg, devoted himself to the perfectionment of a vulnerary balsam. Fracastoro was working at astronomy just then.

Once more the struggle was for Milan, and it was mainly fought upon Italian soil. A French army crossed the Alps and descended by way of Susa to attack Turin. In passing, the fortress of Villaine, which was held by the imperial troops, was stormed. The garrison made a desperate defence, and there were many dead and wounded. The surgeons had their hands full. Passing from case to case, they poured boiling elder oil into the wounds. The poor wretches thus treated yelled in their agony, but they had to submit, for the wounds were "poisoned with gunpowder" and in default of such cauterisation the poison would prove fatal. Such was the teaching of Giovanni de Vigo, surgeon-in-ordinary to the Pope.

The young French surgeon, Ambroise Paré, on his first campaign, was thus engaged when the elder oil ran short. What was he to do? He had with him a salve made of yolk of egg, attar of roses, and turpentine. Smearing lint with this ointment, he used it to plug the wounds. But he had an uneasy conscience. "Last night," he relates, "I could hardly sleep for continually thinking about the wounded men whose hurts I had not been able to cauterise. I expected to find them all dead next morning. With this in view, I rose early to visit them. Greatly to my surprise, I found that those whom I had treated with the salve had very little pain in their wounds, no inflammation, no swelling, and they had passed a comfortable night. The others, those whose wounds had been treated with boiling elder oil, were in high fever, while their wounds were inflamed, swollen, and acutely painful. I determined, therefore, that I would no longer cauterise the unfortunate wounded in so cruel a manner."

As so often happens, chance led to a discovery of prime importance, to the discovery that gunshot wounds are not poisoned wounds, and that the dominant theory was erroneous. But, as always, a man of genius was needed to grasp the significance of this chance happening, to deduce the right inferences, to elaborate and defend the new knowledge until it had become general property.

In Italy during the thirteenth century there had been a great development of surgery, which had spread thence to the adjoining land of France. Surgery must always keep in close touch with life, and can never be so theoretical as internal medicine. Only by practice does a man learn how to operate. A suture holds the edges of a wound together, or it fails to do so. One thing or the other; there can be no dispute about the matter. That was why, even during the heyday of scholasticism, there had been noted practitioners of surgery. Indeed, the prevailing interest in classical and Arabic medical literature was most advantageous to them. They could try this, that, and the other, and hold fast to what was good. Tradition was sifted by practice, and could prove fruitful instead of sterile.

To the surgeons of those days, when most wounds were made with cold steel, "healing by first intention," that is to say a primary, non-suppurative growing together of the edges of a wound, seemed the most desirable ideal. A change came, however, during the fourteenth and fifteenth centuries, when the increasing use of firearms imposed new tasks upon army surgeons. Even "small arms" were then of large calibre, their bullets ranging up to nearly an inch in diameter. These projectiles must have inflicted horrible wounds, most of which, doubtless, were infected from the outset. We can hardly be surprised, therefore, that by degrees the idea gained ground that suppuration was a normal stage in the healing of wounds, and that gunshot wounds were poisoned by the gunpowder. As for suppuration, you may still hear the expression "laudable pus."

Time was needed, however, before Paré's discovery could take effect. Paré was not a man of learning, was not a writer as well as a surgeon. His instrument was the bistoury, not the pen. He sprang from the common people, being a handicrafts-man (as were most surgeons in those days) and devoid of humanist culture. Born in 1510 at Bourg-Hersent near Laval in Maine, he had for a time been a barber's apprentice. Then, going to Paris, he spent several years working at surgery in the Hôtel-Dieu. When the war broke out he was considered sufficiently expert to accompany Marshal Montejan as regi-mental surgeon. His scientific equipment was inconsiderable. Since he had never learned Latin, the writings of the ancients were closed books. But he was endowed with great surgical skill, was a good observer, and was so eager to learn that he would try the recipes of old wives and would pay court to obscure surgeons in order to learn the secrets of their practice. Like Paracelsus, he did not disdain to study the therapeutic lore of the common folk.

Upon this first campaign, his abilities attracted attention. A physician of Turin, who saw him at work, said to Marshal Montejan: "Sir, you have with you a surgeon who, though young in years, is old in knowledge and experience. Take great care of him, for he will do you good service and bring you honour."

After the Peace of Nice in 1538, Paré returned to Paris. He married, and devoted his energies to practice. A few years later, war broke out again between the two monarchs, and Paré was eager to march with the French army. The methodical efficacy of his new way of treating wounds, his marked operative skill, and his successful dealing with the wounds of persons of importance, made him more and more widely known. His colleagues recognised his superiority, and begged him to put his ideas concerning the principles of wound surgery upon written record.

After the Peace of Crespy in 1544, Paré was again in Paris. His fame had reached the ears of Jacques Dubois, whose acquaintance we have already made as one of Vesalius' teachers. Dubois invited Paré to dinner. The two men had a talk about gunshot wounds. Paré warmed to the subject, related his experience, and explained his reasons for believing that gunshot wounds were not necessarily poisoned wounds. Dubois, recognising the outstanding intelligence of his guest, likewise urged him to publish his experiences, in order to counteract Vigo's disastrous teaching. It was under these auspices that, in 1545, was published Paré's first literary work, the little manual upon the treatment of gunshot wounds which has become a classic. This was the first of a long series of valuable monographs.

If anywhere, it was in the field of surgery that the new science of anatomy was to come into its own. Paré had from the first recognised the great importance of anatomy. Even when on active service, he made dissections whenever opportunity offered; and he relates having dissected the left side of a body while leaving the right side intact, as a guide to operative work—a specimen which he took home with him. The years 1545 to 1550 were mainly devoted to anatomical study, with two interruptions for field surgery connected with the siege of Boulogne. Dubois appointed him prosector. Dubois was firmly convinced of the soundness of Galen's teaching, and it was not until the professor died that Paré ventured to acknowledge his acceptance of the new Vesalian anatomy. Then several anatomical works of his own were published. Although they did not contain any new discoveries, we have to remember, when considering them, that they were composed exclusively for practical purposes, were guides for surgeons who needed topographical rather than systematic knowledge.

In 1552 war broke out again. This campaign was of the utmost importance to Paré, for it was now he became aware that, in amputation, ligature was preferable to cauterisation for the arrest of hæmorrhage. The ligature was not a novelty, but an old device which had passed into oblivion, and upon whose advantages it was needful to insist once more. The same year, under orders from the king (whose surgeon-in-ordinary he had become), he managed to make his way into the beleaguered city of Metz, to help the wounded there. When next year he was taken prisoner at Hesdin, he bought his freedom by amazingly successful operations, without disclosing his identity to the enemy. Fresh honours were awaiting him in Paris. In 1554 he was appointed maître-chirurgien at the Collège Saint-Côme— an unprecedented honour for a sometime barber's assistant who had no Latin.

The ensuing years were spent in war service, in accompanying the king upon journeys, and in Parisian practice. In the army, Paré's popularity was unbounded; and after the death of Henry II, Francis II, and then Charles IX, continued to place the utmost confidence in him. He wrote many more books. Whenever a question was topical, he was moved to record his experiences upon the matter. Sometimes these concerned purely medical and surgical matters, but sometimes led him farther afield, and then brought him into conflict with the faculty. He died on December 20, 1590, when eighty years of age.

Paré, also, was a man of the Renaissance, although of a very different type from the physicians studied above. Like them, however, he was a discoverer of new territory and a conquistador. Unencumbered by tradition, he followed his sound instinct. Many of the operations he introduced into daily practice were not new but had been forgotten, and were revived through his authority.

A practitioner above all, nevertheless as a writer he felt the need to provide theoretical grounds for his contentions. He did this with the aid of the medical ideas of Galen, some of whose writings—and especially the *Methodus medendi*—had been translated into French. He was far from being opposed to Galen, as Paracelsus and Vesalius had been. How could he, a mere barber by training, venture to contradict the great master? All the same, the most characteristic feature of Paré's work was that when he found a disharmony between theory and experiment he gave theory the go-by. Experience took the lead; "ratio" and "auctoritas" must bow to it, and were only valid when they confirmed it.

Paré's ways of thinking are admirably illustrated by the following anecdote. When he was on his first campaign, a scullion fell into a cauldron of boiling oil and was horribly scalded. Paré having been summoned, he ran off to the apothecary to fetch the customary cooling applications. There he encountered an old woman who advised him to apply raw onion, chopped and sprinkled with a little salt, for this, she said, as experience had shown her again and again, would prevent the formation of blebs. True to his principles to make trial of every remedy from which good might be expected, Paré followed the old woman's counsel, and the result was satisfactory. He continued experimenting in this direction. A German soldier had his face badly burned, and Paré treated half the face with chopped onion and the other with one of the usual remedies. The result was that on the former half no blebs formed whereas the other half was thickly covered with them. Soon afterwards a number of soldiers, while storming a fortress, were burned by the ignition of a train of gunpowder. Paré seized the opportunity to try the method once more, treating some of the patients with onions and the rest of them otherwise—with the same result as before. These experimental data convinced Paré that the application of raw onion was of great value in the treatment of burns and scalds. But what had theory to say about it? According to Galen, onions are warm in the fourth degree, and are therefore strongly contra-indicated in burns and scalds. Paré did not venture to infer that Galen had been wrong. Yet it never occurred to him to doubt the accuracy of his own observations, and since it was necessary to confirm them "ratione et auctoritate," theory must be adapted to experience. Well, every one knew that it was with Galen as with the Bible. By searching diligently, you could find a text to support whatever you pleased—or you could modify the text to suit your wishes. Paré discovered that onions are indeed potentially, that is to say metaphorically, warm in their effect; but that actually, that is to say as made known to us by our senses, they are damp. By their warm temperament they thin the integument, and by their moistness they loosen its structure. We should infer from this that they would promote the formation of blebs. Paré, however, argued that, thanks to the aforesaid qualities of onions, the inflamed humours were drawn forth, consumed, and dried, with the result that no blebs were formed—this being a sign that Galenic doctrine is extensible, and must not be interpreted too rigidly. Here he had the proof "ratione"; and as for the proof "auctoritate," Galen was himself the required authority. After all, Galen admitted numerous instances in which it was necessary to treat, not contraria contrariis, but similia similibus. For instance, viper's flesh (in theriac) was an antidote to a viper's bite.

Paré's commanding figure stands upon the threshold of modern surgery. It was thanks to him, in the main, that for several centuries France took the leadership in this field.

I must allude to one of his character traits which makes him more congenial than the majority of medical notabilities, one which distinguished him from many of his contemporaries. He was extremely modest, this modesty being the outcome of a profound piety which was untinged by bigotry. For him, as for Paracelsus, the foundation of the healing art must be love.

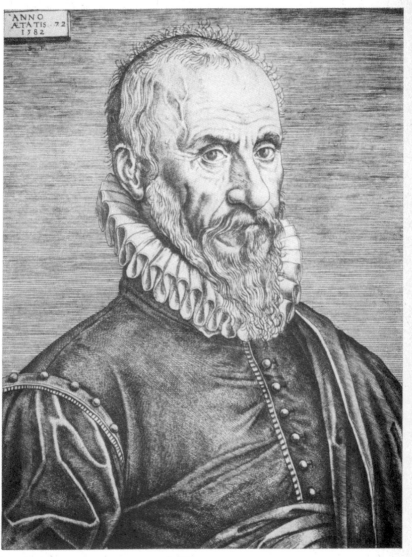

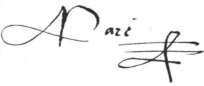

AMBROISE PARÉ, 1510–1590

Again and again we find him adjuring young surgeons not to work for the sake of monetary reward, and to do their duty to the last even in hopeless cases or cases that appeared hopeless. "For nature often brings things to pass which seem impossible to the surgeon." If the surgeon was successful in bringing about a cure, he must not plume himself on this, but must ascribe the happy result to God's grace. The oft-quoted saying of his, "Je le pensai, Dieu le guarist," is the most signal of the great French surgeon's titles to honour, superadding to his manifold services the atmosphere of all that was best in humanism.

CHAPTER SIXTEEN

WILLIAM HARVEY
1578–1657

THE sixteenth century had drawn to a close, and a new century had opened. A profound change had occurred in thoughtful men's ways of looking at the world, in the relationship between the individual and the universe. Michelangelo had broken new trails for art. He and the artists who followed him contemplated the world in its multifarious mobility. They were no longer concerned with, they no longer strove mainly to represent, extant beings, to depict what had happened; they did not gaze at man's eye but at his vision. In their works they broke through the limits imposed by circumscribed forms, and they obliterated sharp outlines, bathing them in chiaroscuro. They direct our gaze towards profundity, towards unlimited distance. Even sculpture, even architecture, was becoming picturesquely mobile. Pillars had assumed a spiral form. Stone itself had come to life.

Galileo Galilei had a telescope made for himself, that he might scan the depths of the skies. He discovered the satellites of Jupiter; the Milky Way disclosed itself to be a numberless multitude of little stars; instead of seven Pleiads, there proved to be thirty-six. Galilei studied the laws in accordance with which bodies fell freely; studied the movements of the pendulum; studied the rotation of the earth. Physics became dynamics.

Let us return to Padua, where Vesalius had taught for a time. The seed he had sown had borne good fruit. One of his successors, Colombo, had succeeded in proving that blood flows out of the heart into the lungs and through the lungs back into the heart; but in this discovery he had been anticipated by Miguel Servetus, the Spanish physician and theologian, burned alive by Calvin at Geneva in the year 1553. After

138

Colombo, Gabriele Falloppio, whose name is immortalised in anatomical nomenclature ("the Fallopian tubes"), had been teacher of anatomy in Padua, and had differed in many respects from Vesalius' teaching, though an ardent admirer of his predecessor. When Falloppio died in 1565, his pupil Girolamo Fabrizio d'Acquapendente took on the work of sustaining Padua's fame as a great school of anatomy, and was brilliantly successful. Becoming a distinguished surgeon as well as an anatomist, he built at his own charges an anatomical institute to which pupils flocked in large numbers, and, in the course of his long life, he was able to enrich anatomical knowledge by numerous discoveries, the most momentous of which was that of the existence of valves in the veins.

Fabrizio was born in 1537 and died in 1619. Among his pupils at the turn of the century, one of the most diligent was a young Englishman, William Harvey by name. It was not chance that had brought him to Padua. At the university of Cambridge he had worked at Gonville College, which had been reorganised by John Caius, at one time a student at Padua and a pupil of Vesalius. (This college is now known as Gonville and Caius, or, for short, simply as Caius.) It was natural, therefore, that Harvey should remove to Padua as soon as he had taken his degree of B.A. at Cambridge. He spent several years in the South, becoming doctor of medicine of the university of Padua in the year 1602.

Returning to England, he engaged in private practice in London, and in the year 1609 was appointed physician at St. Bartholomew's Hospital.

Until then there had been nothing noteworthy about his career. His course of studies was the same as that of dozens of other physicians of the day. But Padua in the late Renaissance had a peculiar effect upon its students, much as Alexandria had had in the days of antiquity. One who had studied in Padua, in that workshop of anatomy, was apt to be haunted by anatomy for the remainder of his life. Thus it was with Harvey. He was practising in the British capital, had many patients, and plenty of superadded occupations at one of the largest hospitals in the metropolis. He was, however, obsessed by anatomical ideas. What enthralled him in the human body? Not that which the doctors of the sixteenth century had been so powerfully impressed by, not its beautiful proportions, its perfection, the harmony of its forms. Those qualities were what had impelled them to study the structure of the underlying organs. The spell that worked on Harvey, the spell which shows that we have entered into a new era, was movement. The starting-point of his original researches was the two elementary movements which persist without cessation in man from birth until death—the pulse and the breathing.

What is the pulse? Obviously it is an expression of the movement of the blood. Now, what is the nature of that movement? The science of Harvey's epoch furnished no satisfactory answer. Galen's theory still held its ground. Galen had taught that the ingested food is elaborated in the liver to become blood, that thence the blood permeates the body, conveyed by the vessels in a mysterious to-and-fro movement, that part of the blood flows into the right side of the heart, thence passing through pores in the septum into the left side of the heart and pursuing its way through the organism. He taught, moreover, that the blood in the liver, the heart, and the brain is tinctured with "spiritus" which controls the vital functions. He also declared that blood flowed from the heart into the lungs, discharging there the residues of the organism, whereas air made its way from the lungs into the heart, keeping the blood sufficiently cool and supplying it with pneuma.

This theory was logically constructed, circumscribed, impressive, and it explained a good deal. It had, however, in many respects been shown to be faulty by the studies of the Renaissance. People had become better acquainted with the structure of the heart. There were not any pores in the septum,

140

after all. Obviously, then, the blood must take some other route than that described by Galen. At this vital point, the theory collapsed like a house of cards, and there had been nothing satisfactory to put in its place. Fracastoro expressed the opinion of many of his contemporaries when he said that the movements of the heart were known to God alone. Other questions, morphological questions, seemed much more urgent than these dynamic problems.

But times had changed since the days of Fracastoro. Function now, instead of structure, stood in the foreground of interest. Fabrizio, already, had refused to be content with purely morphological views, had invariably inquired as to the functions of the organs he described. All the same, he was too much under the spell of tradition to fly in the face of such authorities as Aristotle or Galen, and his subserviency in this respect prevented him from drawing logical conclusions from his discoveries.

The problem of the movements of the blood gave Harvey no rest. Since recorded science could not answer his question, he must question nature herself. Continuing his work for many years, he dissected innumerable animals, and, more important still, animals belonging to no less than eighty different species. He saw and felt the heart beat. Watching the phenomena of its beat, he asked what the causes of its movement could be. By degrees the problem began to clarify itself in his mind. In the year 1615 he was appointed professor at the College of Physicians in London. Next year he delivered his first lecture. His manuscript notes are extant, and show that he had solved the riddle of the movements of the blood. Yet what he had discovered was so utterly different from traditional views, was so incredibly novel, that he did not yet dare to think of publication. It was necessary for assurance to be redoubled. He went on with his work.

Meanwhile his professional reputation was steadily increasing. In 1618 he was appointed physician-in-ordinary to King

James I, and after that monarch's death held the same office in the service of King Charles I. Year succeeded year, until at length, in 1628, he felt sure that the soundness of his theory had been established beyond the possibility of doubt. A brief manuscript written in his crabbed and almost illegible handwriting was sent to a Frankfort publisher, and the famous essay appeared under the title *Exercitatio anatomica de motu cordis et sanguinis in animalibus.*

The publication aroused a storm of anger against Harvey. What had he dared to maintain?

Any one who grasps the exposed beating heart of an animal in his hand will feel how the organ draws itself together and becomes hard. This drawing-itself-together of the heart, the systole, is the active phase of the heart movement. During the systole, blood is driven into the great arteries. How much blood?

Let us pause for a moment to consider this point. The question as to the quantity of the blood driven out of the heart by the systole, the answer to which seems in our days self-evident, was then mooted for the first time. Not merely to answer it, but to ask it was a remarkable innovation. The older physiology had always thought in qualitative terms, had never worked with measuring-stick and numbers, and had never taken the element of time into consideration. But, as has been well said, "The right phrasing of a question is already a great step on the way towards its answer."

Harvey estimated the amount of blood ejected by the heart during the systole at two fluid ounces. If the heart beats 72 times per minute, this means that the quantity of blood ejected by the organ in the course of an hour is $72 \times 60 \times 2 = 8640$ fluid ounces. That is three times the average weight of the adult body. Where does so vast a quantity of blood come from? From the food? By incessant new formation? The figures make it incredible. Impossible that 8640 fluid ounces of new blood can be formed hour after hour. Whither does

the blood go? Does it ooze away into the tissues? This, likewise, is manifestly impossible, for the tissues would become
turgid and would burst owing to the influx of such quantities
of blood. There could, then, be no other possibility than that
the blood must get back out of the arteries into the heart, and
the only channels whereby it could reach the heart were the
veins. The next step in the demonstration, therefore, must
be to prove that the blood-stream in the veins flows always
towards the heart. By simply gripping the hand round a staff,
by laying a finger upon the superficial veins of the forearm,
and by close observation, it was possible to show that the
valves in the veins were actually so arranged as to make a
centrifugal flow of the blood through them impossible.

The circle was complete. The circulation of the blood had
been discovered. From the left side of the heart, it flows
through the arteries into all parts of the organism, makes its
way (obviously, thought Harvey) through gaps in the tissues
into the veins, is conveyed by them to the right auricle of the
heart and through this into the right ventricle. Then the blood
flows through the lungs and back through the pulmonary veins
to the heart again, this time to the left auricle and the left
ventricle.

Harvey was content with this fundamental demonstration.
Such problems as the significance of the air taken into the
lungs, the origin of bodily heat, etc., he passed over, recognising that for the nonce they were insoluble. He did not try
to establish a complete, a circumscribed physiology of the
circulation and respiration, being satisfied to describe what
he could prove by direct inspection. Therein lay his greatness,
and the essential novelty of his outlook.

Harvey was an anatomist. He wrote an anatomical monograph. But in his hands anatomy took on a new shape, became
anatomia animata, became physiology. It became, moreover,
physiology of a very different kind from any that had previously
existed.

143

Thenceforward physiology was inseparably associated with anatomy, and a physiological explanation was only acceptable if it was anatomically possible. Thenceforward investigators, making use of the experimental method, would go on trying to reduce vital phenomena to regular successions, to show that they were subject to the same kind of "laws" observable in inanimate nature.

It is easy, then, to understand why, at first, Harvey's discoveries encountered so obstinate a resistance. His whole train of thought was unfamiliar to his colleagues. Yet the facts were obvious, and in the end they prevailed.

Being physician-in-ordinary to the King, Harvey accompanied his royal master and occasionally some of the courtiers upon journeys which led him through Germany as far as Vienna. In 1642, the Civil War broke out. He had little or no interest in politics, but he was with the princes in the first battle. While the fight was raging, he took a book out of his pocket and read—until some stray bullets drove him from his resting-place. London was in the hands of the Parliamentarians. The court removed to Oxford, and Harvey went with it. He was well received at the university, being made principal of Merton College. His stay at Oxford was not long, however, for the rebels conquered the town in the year 1646. He was then sixty-eight years of age, and yearned for repose. Quitting the royal service, he retired into private life.

There was one more problem in which Harvey was deeply interested. It was embryology, another form of dynamic anatomy. Its theme, likewise, was movement, change. How natural that a man whose mind works dynamically should devote himself to this particular subject.

Investigators had long been keenly interested in the problem of the origin of human beings, of their development in the maternal womb. They had wondered which organs were first formed, and when the "soul" entered the foetus. Now, at length, it was becoming clear that embryology would be an

144

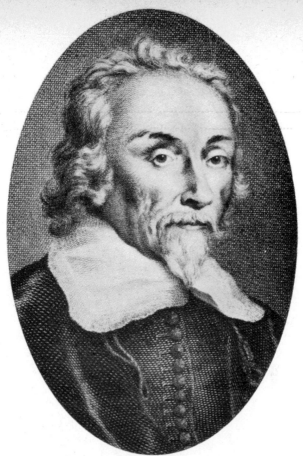

Will Harvey

WILLIAM HARVEY, 1578–1657

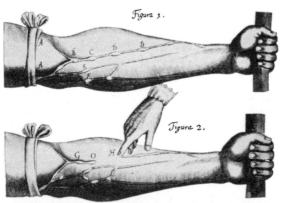

VEINS OF THE FRONT OF THE FOREARM, AN
ILLUSTRATION IN HARVEY'S *Exercitatio*

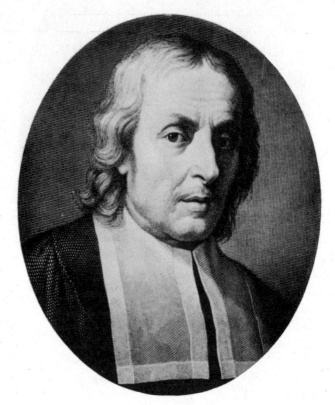

MARCELLO MALPIGHI, 1628–1694

important aid to the understanding of anatomy. This, likewise, was a field in which Fabrizio had been a pioneer.

Harvey's embryological studies occupied him for many years. He opened fowls' eggs at various stages of incubation and dissected the embryos. The royal deer-park was free to him, and there he could study the embryos of other mammals. His book *De generatione animalium* was published in 1651. He had hesitated before giving it to the world, and only did so at last because of the urgent representations of his friends. Whereas in the matter of the circulation of the blood he had felt himself able to supply definitive information, as regards animal development he knew that his work was inchoate. The field to be covered was enormous, and the means for the solution of the problems of embryology were still extremely inadequate. All the same, this book of Harvey's was enormously in advance of anything that had previously been written on the subject. The phrase "Omne animal ex ovo," coined by Harvey, proved to be one of those winged words which guide and fertilise subsequent research.

Thus, in his scientific labours, Harvey was a consistent dynamist. This made him an important factor in the movement I sketched in the opening paragraph of the present chapter.

CHAPTER SEVENTEEN

MARCELLO MALPIGHI
1628–1694

HARVEY'S theory of the circulation of the blood was marred by a notable hiatus. He failed to discover how the blood made its way from the arteries to the veins. Obviously there must be channels of some sort by which the circulating fluid passed, but their nature remained obscure. They were assumed to exist, ex hypothesi—for the hypothesis was indispensable. Its correctness was at length objectively demonstrated by the Italian anatomist Marcello Malpighi. In the year 1661 he reported having seen, in the lungs and in the mesentery of the frog, how the terminal arteries and veins were connected by a network of vessels as fine in calibre as the finest hair, and therefore to be called capillaries. The blood passed from the arteries into the veins, not through vague lacunae in the tissues, but through extremely minute vessels which existed in all parts of the body. Malpighi discovered something more than this. Examining the mesentery of a hedgehog, he saw there, not only the capillaries, but also the blood flowing through them, and in this blood he perceived little red globes (as he thought them) of a standardised magnitude. He believed them to be fat droplets, but they were the red blood-corpuscles.

How had these discoveries been rendered possible? By means of an instrument which opened new horizons to the anatomist's eye—the microscope. In the sixteenth century, anatomical studies had been pursued with the utmost fervour, and the most important items of new knowledge had been acquired. But the powers of the unaided eye were greatly restricted. Although the coarse structure of the organs could be made out, the refinements of that structure eluded examination.

146

Then the Dutch spectacle-makers invented the telescope; and, by a simple modification thereof, Galileo made the compound microscope. Now the eyes were provided with means for plumbing unanticipated depths. Although these early microscopes were primitive instruments as compared with those now in use, many of them could magnify as much as two hundred diameters. The consequent revelations were marvellous. The microscopist examined whatever came to hand. A drop of water would sometimes disclose itself to be a world full of living creatures. A Dutch investigator living in Delft, Antony van Leeuwenhoek by name, who ground his own lenses and was continually improving his instruments, saw bacteria, saw the cross-striation of voluntary muscular fibres, and saw the bone-corpuscles. He made his discoveries known in letters to the Royal Society of London.

But it was Malpighi, above all, who systematically applied the new instrument to anatomical research. Just as Vesalius had been the founder of scientific naked-eye anatomy, so was Malpighi the founder of microscopical anatomy.

To the unaided eye, the frog's lungs appear to be nothing more than membranous sacs. The microscope had disclosed the capillary network in their walls. Malpighi followed the road thus opened up, although the difficulties were enormous. He was breaking entirely new ground. At first it seemed wellnigh impossible to unravel the confusion that presented itself to the greatly intensified vision of the microscopist. The reader must bear in mind that the staining methods which have been of such great help to us in modern times were still unknown. That was why Malpighi found it more profitable to study the simpler forms, the insects, than to continue his investigations upon the higher animals. Even there, however, the conditions were still extremely complicated; so, still in search of simplification, he began to examine the minute anatomy of plants. Here advance was easier, and he worked at the subject for a good many years. In 1671, since he was a member of the Royal Society of London, he sent to that body the first fruit of his studies in the form of a treatise entitled *Idea anatomes plantarum*. Further papers followed, until at length they came to form a comprehensive work upon the microscopical anatomy of plants. Thus Malpighi shares with Nehemiah Grew, secretary of the Royal Society, a man about thirteen years younger than himself, the merit of having founded the study of vegetable anatomy.

Having got as far as this, Malpighi felt himself able to resume the microscopical study of the higher animals. His eyes had been trained by the examination of simpler forms; but even when he turned to the higher animals, he thought it better to avoid complications, and therefore, like Harvey, he devoted himself to embryology. Just as he had studied the buds of plants, so did he now study the embryonic forms of animals. His guiding principle was an advance upon Harvey's; not only "omne animal ex ovo," but "omne vivum ex ovo."

He traced the development of the chicken within the egg, opening one egg after another in a clutch every six hours during the earlier stages of incubation. Being far better equipped than his predecessors, he discovered much more, so that his drawings of the development of the embryo as a whole and of that of the individual organs greatly excelled previous attempts of the kind, and it was long before they were surpassed.

From this he proceeded to his classical investigations concerning the minute structure of the particular organs; the skin, the tongue, the spleen, the kidneys, the various parts of the nervous system. In 1689 there was published in London his monograph upon the structure of the glands, the result of twenty-two years' work. These pioneer investigations served not only to lay the foundations for further anatomical research, but also to fertilise physiology. The more that was known of the structure of an organ, the more easily could its functioning be understood, and the more profound, therefore, was the insight acquired into its relationships with the organism at large.

Malpighi spent the greater part of his life in Bologna, near which town he had been born. There he studied philosophy and medicine. Subsequently, except for a few years spent as professor in Pisa and thereafter in Messina, he retained, until 1691, his post as lecturer on medicine at the university of Bologna. Medicine, be it noted. Anatomical studies were, until far on into the seventeenth century, presided over by men who had remained disciples of Galen, men who looked upon their colleague's microscopical investigations as an idle pastime, who were jealous of the recognition Malpighi had secured in foreign lands, and who molested him in various ways. So serious were these molestations, that on one occasion Malpighi's villa was sacked, his instruments were broken, his papers were burned, and his very life was endangered.

Thus Malpighi was far from happy. He was perpetually harassed, and his worries are manifest in the man's portrait. A summons to Rome as physician to Pope Innocent XII brought relief. From this date his letters grew more cheerful. Still, his increasing practice left him very little time for scientific study nor could he enjoy the happier circumstances long, for he died in 1694.

CHAPTER EIGHTEEN

SANTORIO SANTORIO
1561–1636

MALPIGHI had completed Harvey's work. Let us go back a
little into the opening years of the seventeenth century, the
years to which Galilei's dominating figure gave their imprint,
since his influence was far-reaching. He was one of the first
investigators to practise the modern method of inductive
natural science, and many scientists followed in his track. By
his activities, by the results he achieved, the value of the
new method was much more signally demonstrated than by
the theorising of such a writer as Francis Bacon.

From the seventeenth century onward, the destinies of
medicine were inseparably associated with those of the natural
sciences. A sort of alliance was entered into between medicine
and natural science, so that they developed along parallel lines,
interpenetrated one another, reciprocally fertilised one another.
The ties between them were closer at one time, laxer at another.
Occasionally the natural sciences would become so engrossing
that medicine became a mere branch of natural research, thus
losing sight of its true task—cure. Man seemed no more than
one among many natural objects, so that doctors forgot that
their patients were suffering creatures, equipped with minds
as well as bodies. Then there would be a swing the other way,
the classical idealist contemplation of nature would move into
the foreground, and philosophical trends would predominate.
Ever more plainly, however, in the course of the development
of knowledge, the natural sciences disclosed themselves to be
the indispensable methods for use in effecting medical advances
—invariably fruitful so long as they were kept in their place
as methods and medicine retained its autonomy.

In Galilei's hands, the telescope had been remade into the

microscope, without which no doctor can do his work to-day. Galileo also discovered the thermometer, and the new implement was at once pressed into the service of medicine. From very early days physicians had been aware of the importance of changes in the temperature of the human body. The increased heat manifest in fever was a conspicuous symptom, and doctors detected it by laying a hand upon the patient's body.

When Galilei flourished, there was an attempt in all fields of scientific research to pass from the subjective description of phenomena to their objective measurement. Temperature had become a physical concept, and it could be expressed in numerical terms. Such a view could not fail to bear fruit in medicine. It was not enough to know merely that a patient was suffering from "fever." Essential to a knowledge of his ailment was that the doctor should be able to determine and to record the slightest oscillation in the degree of fever. The newly invented instrument seemed eminently adapted for this purpose.

The first man to invent what we now call a "clinical thermometer" was a physician from Capodistria, Santorio Santorio. Shrewd of intelligence, with a passion for research, he was, besides being well acquainted with the traditional literature of medicine, inspired by the new methodology of the exact sciences.

Santorio had taken his medical degree at Padua in the year 1582. He was generally esteemed for the breadth of his knowledge, for his trustworthy character, and for his zeal. When the court of Poland needed a competent physician, and applied to Padua, Santorio was recommended for the post. It was offered to him, he accepted it, and went to Poland in 1587. Ere long he had an extensive practice, being summoned in consultation to different places in Hungary and Croatia. Returning to Italy in 1611, he became professor of theoretical medicine in Padua. In 1629 he resigned his professorship, and, despite offers from various universities, he settled down in Venice to devote himself to practice and to scientific study.

Santorio wrote seven treatises, which comprise two thick volumes. He began his career as a medical writer with a comprehensive work upon the way of avoiding mistakes in medical practice. Still following the scholastic method, he fortified his statements by quoting as many authorities as possible, yet justified himself, not only "ratione," but also "experimentis." This treatise, and also the following one (a commentary running to 763 pages upon Galen's brief *Ars medicinae*), are medieval in form, but are animated by a new spirit. Both of them contain a great deal of original experience. Nuggets of gold are scattered through them, but are often hard to find amid the sand in which they are embedded.

Of a very different character, even externally, is the book upon which Santorio's title to fame mainly rests. It appeared in 1614 under the somewhat obscure appellation *Ars de statica medicina*, a slender booklet, penned in aphorisms, the upshot of thirty years' experiments. Even in this case, Galen had been the starting-point. Galen had assumed that the skin "breathed" to some extent as well as the lungs; that volatile substances left the body by way of the skin. To what extent did this "perspiratio insensibilis," this invisible sweating, take place? Santorio mooted the question, and he answered it, not speculatively, but by the use of the scales. He weighed the body, weighed what was ingested, and weighed what was passed in the excreta. He constructed a big balance, sitting in one of the scales on a chair with a table in front of him. He recorded the changes in figures, was able to provide his "perspiratio insensibilis" with a numerical expression. He traced its variations under the influence of air and water, of food and drink, of sleeping and waking, of movement and repose, of sexual activity and emotional excitement. He came to the conclusion that the organism gave off several pounds every day by way of insensible perspiration, and he believed

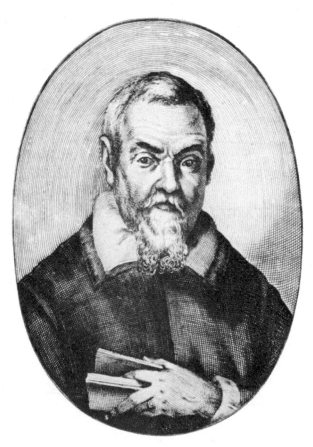

SANTORIO SANTORIO, 1561–1636

that its amount furnished a guide to the diagnosis of various diseases and indications for treatment.

Santorio was well aware that his researches were "new, and unprecedented." He was prepared for attacks, which were, indeed, forthcoming. He sent a copy of his book to Galilei, with a letter from which some extracts may be made: "Obviously this method I have discovered is of great importance, since it enables us to ascertain the precise amount of that insensible perspiration interference with which is, according to Hippocrates and Galen, the cause of all diseases. The ground for believing this is that the insensible perspiration is more extensive than all the visible and palpable excreta taken together." Nor, indeed, would it matter, if Galen had known nothing about insensible perspiration, "for that this secretion actually exists is sufficient."

Having thus entered upon the path of clinical experiment, Santorio continued to advance along it. Other physiological and pathological phenomena must be capable of exact measurement. It is plain enough to us why the invention of the clinical thermometer followed upon the use of the scales to determine the amount of insensible perspiration.

This first of clinical thermometers was a primitive instrument. The globular expanded end of a convoluted capillary glass tube (graduated) was placed in the patient's mouth. The other end of the tube dipped into a vessel filled with water. The temperature was estimated from the amount of warmed air that was expired.

It was likewise necessary, however, that a quantitative determination of the pulse should be taken. According to the hitherto accepted doctrine of the pulse, it was enough to describe the qualities of the beat, which were examined in the utmost detail—often with a good deal of hair-splitting. But, said Santorio, it was much more important to determine the frequency of the pulse, to count the number of beats within a specified time. This is done to-day with the aid of a watch. But the timepieces that existed at the end of the sixteenth century had no second-hand, nor indeed a minute-hand. Santorio, therefore, constructed a special instrument for readings of the pulse, a "pulsilogium." It was merely a pendulum, a thread by which a leaden ball was suspended. The length of the thread was increased or diminished until the pendulum swung synchronously with the pulse. Its length then gave an objective measure of pulse-rate.

Santorio made another instrument, a hygroscope, designed

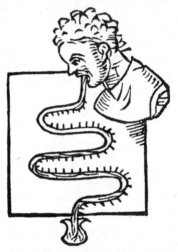

SANTORIO'S CLINICAL THERMOMETER

to record the amount of moisture in the air. Still more remark-able apparatus were designed by this fertile brain: for instance, a suspended couch; an arrangement by which a patient could have a bath while remaining recumbent and making no exertion. Naturally a doctor with such outstanding technical equipment would enrich the surgeon's instrumentarium as well. The most important of his inventions in this field were a new trocar, an instrument for the performance of tracheotomy, and an instrument for the extraction of stones from the bladder.

Santorio's ideas ran along similar lines to Harvey's. He

154

made the same steps from qualitative to quantitive observation. His method, like the Englishman's, was that of experiment. Both of them thought in mechanical terms. Both of them tried to bring biological phenomena into touch with the fixed laws that prevail in the world of inorganic matter. They were contemporaries, but Santorio was about fifteen years older than Harvey, and his chief work was published fourteen years before the *Exercitatio*.

Their successors, however, gave the palm to Harvey, and regarded Harvey as the founder of modern physiology, of exact biology. There were various reasons for this. Harvey had chosen a more engrossing theme. The problem he investigated was one of extreme actuality; he solved it effectively with the aid of the new methods; and he replaced an erroneous theory which had been dominant for many centuries by a new and sound one. Moreover, he developed his ideas in a work which was a model of clarity, in which nothing of importance was omitted, and which covered the whole field.

Santorio used like methods, but his chosen field, that of insensible perspiration, was of much less interest to the doctors of his day than the problem of the circulation of the blood. Besides, it was far too complicated for full and definitive solution by the light of those days. There were inevitable and numerous discrepancies in the figures he recorded. Centuries had still to pass before precise calculations were to become possible in this domain. Harvey was a master of condensation, of restriction. He made no allegations except concerning matters for which he could provide solid foundations. Santorio deduced from his observations conclusions that were far too comprehensive. He made insensible perspiration the basis of all pathological happenings.

Finally, Santorio chose a most unhappy form in which to make the result of his investigations known to the world. His *Statica medicina* is penned in aphorisms. Valuable as brevity is, if injudiciously used it leads to obscurity, and that was what happened in Santorio's case. His account of the way his experiments were organised, and his calculations, lacked detail and precision. His observations and his descriptions of his new instruments, as contained in his other writings, are buried in prolix commentaries upon Galen and Hippocrates, and, pre-eminently, in a commentary upon the first section of the first book of Avicenna's *Canon*. He was a man of genius who made great discoveries, but he did not know how to turn them to account, and it was not till long after his death that his instruments, modified and greatly improved, were revived to enrich the science and practice of medicine.

These defects notwithstanding, Santorio takes honourable place among the constructive geniuses to whom the development of modern medicine is due.

CHAPTER NINETEEN

JAN BAPTISTA VAN HELMONT
1577–1644

HARVEY'S work marks the change from a static to a dynamic outlook. A new science was being born. This period, which in art corresponded with the change from the Renaissance to the Baroque, was one of formidable tensions, cleavages, and oppositions. It was the epoch of the absolutist State, but also that of the great democracies. It was the Age of Reason, of a cold and calculating realism. Investigators were trying to understand, to measure, and to control the realities of life. But it was likewise the period of fanaticism and bigotry; the period in which such men as Campanella were racked; such as Giordano Bruno were sent to the stake; such as Galilei were forced to recant their scientific teaching. On all hands, groups of religious sectaries were winning their way to power. In Germany, the Thirty Years' War was raging, so that the whole field of scientific life lay fallow; in England, the Great Rebellion was in progress, and a king was decapitated by the public executioner; in the Low Countries, after almost interminable struggles, the Dutch and Flemish Protestants freed themselves from the Spanish yoke. In the South, the Counter-Reformation was in progress, and the Jesuits were triumphant. Maladies due to defect and maladies due to excess, gave the pathology of the time its peculiar stamp.

Turning our gaze northward, we see a doctor in whom all the cleavage of the Baroque period became manifest—Jan Baptista van Helmont. In him, scepticism and faith were united. For him, as for Descartes, doubt was the starting-point of thought. He was a sober-minded investigator, whose lucid intellectual faculties enabled him to enrich the natural sciences.

Yet, at the same time, he had an ardent religious faith. In most respects he diverged sharply from the traditions of the past; he wanted to be creative, to discover new paths for medical science and art. There was but one of his predecessors whom he regarded as mentally akin—Paracelsus.

Vesalius, Harvey, Santorio, Malpighi, these men had become great by specialising, by the study of particular provinces of knowledge, by attacking specific problems which they dealt with along novel lines, and they thus arrived at entirely new results. Such men as Paracelsus and van Helmont, on the other hand, would not confine their energies to any limited task. Their thoughts embraced the whole cosmos. Incessantly they contemplated a whole, excogitated systems which were to embrace all phenomena. The upshot was that they often over-shot the mark, hurried to points which were miles beyond their goal. Both of them, too, remained solitaries. Yet they are still extraordinarily alive to us to-day after the lapse of centuries. No one among us who is competent to overcome the linguistic difficulties that attach to their writings can fail to be impressed by the extensive grasp of their intelligence, by the wealth of their intuitions.

Van Helmont was a man of good family. Born in Brussels, he studied at the university of Louvain. Restlessly, discontentedly, he passed from one faculty to another. Botany led him to materia medica. Then he worked as assistant to a physician. "Soon, however, I became extremely rueful because in the curative art I found nothing to expect but dissatisfaction, uncertainty, and surmise. I could dispute concerning the medical art in connection with every disease, and yet I had no fundamental knowledge how to cure a toothache or the itch." A dream moved him to qualify as a doctor, and in this dream he was promised the acquisition of the powers of the archangel Raphael and the gift of divine methods of healing. With fiery zeal he flung himself into these new studies, acquired a vast amount of knowledge, and lectured on surgery in Louvain.

Medical science, however, was a disillusionment. Abandoning the profession for a time, he travelled to Switzerland, Italy, France, and England. On his journeys, he met alchemists, for in those days there were many of them, bold adventurers, continually on the road. They taught him the secrets of the use of fire. A new world opened to him. At this juncture, likewise, he made acquaintance with the writings of Paracelsus, to whom, as he tells us, he owed much, although he did not hesitate, often enough, to criticise his predecessor. He decided to become a student of natural science. Chemistry would provide true and effective remedies; but, more than this, it would provide a key to the understanding of nature.

Marriage to a wealthy lady of Brabant put him in possession of an estate at Vilvorden near Brussels. Settling down there in 1609, for the rest of his days he lived a lonely life, devoted to his studies. Whither did these lead him?

The vivifying principle of matter is the "archeus." This archeus (a Paracelsian concept) is the dynamic, the effective principle of matter. It does not act directly, but, in order to influence matter, avails itself of a "ferment," an extremely subtle form of matter, regarded, like the archeus, as gaseous. Whereas the archeus is immanent in the body, the ferment is superindividual. It has been created by God for all eternity. In the seed (Same, semen), the archeus generates itself through a process analogous to putrefaction. In the last analysis, matter, of whatever kind, arises out of the element water. There are only two basic elements in all bodies: water as the material substratum, and the ferment or seminal substance as the dynamic substratum. The individual human being consists of archeus, anima sensitiva, and mens. Mens, the soul or mind or spirit, is the divine part of man. The anima sensitiva comprises the psychical functions. It is the individual part of human beings, that upon which health or illness depends, and the source of the "vis medicatrix naturae."

Under the working of the archeus, the semen or seed develops into the body. The body divides itself into organs; and through-out, in every organ, there is an archeus, the organ-archeus (archeus insitus) upon which the activities of the organs depend. It is the ruler, the guardian of the organs. It regulates the change of substances (what we now call the metabolism) in the organs, taking care that this shall run a normal course. The archei of the separate organs are controlled by the archeus of the organism at large, by the archeus influus.

Now, what is illness or disease? Disease, also, is life. It is something thoroughly real, a positive and substantial vital process, an "ens reale subsistens in corpore." The causes of disease take effect upon the archeus of the organism. "Ideae morbosae," morbid ideas, arise by making their imprint upon the organ-archei. Thus the dynamic principle of the organ is disturbed. Thereby the ferment is changed, and the change takes effect upon the matter of which the organ is composed. Precipitates are formed. The malady becomes a disturbance of tissue-change, arising in this organ or in that, and mani-festing itself by local changes of which we are made aware by the precipitates that occur.

Treatment, therefore, must not be a vague general treatment, but must be directed against the specific disease that is in progress, against the "idea morbosa." The most effective remedies are chemical, the arcana of Paracelsus.

We see that van Helmont's system is a hotch-potch of idealistic-spiritualistic and empirical-scientific ideas. His doc-trine of illness was essentially dynamic, and it directed the attention of the physician to the organs—above all to the morbid processes going on in particular organs. The trans-formations which went on in the organs in the course of disease were, he maintained, chemical processes. The application of these notions to particular diseases proved extremely fruitful, especially in respect of the doctrine of catarrhs, asthma, and lung-diseases in general. Chemical remedies, which had been advocated by Paracelsus, although their introduction had

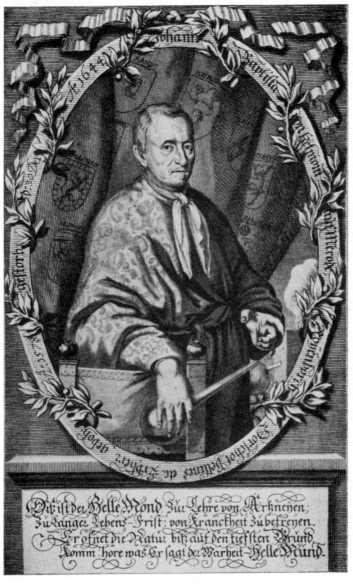

JAN BAPTISTA VAN HELMONT, 1577–1644

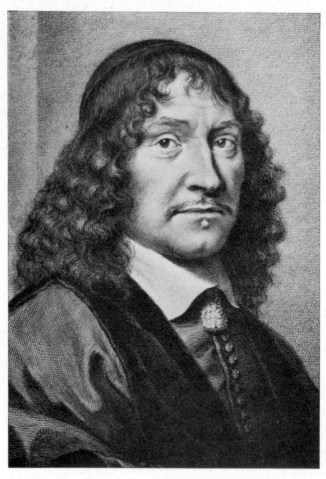

FRANZ DE LE BOË [SYLVIUS], 1614–1672

encountered a stubborn resistance, were given a new impetus by van Helmont.

The domain of chemistry was very variously enriched by van Helmont's studies. He investigated the various substances having the physical qualities of air, and coined for them a new general denomination, gas. He disclosed their difference from (visible) steam; and he discovered carbonic acid, thus becoming the founder of pneumatic chemistry.

The closing years of van Helmont's life were harassed. A small work of his in manuscript, directed against a Jesuit and discussing the magnetic treatment of wounds, fell into the hands of a stranger, was printed against his wishes, and attracted the unfavourable attention of the Inquisition. A charge was brought against him, and for a time he was imprisoned. An interminable trial dragged on. Van Helmont recanted, but this was of no avail during his lifetime, and he was not acquitted until two years after his death, the ground for the acquittal being that he had always led so pious a life.

His opus magnum, the *Ortus medicinae,* was a posthumous work, published by his son in 1648. In part owing to difficulties of style, and in part because of the nature of its contents, it was very difficult to understand, and therefore for the time had but little effect upon professional thought and practice. Medicine was pursuing the road of anatomy and of mechanistic physiology. That was why van Helmont, like Paracelsus, stands apart from the general forward movement of medical science.

CHAPTER TWENTY

FRANZ DE LE BOË [SYLVIUS]
1614–1672

ALTHOUGH van Helmont's system was little understood, and
to his contemporaries and immediate successors seemed
extremely complicated, it was plain that he worked with
chemical concepts. Many of the classical physicians had held
that health was a state of equilibrium, and that illness was
a disturbance of this equilibrium. They believed that the
equilibrium of health was sustained by various forces; by the
qualities, the atoms, the juices, and especially the four cardinal
humours. The motive forces were the intrinsic warmth of the
body, the pneuma, and the vital spirits. In the beginning of
the seventeenth century, however, a remarkable growth of the
exact sciences had taken place, especially in the realms of
physics and chemistry. Speculation was being driven more
and more into the background by experiment and by the
records of observations that could be numerically stated.
Harvey had given a striking demonstration of the way in
which mechanical considerations could enrich biological
science. Santorio had shown that even the problems of tissue-
change or metabolism could be numerically considered.

It was natural that physicians' thoughts, at this date, should
turn farther and farther away from the classical concepts of
disease, that they should endeavour, more and more, to explain
health and illness with the aid of the new physical and chemical
outlooks.

Paracelsus and van Helmont pressed chemistry into the
service of medicine. It was obvious that changes must occur
in the animal body akin to those which could be observed in
a chemical retort. In the body, too, there were acids and
alkalis. Who could doubt that disturbances of the body-

chemistry must manifest themselves in the form of morbid phenomena? The salts which were sometimes found in the urine, the gall-stones and the vesical calculi which were occasionally found at post-mortem examinations, must be the terminal products of abnormal chemical reactions.

Thus by degrees in the medical science of the seventeenth century there came into being a trend characterised by the fact that those who were involved in it worked predominantly with chemical ideas. For that reason we speak of iatrochemistry, and of iatrochemists. The chief of this school was Franz de le Boë, the Leyden clinician who is best known under his Latinised name of Sylvius.

Sylvius sprang from a French Huguenot family which had originally been known by the name of Dubois, and had migrated into the Low Countries. War had driven his parents thence into Germany, so that Sylvius was born at Hanau. He studied in German and Dutch universities, and took his degree in medicine at Basle in the year 1637. To be near his parents, when twenty-three he settled down to practise in Hanau, receiving an appointment in that town from the municipal council. Within two years, however, the craving for a less restricted environment mastered him. He went to Paris to improve his medical education, removing thence to Holland, where he gave botanical and anatomical lectures in Leyden, attracting many students. It was especially as an anatomist that he excelled.

Sylvius, indeed, was firmly and lastingly convinced of the fundamental importance of anatomy to medicine. He wrote an anatomical work, and a fissure in the brain bears his name. Above all, however, he was enthralled by the newest physiological investigations. In the campaign that was still raging about the circulation of the blood (Harvey's *Exercitatio* had been published, it will be remembered, in the year 1628), he passionately espoused the views of Harvey, promulgated

163

the Englishman's teachings at Leyden, and fortified them by experiments which convinced even the most incredulous.

Still, Sylvius had no regular post at Leyden. He merely gave lectures there as any doctor might. When his friends urged him to start a practice in Amsterdam, he followed the call, and soon became one of the most highly esteemed physicians in that city. His contemporaries describe him as an extraordinarily handsome, imposing, witty man, who could laugh merrily on occasion, thus fulfilling his favourite motto of "bene agere ac laeteri." All the same, he was a man of exquisite manners. His jokes were never offensive; and, one of his biographers tells us, he was never seen intoxicated—which was not to be said of many men in seventeenth-century Holland. Nor was he a stickler for fees, being ready to do his best gratuitously on behalf of the poor who were members of the Protestant Walloon Church.

Sylvius carried on a successful practice in Amsterdam for seventeen years. Then, in 1658, when the chair of medicine fell vacant in Leyden, he was unanimously appointed professor. His first impulse was to refuse the call. He had all he wanted in Amsterdam: work he delighted in, a large income, honour, friends. What awaited him at the university? The slavery of academic life; controversies with his professional colleagues. He would have to assume that air of omniscience expected of a professor. In the end, after many hesitations, he accepted. What was the lure? That which invariably acts upon those who are most attracted by an academic career: the possibility of being surrounded by a circle of young men; the possibility of unfolding his favourite ideas, of testing them by noting their reaction upon fresh, vigorous, and youthful minds; the possibility of expounding his own doctrines far more effectively than could ever be done by the printed word.

During the years spent in the practice of his profession, Sylvius had gathered much experience. He knew well enough that many of his views were original. Himself firmly convinced of the importance of chemistry, he could not fail to know that few of his colleagues shared his opinion in this respect. He had, therefore, a mission to fulfil. Dormant memories awakened in him. He had long before enjoyed the intoxication of the crowded lecture-theatre, the mute but thrilling response of an attentive audience. Stifling his objections, he returned to Leyden and stood one day before the students, no longer a youth, but a man of mature years. He lectured, and once again he delighted and convinced his hearers. His reputation, and therewith the reputation of the university, spread quickly and far. Students flocked to Leyden from Hungary, Russia, Poland, Germany, Denmark, Sweden, Switzerland, Italy, France, and England. Such international repute was easier then than now. Science in those days had an international tongue, for throughout western and central Europe lectures were given in Latin. The same academic customs prevailed everywhere. A student who had passed his examination in Leyden could practise wherever he went, and his degree entitled him to teach in any university.

The Leyden faculty was the first to give clinical instruction northward of the Alps. The idea of utilising the hospitals for teaching purposes had been born in Italy. In Padua (always Padua!) already in the sixteenth century da Monte had been accustomed to take his students to the Ospedale San Francesco and to lecture to them at the bedside of the sick. After da Monte's death, the practice had fallen into desuetude, but it had not been forgotten, and the students at Padua, especially the German students, demanded its revival. In 1578 it was reintroduced at the same hospital by Bottoni, who demonstrated upon male patients, and by degli Oddi, who lectured on the cases of women. When these two teachers died, there was once more an arrest of clinical instruction. Ere long, however, certain Dutch doctors who had worked at Padua, Heurnius and Schrevelius by name, transplanted the method to Leyden. At first the Dutch students revolted against this innovation.

Then, as now, questions were put to students at the bedside, and the young men found it disagreeable to have their ignorance disclosed before the sick. However, the superiority of practical over purely theoretical instruction was plain, so the practice of clinical demonstration became established in Leyden after all. Then came Sylvius, whose worldwide fame lent renown to the Leyden clinic, who attracted a large following from distant parts, and became head of a school.

What was the secret of Sylvius' success? His medical system was extremely simple, and he worked with topical concepts, with such as were congenial to his time. He was a declared mechanist. His inclination was to attach especial importance to anatomy and physiology; but with the anatomy and physiology of that time the phenomena of health and disease could not be adequately explained, and therefore his speculations ran also into other fields, such as that of chemistry, for which he showed a predilection.

Fermentation was the process by which one substance changed into another. By such a process, by fermentation, through the influence exerted by the glandular secretions, what was ingested as nutriment was converted into blood. The ultimate products of these changes were acids and alkalis. If the balance between the acids and the alkalis was rightly maintained, the individual was healthy. On the other hand a disturbance in body-chemistry led to the formation of "acrimoniae," which might be either acid or alkaline, which made their way into the blood, and there gave rise to illness. The aim of treatment must be, "to maintain the energies of the organism, to drive away the illness, to remove the causes, to mitigate the symptoms." Acids were counteracted by alkalis, and alkalis by acids. The bodily juices—bile, mucus, etc.—were evacuated by emetics and purgatives both of vegetable and of mineral origin.

Sylvius' writings, his *Disputationes medicae*, 1663, his *Praxeos medicae idea nova*, 1671—whatever appeared during this period was novum or inauditum—contain numerous and extremely valuable observations. For instance, he gave an admirable description of tubercles in the lungs, which he had frequently seen, and which he regarded in many cases as the causes of consumption.

Sylvius found enthusiastic adherents, especially in the Netherlands, but also in Germany and England. Among the most noted of his British followers may be mentioned Thomas Willis (1622–1675).

Van Helmont and Sylvius both thought in chemical terms, and both turned chemistry to account for the purposes of medicine. Yet how different were the two men. Van Helmont was a Catholic and a mystic; Sylvius was a Huguenot and a rationalist. Van Helmont lived a lonely life, was misunderstood, and ultimately prosecuted. Sylvius was a cheerful fellow, surrounded by thankful patients and admiring students, and secured immediate success. Still, van Helmont's work has been more enduring; the problems he mooted are those which still exercise our minds to-day. Sylvius' mission has become no more than a memory of a distant past. Short-lived is the work of the happy man. He only who has eaten his bread with tears, knows the heavenly powers.

CHAPTER TWENTY-ONE

GIORGIO BAGLIVI
1668–1707

WHILST in the North, as we have seen, it was chemistry which took pride of place in the minds of scientists; in the South physics was dominant. Galilei's work and methods continued to exert a dominant influence. Santorio's experiments, Harvey's theories, had pointed out the way. Philosophic trends fortified these inclinations. The philosophers of the time had graduated in the schools of natural research. Mathematics had replaced scholasticism. Descartes declared that the human body was a machine regulated by mechanical laws. All the phenomena of the organic world could be mechanically explained. Movement was the pre-eminent characteristic of the manifestations of life. What was the origin of muscular contractions? They depended upon the influx of a vapour, a spiritus, and they too were mechanical. The vital spirits, the essences of life, were formed by rarefaction of the blood. The idea of "l'homme machine" was widely prevalent before the eighteenth century, long before the birth of Lamettrie.

This complicated and delicate machine had to be studied. The method of study was experiment. But experiments of the kind could only be made with the aid of instruments, of apparatus, often of a very costly kind. The universities, which with few exceptions clung to tradition and stood upon the old ways, would not provide means for these new studies. That was one of the main reasons for the foundation of learned societies, of academies, which became centres of experimental research.

In the opening years of the seventeenth century a few men of learning, having met in Duke Fredrigo Cesi's palace, joined to form the Accademia dei Lincei (the Lynxes). The duke

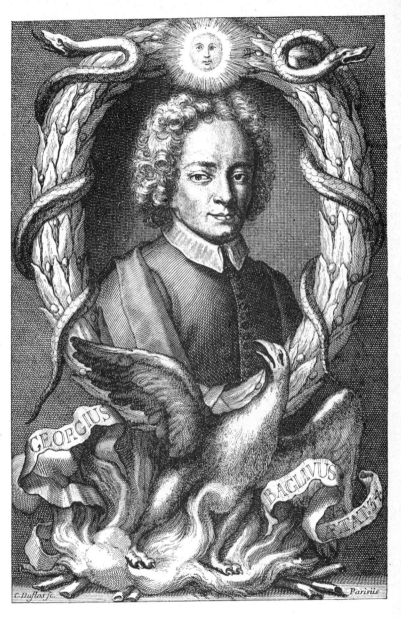

GIORGIO BAGLIVI, 1668–1707

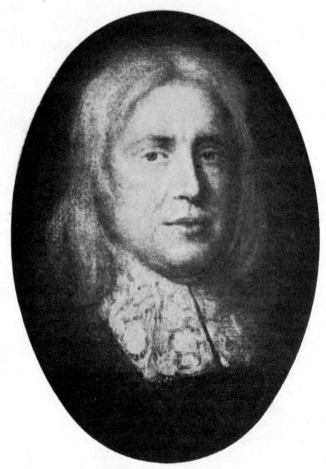

THOMAS SYDENHAM, 1624–1689

was himself devoted to natural science, had a cabinet of specimens, and a botanical garden, studied bees and plants, and was an able experimenter. The society grew until it numbered thirty-two members, among them Galilei. A new form of labour community was to be created, an intimate league of men having like aims. The founders had the vision of an order of scientists, with branch academies throughout the world. This order was to supply all the requisites for research: laboratories, instruments, collections, libraries. It was to have its own printing establishments to diffuse the acquirements of research, and there was to be a vigorous exchange of ideas among the different academies.

Although these far-reaching plans were not destined to be realised, the Accademia dei Lincei did excellent work for more than half a century, and it became a model for similar organisations.

At Florence the Medici princes, Ferdinand II and Leopold, both of whom were greatly interested in natural research, assembled around them a staff of scientists, most of them pupils of Galilei, to form an Accademia del Cimento, whose experimental methods were to set an example for all the world.

In other countries like bodies came into existence. In England there was founded in 1662 the Royal Society of London for Improving Natural Knowledge (commonly known for short as the Royal Society), of which, as we have learned, Malpighi was a member. In 1666 there came into existence the French Académie des Sciences. In Germany, too, unfavourable though the times were, the spirit of the new research was astir. As early as 1622, in the opening years of the Thirty Years War, Joachim Jungius founded in Rostock the Societas Ereunetica, whose motto "Per inductionem et experimentum omnia" gave concise expression to the aims of natural science. Unfortunately it died in infancy, surviving no more than two years. But there still exists, though its name has changed, the Collegium Naturae Curiosorum (founded 1652), which in 1677 became the Sacri

Romani Imperatoris Academia Naturae Curiosorum; and in 1687 the Academia Caesarea Leopoldina, centred in Halle and still extant. At first this was no more than a group of physicians interested in the study of science, but in course of time it tended more and more to become the centre of natural research in Germany, and acquired important privileges.

Several doctors were members of the Accademia del Cimento. One of them, a Dane named Stensen (1638–1686), was a noted anatomist and physiologist who, influenced by Bossuet, became a convert to Catholicism and in due course rose to the rank of bishop. He was the discoverer of the duct of the parotid gland, called after him Stensen's duct (also Stenson's duct, Steno's duct, and the Stenonian duct), and did valuable work in the field of the physiology of the muscles. Another member of the Accademia del Cimento was Francesco Redi (1626–1694), equally famous as poet, zoologist, and physician, author of *Esperienze intorno alla generazione degli insetti*. By a simple experiment, he refuted the theory of spontaneous generation. Down to his time, people had believed that maggots came into existence in putrefying flesh without extraneous aid. Redi, protecting pieces of meat from the access of blow-flies by gauze, showed that the meat putrefied without any development of maggots in it. Blow-flies were attracted by the smell, crawled over the gauze, and laid their eggs upon it. The eggs hatched out there, and not in the meat.

The most noted member of the Accademia del Cimento was Alfonso Borelli (1608–1679). Primarily, he was a mathematician, and was for a time professor of mathematics in Pisa. In addition however, he was a physicist and a physiologist. Advancing along the paths opened up by Harvey, he did his best to explain vital manifestations in physical terms, and to show that they were subject to physical laws. In a famous book (published posthumously) *De motu animalium*, he showed how the movements of animals were effected in accordance with the laws of mechanics. Studying the movements of the muscles and that of the heart (which is a muscle, though a peculiar one), he proved that the movements of this organ and the work it did could be expressed in numerical terms. He also studied the mechanics of respiration. The thorax, he said, enlarged itself actively through the contractions of the intercostal muscles; and the lungs, which were extensible, passively followed this expansile movement. Expiration, on the other hand, was a mere process of relaxation. This view of the respiratory process is the one which has prevailed down to our own day. Digestion, likewise, said Borelli, was a mechanical process, not, as the iatrochemists supposed, a fermentative one. The gastric secretion was poured out in consequence of blood pressure. In this way, thanks to the working of physiological factors, the stomach was enabled to rub down the food, mixed with the gastric juice, into a thin pap.

If, however, the normal processes of life could be interpreted mechanically, similar explanations must apply to morbid phenomena. What were fevers, pains, convulsions, etc., other than disturbances in the movements of the nervous juices? If the apertures of the nerves were blocked, morbid manifestations were inevitable. The same thing when the blood underwent stasis in the capillaries. The heat of inflammation was produced by friction of the blood against the walls of the vessels.

Thus by degrees there arose in Southern Europe, as a counterpart to the iatrochemists of the North, the school of iatrophysicists, iatromechanists, or iatromathematicians, whose views gained wide acceptance.

The iatromechanical doctrines attained their climax and reached a critical turning-point in the teaching of Giorgio Baglivi.

Baglivi was born in poor circumstances at Ragusa—born at sunrise on September 8, 1688. The name of the family was not

Baglivi, but Armeno, which perhaps gives a clue to its origin. Unable to make a living in Ragusa, the Armenos removed to Lecce in Apulia. Young Giorgio and his brother Giacomo attracted attention there by signs of lively intelligence. A Jesuit who was a fellow-countryman of theirs recommended them to a wealthy physician, Pierangelo Baglivi, who adopted the two lads, gave them his name, and left them his property. Giacomo became a priest, but Giorgio espoused the profession of his adoptive father.

After studying at the university of Naples, he travelled for several years in various parts of Italy, arriving at Rome in the spring of 1692, and settling down there for a long time. In Rome, Baglivi struck up a friendship with various persons of note, such as Lancisi, Trionfetti the botanist, and Pacchioni the anatomist. Malpighi, too, had been for a year in Rome. Him Baglivi knew already, having attended Malpighi's lectures in Bologna for a time. True, by this date Malpighi was an old and broken man, so that there could be no intimacy between him and Baglivi, who was forty years younger. Still, when in July 1694 Malpighi had a stroke of apoplexy he sent for Baglivi, thus showing that, young though Baglivi was, he already enjoyed a considerable reputation as a practitioner. The same year, Malpighi succumbed to a second attack of apoplexy. Baglivi made a post-mortem examination, and then wrote a clear, simply worded, and effective report concerning the illness and the result of the autopsy.

Baglivi was now inclined to quit Rome and to return to Lecce, but Pope Innocent XII induced him to stay on for a time, and soon a vacancy occurred which bound him to Rome for the remainder of his life.

Lancisi, who up till now had been professor of anatomy at the Sapienza, the papal university, was in 1696 appointed professor-in-chief of practical medicine. He had, therefore, to leave his anatomical chair. A competitive examination took place, and Baglivi got the best marks among thirteen candidates.

He was professor of anatomy at the Sapienza for five years, and then, in 1701, he was appointed professor of theoretical medicine.

Thus it was that Baglivi remained in Rome until his premature death before reaching the age of forty. In his brief career he did a great deal of practical and literary work. At the age of twenty-eight he penned two books, *De praxi medica*, which made his name widely known, and brought him the membership of various academies. There followed theoretical writings: *De fibra motrice et morbosa*, and various lesser monographs.

As far as theory was concerned, Baglivi was a declared iatromechanist, and, indeed, pushed the doctrine of this school to an extreme. He regarded the human organism as a sort of tool-chest. The teeth were like scissors, the stomach was a bottle, the intestines and the glands were sieves, the vessels were but a system of tubes, and the thorax was no more than the box containing a pair of bellows. The tools of which the body was made up were moved by the fibres, in virtue of their tone. A normal tone determined health, whereas if the tone were too high or too low illness was the result.

When we turn to watch Baglivi as a working practitioner, we are overtaken by surprise. Although as far as theory was concerned he was a dogmatist, in his practical work he was free from preconceptions. He was a great clinician, a remarkably able observer, and highly skilled in treatment. He did not draw any inferences from his theories, did not allow his practice to be determined by them. Indeed, his practical principles gave the lie to his theories. Let me quote at random a few sentences from the introduction to his *De praxi medica*:

"The doctor is the servant and the interpreter of nature. Whatever he thinks or does, if he follow not in nature's footsteps he will never be able to control her. The origin and the causes of disease are far too recondite for the human mind to unravel them."—"The two fulcra of medicine are reason and observation. Observation, however, is the clue which must guide the physician in his thinking."—"Up till now we have been far too readily satisfied with brilliant hypotheses, with subtle logical distinctions and definitions. They are doubtless a great ornament to our art, but they do not make it practically effective."—If theory had made advances, this had been exclusively owing to the experimental science which had developed during the seventeenth century. All the same, the man who failed to read Hippocrates was a blockhead. There had been no greater physicians than he in the past, nor would be in the future.—"If only physicians would at length come to their senses, would awaken from their slumbers, and would realise how sharply the old virile medicine of Hellas is distinguished from the speculative and vacillating medicine of the moderns!"

These are unmistakably reactionary notes. They give expression to a profound dissatisfaction. One who writes in such a way is disappointed with the recent acquisitions of science. He directs his gaze backwards, and the figure of Hippocrates looms large before his gaze. The healing art of the Hippocratists, that of days when theory occupied a secondary place and when practice was the main thing, seemed to him the most desirable ideal. Yet Baglivi was a man of science. He made post-mortem examinations, and he experimented like his colleagues. Nay, he even excelled them in the speculative inferences he drew from his researches.

A gulf yawns in Baglivi's work. There is a chasm in it between theory and practice, between his science and his art. With him, theory no longer determined practice, had become valueless for practice, which sought other guidance. Conversely, theory was no longer the outcome of practical experiences. Science and practice had parted company.

Baglivi was himself aware of this cleavage, but he was too deeply involved in the mechanistic atmosphere which prevailed in Italy at that date to escape from it. The new trend was to come from a different side.

CHAPTER TWENTY-TWO

THOMAS SYDENHAM
1624–1689

WHEN Sydenham died, at a date when Baglivi was still a student at Naples, he was buried in St. James's Church, Westminster. On his tombstone he was described as "medicus in omne aevum nobilis." Posterity conferred upon him a supreme title of honour by speaking of him as the English Hippocrates. Those who wished to pay honour to Baglivi described him as the Italian Sydenham. Sydenham was not a distinguished man of science, had not been a professor at a university, nor a voluminous writer. His collected works comprise no more than one volume of moderate size. He was merely an able London practitioner.

The great doctors of the seventeenth century, so far as we have hitherto made their acquaintance, were distinguished investigators and profound thinkers. All of them, indeed, were likewise practitioners, more or less successful, for pure theoreticians did not yet exist. The time has come, however, for us to ask what kind of a man was the average practitioner of those days. Had the newer researches begun to take effect on practical medicine? Had they improved the technique, had they raised the level, of the ordinary doctor?

The answer must be that in most countries, well on until the middle of the seventeenth century, the average practitioner was a poor creature. In this respect, the satires of Molière are not so exaggerated as they may appear. The doctor felt that he had been uprooted. Recent research had undermined the edifice of classical and medieval medicine, which had seemed to be established on such firm foundations. What had taken its place? Not one doctrine, but many. Whom was the practitioner to follow; Paracelsus, van Helmont, the iatrochemists, or the iatrophysicists? They all contradicted one another, and often vilified one another. No doubt anatomy and physiology had brought important contributions to medical knowledge; but anatomy and physiology were not a new healing art. They were no more than the road to such an art—a long, long road which it would take centuries to traverse. Practice could not wait. It needed immediate directives.

Chemistry and physics, likewise, had plainly demonstrated their importance to medicine; but the zeal for discovery which inspired the iatrochemists and iatrophysicists had outstripped discretion. There was one thing they had not learned, the need for moderation, for restriction. They wanted to explain everything. Even though their concepts were substantially those of modern natural science, their systems as yet, when closely scrutinised, are seen to have been nothing more than speculations upon natural philosophy, not differing greatly from the Galenic system. How little use the new teachings were in practice, at the bedside, is plainly disclosed by the behaviour of Baglivi who, in his clinical work, advised a return to the principles of the Hippocratic writings.

There thus existed an unhappy cleavage in medicine throughout the seventeenth century. Practitioners were aware that the old traditions had been discredited, but they could find nothing trustworthy by way of substitute. It is easy to understand that most of the universities were conservative; that the faculties regarded it as their duty, not merely to teach, but also to defend, the old doctrines. Down to the time of the French revolution, the faculty of Paris remained ultra-conservative. It resisted innovations with all its might, rejecting, for instance, the new chemical remedies. It actually expelled one of its members for recommending the use of preparations of antimony.

The upshot was that in most "centres of learning" instruction remained true to tradition and purely theoretical. The classical and Arabian authors were taught, expounded, and subjected to

176

comment. "Disputations" went on just as in the Middle Ages. The physicians turned out by these schools were learned enough, but their scientific ideals were those of a past era. The wheel of history cannot be turned backwards. It was preposterous for any one to remain a scholastic when he was a contemporary of Descartes, Francis Bacon, Galilei, and Harvey. That is why the doctors in Molière's plays produce so irresistibly comic an impression. They are fossils, physicians who have survived from a remote past. The epoch in which they lived had adopted a new scientific ideal, in spite of the fact that their ideal was alien to most medical practitioners of the time.

The result of this conflict in their minds was that the more intelligent among the doctors escaped from medical practice into natural science or into other fields. For instance, there was Guy Patin, who played a part in political life; and there was Théophraste Renaudot, who became historiographer to the king, and who in 1631 founded the "Gazette de France," the first political newspaper in his country. Renaudot also established a pawn-shop, and he gave gratuitous medical advice to the poor. Medical practice was becoming hopelessly confused.

Yet the progress of the healing art can never be arrested. Every sick person who consults a doctor is an exhortation to him to improve his knowledge. Every physician who loses a patient has an uneasy conscience. The requisite change came, and it came from the field of practical medicine. The man who brought it about was Sydenham.

The story of his life can be briefly told. He was the son of a landed proprietor, and in 1642, when he was eighteen years old, he was sent to Oxford. Then the Great Rebellion broke out. Since his family was of a Puritan way of thinking, he took service with the Parliamentary army. On the other side, in the royal camp, was William Harvey, already an old man, and in truth little interested in this political dispute. The King's armies were defeated, and the Parliamentarians seized Oxford in 1646. The first act of the Civil War was over. Sydenham was freed from his military occupations, and was faced with the need for choosing a profession—a difficult matter after four years wasted as a soldier. At this time he was in London. His brother fell sick, and was treated by a well-known physician named Thomas Coxe. This gentleman had a talk with young Thomas Sydenham, and strongly advised him to enter the medical profession. Why not? Sydenham returned to Oxford, now under Puritan control, in order to study medicine. The work came hard to him, for while in the field he had completely forgotten his Latin. However, in 1648, thanks to patronage, he was granted the degree of bachelor of medicine. He stayed on in Oxford. War broke out again. Cromwell had subjugated Ireland and was campaigning in Scotland against Charles II. There was dread of a rising against the parliament in England. A militia was established, and Sydenham was enrolled in this, not as surgeon, but as captain of horse. After the defeat at Worcester, Charles II escaped to foreign parts, and in 1653 Cromwell became Lord Protector.

Now Sydenham settled down at Westminster in general practice. Owing to the disorders of the time, his medical education had been defective, and he does not seem at first to have displayed much enthusiasm for his profession, being far more interested in politics. He stood for parliament, and was defeated. Then he applied for an official post, which was granted him by Richard Cromwell in 1659, Oliver Cromwell having died the year before. But in 1660 came the Restoration, and Sydenham was deprived of his post.

Now he had no resource but to devote himself seriously to medicine. Aware of his own deficiencies, he went to Montpellier to complete his medical education. In 1661 he returned to London, and, at the age of thirty-seven, devoted to the healing art all the energy which he had hitherto given to party struggles. He was not weighted by academic ties, and had felt the pulse of life. In actual fact, he was not even yet legally qualified to practise. For this it was necessary to have passed an examination by the Royal College of Physicians. With considerable difficulty he got the necessary papers together, passed his examination, and received the licentiate in 1663. He was not yet doctor of medicine, but that could wait. In 1676, when he was fifty-two, he took his medical degree—not at Oxford but at Cambridge. What did these externals matter? Medicine, to his way of thinking, was concerned with far more important things.

What mattered, considered Sydenham, was that a doctor should come to know diseases, should learn the conditions out of which they arise, should be aware of the means by which they can be cured. Little need for so much theorising! We have before us a sick and suffering human being. That is our object of study; the symptoms, their changes, the cause of illnesses.

What is illness? It is a struggle between the physis, the nature, of the sick person and the noxious influences that have produced the illness. The symptoms are the expression of this struggle. Noxious influences act upon a human being. Disturbances arise which manifest themselves as "symptomata essentialia." The organism reacts against these influences, tries to overcome their evil effects through its native healing power, tries to make good the disturbances. The manifestations of this reaction are the "symptomata accidentalia." Illness is a natural process, is for the main part nature's healing activity. One of the mightiest weapons of the organism in its defensive struggle is fever.

The doctor's business is to assist nature in its struggle, to guide and to intensify the healing power of nature. Now, if the doctor is to intervene to good purpose he must know the particular diseases as well as possible. Particular diseases exist. There are "species morborum," various kinds of illness, just as there are species of animals and plants. Even as the zoologist and the botanist learn how to distinguish animal and vegetable species one from another, so must the physician endeavour to distinguish the various diseases. As compared with the illness, the individual sufferer passes into the background. The nature of the disease determines the individual's morbid experiences. The way to an understanding of particular diseases is their clinical observation from the appearance of the first symptoms to the disappearance of the last.

Sydenham followed up this line with all the zeal of a scientific investigator. From the age of thirty onwards he had been tormented by gout, and we owe to him a classical description of this disease. In the district where he practised, various febrile disorders were prevalent, and he studied them. From 1666 onwards he published a number of monographs, mainly concerned with epidemic diseases observed by him during his practice since 1661. In these monographs we find admirable descriptions of smallpox, measles, dysentery, and syphilis. The constitution of the individual, he held, was of minor importance, but there certainly existed an "epidemic constitution." One who had this epidemic constitution fell sick in a specific way. There were also certain "telluric influences," working in accordance with fixed laws, and determining the appearance and the decline of epidemics.

It was the particular disease that was present upon which the choice of remedial measures depended. Each illness had its appropriate treatment. Since, however, the illness was never a purely local process, but was a reaction of the whole organism, the doctor had to treat, not a single organ, but the sick man as a whole.

The problems concerning the intimate mechanism of disease, concerning the forces upon which the normal and pathological vital manifestations depended, passed into the background. Sydenham adopted the humoral pathology, but worked with more modern humoral concepts than those of Galen. Still, he laid little stress upon such theoretical considerations. For him the particular diseases were the main thing.

Therein lies Sydenham's historical importance, that he turned physicians' attention in a new direction, towards particular illnesses; that he brought doctors out of the laboratories into the sick-room. Whereas for a century investigators had been studying man in general, had been studying illness in general, had been trying with the inadequate methods and instruments of the day to solve the problems of general pathology, Sydenham proclaimed the importance of special pathology. First, he said, let us study particular diseases, let us learn how they make themselves perceptible to us in a particular patient. Let us seek to learn from experience what remedies are best in particular diseases. General conclusions can wait.

Thus it was that Sydenham came to seem to his contemporaries "the English Hippocrates." Unquestionably his medical art and science had in many respects the characteristics of a reaction, and Sydenham regarded himself as a Hippocratist. Like Hippocrates, the basic principle of his medical thinking was the humoral pathology, and like Hippocrates his general outlook upon illness was that it was a natural healing process. Nevertheless there lay a whole world between the two. The decisive difference between them becomes plain in respect of their divergent outlook upon illness as soon as they quit the domain of the general. Hippocrates recognised only disease, not diseases. He knew only sick individuals, only cases of illness. The patient and his malady were for him inseparably connected as a unique happening, one which would never recur. But what Sydenham saw above all in the patient, what he wrenched forth to contemplate, was the typical, the pathological process which he had observed in others before and expected to see in others again. In every patient there appeared a specific kind of illness. For him maladies were entities, and his outlook upon illness was, therefore, ontological. Hippocrates wrote the histories of sick persons, but Sydenham wrote the history of diseases.

Here was a new outlook, and one which lifted Sydenham far above the platform of antiquity. He was not a reactionary, was not a man with his gaze fixed on the past, but was a pioneer who looked continually forward. Already in the early days of the Renaissance, indeed, this new outlook upon illness began to disclose itself, gradually taking shape in the writings of Paracelsus and van Helmont, though imperfectly. Now, in Sydenham, it was clearly discerned and succinctly formulated.

It proved amazingly fruitful. Other physicians set to work to study particular diseases. They endeavoured to establish order, to delimit groups, in the vast ocean of symptoms and symptom-complexes. No doubt there were plenty of atypical cases, but these were deviations from a type, from a norm. The type or norm existed, even though it was sometimes difficult to understand why divergencies took place. The upshot was the writing of numberless monographs upon particular diseases: upon apoplexy (Wepfer), upon pulmonary consumption (Morton), upon rickets (Glisson). Doctors began to study heart diseases apart from other maladies (Vieussens, Lancisi), and to note the peculiarities of the diseases that tended to affect those who followed particular occupations (Ramazzini). The more extensively this method of research was used, the larger was the number of diseases discovered.

The new outlook upon disease speedily influenced practice. Henceforward, when a doctor was called in to a patient, his first task at the bedside was to make a diagnosis; that is to say, to recognise the nature of the illness with which he had to deal. His treatment would in great measure be determined by his diagnosis.

In most essentials, Sydenham's principles are still our own. He stands upon the direct line of development of modern medicine. As we shall see, his successors brought his notion of disease into touch with anatomical ideas, gave it an ideological foundation, and resumed the study of physics and chemistry. In this way, not speculatively but experimentally, carefully feeling their way, they attacked the problems of pathogenesis.

Thus once more it was practice, actual life, which kept medicine from running off the rails, which reminded the doctor of his proper task, which kept his true goal before his eyes.

There was a further reaction against iatrophysics and iatrochemistry, in a different direction. This was a movement chiefly directed against the materialism of the age, an indignant revolt against the notion that human beings were mere machines, consisting of tools, retorts, and elastic bands. The same movement was manifested in other domains of the mind as well as in medicine: in philosophy, through the development from Descartes to Leibniz; in jurisprudence, through the advance from Roman law to natural law; in theology, through the appearance of pietism.

As far as medicine was concerned, this movement found its most vigorous expression in the animism of Georg Ernst Stahl (1660–1734), professor at Halle. Why, he asked, does the organism not fall to pieces or decay, why does it not putrefy so long as it is alive? The energy which holds it together, that which makes the living alive, is the soul. The whole century had had faith in the soul; but, energetically dualistic, it had established a very sharp distinction between the spiritual and the bodily. Many of the investigators of the Baroque period, many of those whose names we have already learned, were affected by this cleavage, were men of the spirit and men of the body—materialists as investigators, but at the same time believing Christians. They thought, on the one hand, and they prayed, on the other. Science and a man's general outlook on the universe were pigeon-holed apart. People did not deny the existence of the soul. Far from it. But the soul had nothing to do with the domain of science. Consideration of the soul was the province of the theologian. The Enlightenment was to break away from this dualism, was to fuse philosophy and science into a united structure, permeated in every corner by the light of reason.

Stahl followed a different path. He, likewise, bridged over

dualism; but he did so by turning the soul to account for the understanding of biological happenings. The soul which gave life to dead matter! It was, he said, actively at work, not only in consciousness, but also in the unconscious and vegetative realm. All vital processes were under the dominance of the soul, morbid processes not excepted, since they too were vital. All vital processes were purposive, and morbid processes came within the same category.

Such a view had momentous results for the practice of medicine. If the soul, if "nature" (as Stahl sometimes phrased it), induced fever and inflammation, the physician must not try to counteract nature's purposes in these matters. He must not treat intermittent fever with cinchona bark, which cuts the fever short. He should avoid using powerful narcotics like opium, and should try to carry out nature's purposes, to assist nature, by the use of milder remedies. No doubt circumstances arose in which the soul seemed bewildered. Then processes occurred which we are unable to recognise as purposive.

Stahl occupies a notable place in the history of chemistry, as the founder of the theory of phlogiston. If he also secured a considerable number of followers in the medical field, this was mainly because his general outlook on disease followed along the lines laid down by Sydenham, while, with his doctrine of animism, he gave to it a visage congenial to those physicians who were in revolt against materialism.

The reader will realise that such a doctrine as Stahl's must have stimulated the study of psychiatry, and must have prepared the ground for the spread of vitalism.

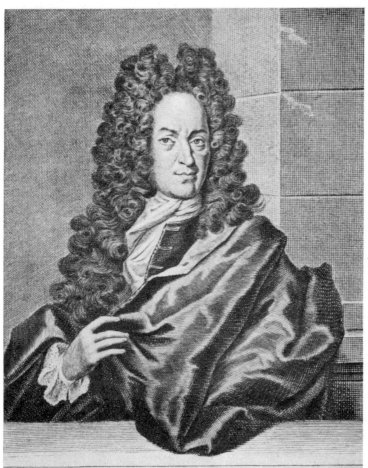

Georg Erneſtus Stahl, Onoldo Francus,
Med. Doct. h. t. Prof. Publ. Ord. Hall. —

GEORG ERNST STAHL, 1660–1734

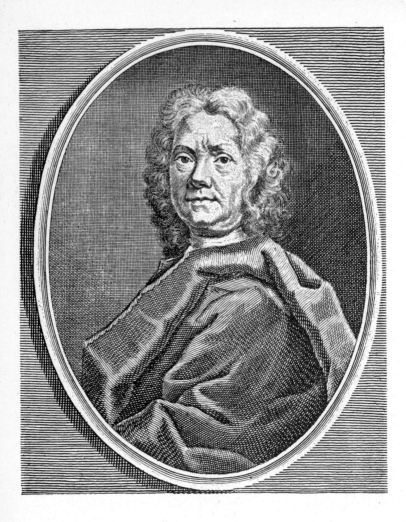

HERMANN BOERHAAVE, 1668–1738

CHAPTER TWENTY-THREE

HERMANN BOERHAAVE
1668–1738

ALBRECHT VON HALLER writes of his teacher Boerhaave: "Communis Europae sub initio huius saeculi magister." In actual fact, at the beginning of the eighteenth century Boerhaave exerted an unexampled attractive force upon all young doctors and students of medicine. Thanks to him, the university of Leyden, where he worked, became the focus of medical life. In Leyden to-day we encounter his traces at every turn. His tomb is in the St. Pieterskerk. Near the old hospital is his monument. Whenever a medical congress is held in Leyden, this monument is bedecked with flowers. The magnificent new buildings in which the medical faculty is housed are known as the "Boerhaave-Kwartier." There is an active cult of his memory.

To what did he owe his extraordinary fame? His writings do not suffice to explain it. He wrote comparatively little: two rather short works; one of them entitled *Institutiones medicae* (1708); and the other *Aphorismi de cognoscendis et curandis morbis* (1709). Apart from these, there were a few botanical and chemical papers, some clinical histories, and a number of academic orations. No doubt it is still a great pleasure to read his thoughtful speeches. His clinical histories are masterpieces. As for the two books already mentioned, their conciseness, their clarity, and their sobriety make them contrast very agreeably with much of the literature of the day, which was apt to be prolix and obscure. Sustained by their author's repute, they ran through numerous editions and were translated into various languages, even into Turkish. We see that Boerhaave's name must have been widely known in his lifetime.

Still, when we read his writings we find nothing revolutionary

185

in them. He made no discoveries, he did not contribute any new ideas of moment to medicine. Nor did he belong to any school, being an eclectic. Yet that was what gave him his strength. He adopted what seemed to him good, no matter the source. He was firmly and enduringly convinced of the importance of anatomy and physiology to medicine. He knew that physics could make important contributions to medicine, and he was therefore strongly inclined towards iatromechanics. Nor was it surprising that in Leyden, where the tradition of Sylvius was still alive, he should have recognised the value of chemistry. Among more recent physicians, however, Sydenham seemed to him by far the weightiest. "I should blush to mention his name without extolling him," he said in one of his speeches.

It is out of these elements that modern medicine has been upbuilded. But in the opening of the eighteenth century, considering how elementary as yet were the sciences named, it would have been overbold to attempt a synthesis of these elements, and would merely have led to the construction of an artificial system. Boerhaave, therefore, wisely renounced the idea of establishing a circumscribed system. He made no attempt to explain all morbid phenomena. He was much less interested in theory than in the patient and the cure—in medical practice.

The secret of Boerhaave's successes is to be found, not so much in his scientific writings, as in his personality, in his alluring personality as physician and clinical teacher. Any one who had come into close contact with him, any one who had seen and listened to him at the bedside, would never be able to shake off his influence, would burn for the rest of life with a sacred fire, and would persistently have the picture of an ideal physician before his eyes. All Boerhaave's pupils were at one upon this matter; they were grateful to him and remained deeply attached to him, describing him as extraordinarily kindhearted, and ever ready to give help. Haller writes of him: "In respect of learning he had equals, though perhaps not many; but hardly any one was worthy to rank with him in his truly divine character, in his goodness to all, in his benevolence even to the envious and to his rivals. No one ever heard him say a disparaging word."

Boerhaave was the son of an impecunious country clergyman, and was himself destined for the Church. In Leyden he was, to begin with, a student of theology. Soon, however, he found that mathematics, chemistry, botany, and medicine were far more to his taste, and in the end he made up his mind to transfer to the medical faculty. Not wishing to attract attention to this change of plan, he removed to another university and took his degree in medicine at Harderwijk. Then, returning to Leyden, he settled down there as a doctor. Not having many patients to begin with, he had plenty of time for wider education, especially in mathematics. In 1701 he was appointed lector of theoretical medicine, and was so successful in this post that two years later he received a call to Gröningen. Leyden, however, did not want to lose him. The university raised his salary, and promised him the next vacant chair. Even in those days professors were long-lived men, and Boerhaave had to wait six years for his promotion. When Hotton died in 1709, Boerhaave became professor of botany, and the post carried with it the direction of the botanical gardens. "No explorer," writes Haller, "ever made his way into more unknown country than this new professor, who knew almost nothing about plants, however much he might have excelled in other departments of knowledge. He applied himself so diligently, however, that, in spite of the severe winter of 1709, in 1710 he was able to publish a list of his plants which excelled that of any of his predecessors." Haller makes repeated mention of Boerhaave's devotion to the botanical gardens. Every morning at seven o'clock he demonstrated plants to the students, "generally pointing out to them on each day hundreds of plants and giving supplementary names without making use of notes." The botanical gardens of Leyden soon became among the finest in the world, for Boerhaave, corresponding freely with men in similar positions, secured seeds from far and wide. "The finest feature of the place is," writes Haller, "that everything is purposively arranged, so that a stranger with Boerhaave's list in his hand can recognise all the plants in accordance with their serial order and by means of the ticketed staves."

In the winter Boerhaave lectured on chemistry. His importance in this specialty is for the most part over-estimated, for indeed there is a tendency to describe him in somewhat exaggerated terms as a man of overwhelming ability in all the fields he tilled. No doubt he was a brilliant experimenter, and his marked capacity as a teacher did not fail him in the chemical laboratory or lecture-theatre; but he was not an originator here, being content to follow in the footsteps of his predecessors, especially those of Robert Boyle.

Where Boerhaave was incomparable was in the domain of clinical instruction, which he took over in 1714 after the death of Bidloo. At the bedside of the sick, the full powers of his personality were unfolded. Here he was not a mere iatro-mechanical theoretician, but a great physician in the profoundest sense of the term. He approached his patients with the keen insight of the born diagnostician, treated them with affection as well as with medicine and good advice, and carried his hearers with him, when lecturing or demonstrating, by the rigorousness of his logic. In the hospital behind the Vrouwen Kerk there were two rooms, each containing six beds—a ward for men and a ward for women available for clinical instruction. Half the doctors of Europe were trained beside these twelve beds! Day after day, Boerhaave went from case to case, explaining them to his students. The senior students were asked to give practical advice, just as they are in our modern hospitals. If we wish to form an idea of the abundance of material dealt with by Boerhaave in his clinical demonstrations, we must turn to the editions of the *Institutiones* and the *Aphorismi* that were edited with commentaries by his pupils van Swieten and von Haller, for the commentaries consist mainly of Boerhaave's own observations, as noted down by these two students. Van Swieten, whose acquaintance we shall make in the next chapter but one as the reformer of medicine in Vienna, was a good shorthand writer. His notebooks are extant. They have been deciphered, and show us in the liveliest possible way how clinical instruction was given by Boerhaave.

Although the roots of the new method reach as far as Padua, it was Leyden, it was Boerhaave's hospital, which was the cradle of modern clinical methods. Here a sound method for the examination of the sick was first worked out. To begin with, the anamnesis (clinical history) was fully recorded; and then the present condition of the patient was ascertained. The investigation was not as yet anatomical. The doctor did not ascertain the condition of the organs, but that of the malady. Thereafter a diagnosis and a prognosis were made, and a course of treatment was laid down. The seed sown in this way at Leyden was soon to sprout in many other places.

Students at Leyden in Boerhaave's day had the advantage of learning, not only from that famous clinician, but also from a distinguished anatomist, Bernhard Siegfried Weiss, who Latinised his name as Albinus.

Boerhaave's practice increased from year to year. Haller writes: "From ten till twelve his consulting-room was thronged by those who sought his advice, for pressure of work now made it impossible for him to visit patients in their homes. Often enough the morning consultations outlasted the fixed hours, so that lecture time had come before he had had a moment in which to eat his dinner. At three in the afternoon additional patients began to arrive. What remained of his day was spent in an extensive correspondence and in his long-continued labours upon the writings of the Greek physicians—unless some distinguished patient dragged him away from his work." Elsewhere in Haller's journal we read: "So widely known did Boerhaave's name become, that students from all lands assembled to hear him, and there was no patient of high degree who did not seek his advice. I have myself seen Monsieur Fénelon, ambassador at The Hague, waiting to catch him as he came out of the lecture-theatre. We students numbered about 120, half of whom were from foreign lands. I doubt if any medical professor's lecture-room was ever before so well-attended as Boerhaave's. Wealth flowed to him from all parts, and it was supposed that his only daughter would inherit a few tons of it. In 1725, not long before my arrival, he had suffered from severe inflammation of the joints, which deprived him completely of sleep."

These attacks of gout became so violent and so frequent that Boerhaave had to cut down his work, and in 1729 he resigned the professorships of chemistry and botany. He continued, however, to give clinical instruction until in 1738, in the seventieth year of his life, he was finally relieved of his sufferings.

CHAPTER TWENTY-FOUR

ALBRECHT VON HALLER
1708–1777

As poet of the Alps, Haller occupies a distinguished place in the history of German literature. His *Versuch schweizerischer Gedichte* was published anonymously in 1732, being manifestly the work of a lyricist endowed with a strong feeling for nature. His poems are tinged with vigorous emotion, but he knew how to avoid the turgidity of other poetic writers of his time. A native of Berne, he had grown up in close touch with the Alps, had wandered far and wide among them, had been profoundly impressed by their majesty. Now he sung them, and described their inhabitants, whose simple ways, he declared, were a warning to town-dwellers. He looked for and found the Deity in nature, writing:

> Enough, there is a God, and nature is His scrip.
> The mighty world's whole structure shows His workmanship.

He discerned the traces of God's handiwork, not only in nature on the grand scale, as disclosed in the Alps, nor only in the human heart, whose depths he tried to plumb. He discerned these traces likewise in nature on the small scale, in the stamens of plants, for instance—being a botanist; in the contraction of the muscles—being an anatomist and a physiologist. He contemplated nature through the microscope, as well as with the poet's gaze. There is no clash between his poetical and his scientific creations. Both are animated by the same ethical feeling.

In youth Haller was a poet, but he remained a scientist all his life long. His contemporaries regarded him as a man of universal learning, as one who was interested in every domain of human knowledge. He was one of the last naturalists in the old sense of the term, such a man as Conrad Gesner or J. J. Scheuchzer; one of those investigators whose observations embraced the entire field of nature both animate and inanimate; one of those who, moreover, tried to turn their scientific acquisitions to practical account in agriculture, stud-farming, medicine, and technique.

Haller was a precocious boy. His father died when he was very young, he was of a weakly constitution, and was hampered by illness throughout his life. He had nothing in common with the vigorous young associates of his own age, and for this reason he early took his own path, gratified his hunger for learning, devoted himself to great tasks, such as the compilation of dictionaries and grammars, and the writing of no less than two thousand brief biographies. His encyclopaedic leanings were already manifest. At school he was extremely ambitious. "It was a great distress to him unless he was regarded as excelling his schoolmates in diligence and ability." His relatives wanted him to study theology, considering that his bent lay in that direction, but he expressed a strong desire to become a doctor, and at the age of fifteen, with that end in view, was enrolled as a student at the university of Tübingen.

There was, he said, not much opportunity for profound study at that seat of learning. True, Duverney, a very able anatomist, taught at Tübingen. But no human bodies could be obtained for dissection, and the students had to rest content with the corpses of dogs. There were botanical excursions, but the students returned home "without any specimens, and usually more than half-seas-over." It need hardly be said that there was no question of clinical instruction. Nevertheless, the sixteen months Haller spent at Tübingen were useful to him. The merry life of the students, the influence of frivolous comrades, and association with the pretty ladies of Tübingen "who were by no means coy," combined to break down the barriers between young Haller and the life of the everyday world. Hitherto he had been like a fish out of water. Hence-

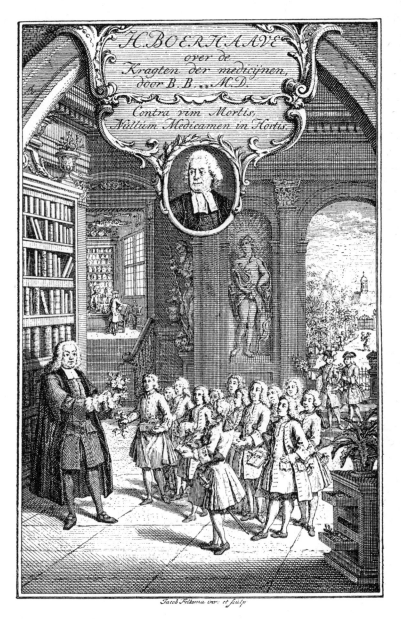

Within the illustration:

H. BOERHAAVE
over de
Kragten der medicijnen,
door B. B . . . M.D.

Contra vim Mortis,
Nullum Medicamen in Hortis.

Jacob Folkema inv: et sculp

BOERHAAVE LECTURING ON BOTANY

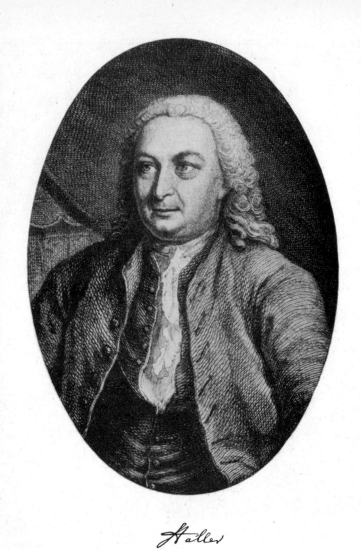

ALBRECHT HALLER, 1708–1777

forward he was less of a solitary, and, as we should say nowadays, less of an introvert.

Tübingen, however, was not a place for serious studies, so in the spring of 1725 Haller removed to Leyden. There he found all that his heart could desire: a dissecting-room in which there were human bodies; a botanical garden; a clinic. Above all in Albinus and Boerhaave he found teachers who were to exert a decisive influence upon his career. It was in Leyden that he received the impetus which made him a man of science. Devoting himself to his medical training with the utmost zeal, he was able as early as 1727 to take his degree as doctor of medicine with a dissertation upon an anatomical topic.

Next came a journey to London and Paris, for medical study in both these capitals. He visited hospitals and museums, attended operations and post-mortem examinations. More and more his interest in anatomy grew. At Paris he found in Winslow a highly skilled anatomist, whose method of studying the organs in situ instead of cut loose from their surroundings was henceforward adopted by Haller. For further training he went to the university of Basle, where he came into contact with an extremely stimulating circle of aspiring young physicians, and also studied mathematics diligently under Jean Bernoulli the elder.

The chief importance of Haller's sojourn in Basle was that there he began to specialise in botany. Before this he had studied botany, just as he studied all the sciences ancillary to medicine; but he had never preserved plants, he had no herbarium. Now, in Basle, stimulated by the wealth of the Swiss flora and surrounded by friends who were enthusiastic botanists, he was fired to make a thorough study of plants. On numerous excursions, he culled them, and, having brought home his specimens, he classified and described them. In view of his character, which invariably led him to strive after completion and to work at far-reaching schemes, we can hardly doubt that already at this early date (when he still had leisure to study the commoner plants) he must have conceived the plan of his great work upon the flora of Switzerland.

It was, therefore, primarily for botanical reasons that in the summer of 1728 Albrecht von Haller, accompanied by his friend Johannes Gesner, made that journey through the Alps whose finest fruit was the poem *Die Alpen*.

After an additional term at Basle, spent mainly in anatomical studies, in the spring of 1729 Haller returned to Berne and settled down there as a doctor. It is easy to understand that in the narrow surroundings of the Swiss capital he felt extremely unhappy. For five years and a half he had had multifarious experiences in a wider world; had dwelt in the foci of research, in Leyden, London, Paris, and Basle; had himself become a scientist, a man devoted to original investigation. Now, at the age of one-and-twenty, he had a keen desire to continue these creative activities, but on all hands he was faced by impeding walls. His fellow-townsmen had no more than a compassionate smile for his enthusiasms. As in childhood, so now, he was isolated.

All the same, he was unremitting in his exertions. He in whom the sacred flame of science has once been kindled can be intimidated by no opposition, which, indeed, serves only to stimulate zeal. Year after year, Haller made expeditions into the Alps, returning each time with an abundance of botanical plunder. He succeeded, moreover, in obtaining permission to make post-mortems at the hospital from time to time. Although the material was scanty, he was able to make a good use of it for scientific purposes. Returning to the study of Boerhaave's *Institutiones medicae,* he began a detailed commentary upon that important work. But this was a toilsome undertaking, devoid of stimulating reverberations, in a backwater (so to say) apart from the main current of research. Then, when he was beginning to lose heart, in the spring of 1736 he received a call to the recently founded university of Göttingen as professor of anatomy, surgery, and botany.

What minister of State to-day would venture to summon from foreign parts to fill so responsible a position a general practitioner of no more than eight-and-twenty, who had only written a volume of poems and a few small monographs? In those days, however, the works of a candidate were not adjudged by their weight or their bulk but by their intrinsic value. The authorities made exhaustive inquiries. No doubt Haller had written very little, but his inaugural dissertation or thesis, in which he had refuted a current anatomical error, sufficed to show his intellectual calibre. Münchhausen, minister to George II, King of England and Elector of Hanover, had, in this appointment (as chancellor of the new university), made a happy selection. It is hardly too much to say that Haller himself was the making of Göttingen. On the other hand, at Göttingen Haller had a field of activity in which he could develop his powers to the full.

A great task awaited him there. As a member of the faculty, *primus inter pares*, it behoved him to help in the creation of a genuinely modern university. There were no old traditions claiming respect at all costs, and ready to stifle innovations in the germ. As regards the relationships of the medical faculties to the State, since the close of the Middle Ages a profound change had taken place almost everywhere. The medieval faculty had been the expert adviser of the State in all matters that concerned the healing art, and was continually being asked to give formal opinions. As we have already seen, it had not merely to enunciate and to transmit a doctrine, but also to maintain that doctrine's pristine purity. Opinions concerning innovations concerning new theories and new remedies, were powerful weapons in this respect. The faculty, likewise, was supreme in deciding who had the right to trust it, supervising in many places the apothecaries as well as the physicians—the whole field of medicine. Its power, therefore, was immense.

When, during the Renaissance, a new science began to develop, many of the universities held stubbornly aloof.

Evolution left them marooned on desolate shores. A number of the governments, absolutist in theory and practice, established medical councils or boards, State instruments of medical administration. These became advisers to the State. They had the right of approval or disapproval, and the right of supervision. The new councils or boards robbed the faculties of many of their privileges. The upshot was that the faculties, like Achilles, sulked in their tents, and grew more and more estranged from the busy life of a reawakening world. A few of them, however, with Leyden in the van, devoted themselves ardently to medical research. By degrees, throughout the eighteenth century and still more during the nineteenth century, the universities became, not merely places of instruction, but centres of research.

The university of Göttingen was planned as one of these new foci of research. For Haller, Leyden was the exemplar. Göttingen was to become a German Leyden. Certain accessories are indispensable to research, and these were provided: a library, which soon became world-famous; a dissecting-room; a botanical garden; a clinic. For investigation, if it is to bear fruit, there are also requisite means whereby the newly acquired data can be made public, and instruments for the exchange of news with those who are carrying on research elsewhere. In 1739 was founded the "Göttingische Zeitungen von Gelehrten Sachen" which Haller edited for twenty-five years, and to which he contributed 12,000 articles, critiques, etc. In 1751, he founded the Königliche Gesellschaft der Wissenschaften, which, under his presidency, became one of the most highly esteemed among academies, and whose publications likewise contain valuable papers by Haller.

He was thus able to work under the most favourable conditions imaginable, and he made full use of his opportunities, displaying a scientific activity unexampled in its comprehensiveness. First of all, he continued his botanical studies. His work on the flora of Switzerland was published in 1742, being

196

arranged in accordance with a system of his own, differing from that of Linnaeus. He published also a considerable number of anatomical studies, the most valuable of these being an atlas of the anatomy of the blood-vessels, illustrated by beautiful copper-plate engravings. In 1747, Albinus published a large folio containing plates of the bones and the muscles, illustrations far more carefully finished than any that had hitherto appeared, this atlas being a milestone in the history of anatomical depiction. Haller's plates of the vascular system were the counterpart to the work. It is still a delight to-day to study these illustrations, wherein fidelity to nature is conjoined with true artistic feeling. Whereas modern photography can only reproduce for us a single preparation, the burin of the copper-plate engraver could represent the common elements of a number of preparations, could elucidate the typical, could by his artistry disclose essentials. In this way were obtained illustrations that had an outstanding didactic value. Haller was a master of the technique of vascular injections, and was thereby enabled to throw light upon numerous obscure problems in the anatomy of the blood-vessels. For instance, he made plain the complicated relationships of the portal system, with the result that the tripus Halleri (the branching of the coeliac axis) bears his name.

More and more, however, Haller's interest turned towards "anatomia animata"—towards physiology. How did the organs work, what functions did they subserve? He had no thought of establishing a "system." The trend of his day was practical and concrete. People were weary of the speculations of the seventeenth century. They wanted to solve specific problems, by means of precise experiments. A controversy about the mechanics of breathing was in progress. What forces determined expiration? Hamberger, professor at Jena, declared that expiration was due to the pressure of air in the pleural cavity. Haller would not accept this view. He opened an animal's thorax under water, and since no air bubbles emerged it was obvious that there could be no air in the thoracic cavity between the lungs and the chest wall. It was (and is) still possible to make important discoveries by extremely simple experiments.

This particular experiment was mechanical, and mechanical likewise were a great many of the other experiments performed by Haller; yet he was anything but an iatromechanist. He was furious when Lamettrie, in order to annoy him, dedicated *L'homme machine* to him. Life, thought Haller, had laws peculiar to itself, differing from those which ruled in the domain of inanimate nature. Still, he did not put this opinion forward as a mere axiom, holding that it must be proved by experiment. For a number of years he was engaged in researches along these lines. A fellow-countryman of his assisted him in the work, one of his students, Johann Georg Zimmermann, by name, in later days physician-in-ordinary to the Elector of Hanover. It was Zimmermann who attended Frederick the Great during the latter's last illness, and whose book *Von der Einsamkeit* still brought tears to our grandmothers' eyes.

The starting-point of these investigations was the problem of muscular movement. Haller was led to the conclusion that irritability and sensibility are the basic phenomena of animal life. He had been forestalled by the Englishman Francis Glisson in the formulation of the concept of irritability, Glisson meaning by this the general tendency of the animal body to react to environmental influences. Haller's definition was more precise. For him irritability was the characteristic possessed by certain organs, and especially by the muscles, to react to stimuli, that is to say, in the case of muscles, to respond by contraction to mechanical, thermic, chemical, and electrical influences.

These outlooks were greatly to modify those of the near future. On the one hand they led towards vitalism, as it found expression in the school of Montpellier. In 1752, Théophile de Bordeu insisted that the function of the glands was also a vital process. The glands, he said, were something more than filters, something more than retorts. When they withdrew certain substances from the blood and elaborated these into secretions, this was effected in virtue of an energy peculiar to themselves. Sensation and active movement were the basic phenomena of life. Bordeu's disciple Barthez assumed the existence of yet a third principle, which he spoke of as "la force de situation fixe," meaning thereby the capacity possessed by all the parts of the body to preserve their respective shape, position, size, etc., including a power of recuperation in case of disturbance. How far this capacity of regeneration went was shown by investigations upon freshwater polyps made in Göttingen by the biologist Johann Friedrich Blumenbach (1752–1840). This investigator recognised that each type of living creature developed in accordance with a specific constructive design, that a "nisus formativus," a formative impulse, was at work in them. For him, the basic physiological phenomena were irritability, sensibility, contractility, in addition to this formative impulse. Promulgating these doctrines, he became the leader of the German vitalists.

In this way Haller fertilised the theory of biology for a long period. But in practical medicine, as well, his doctrine bore rich fruit, especially in a trend that originated in Scotland. The medical faculty of Edinburgh was greatly influenced by that of Leyden. Alexander Monro, one of Boerhaave's pupils, played a notable part in the Scottish capital as anatomist, surgeon, and accoucheur. A man of equal moment was William Cullen (1710–1790), founder of a pathological doctrine wherein the main stress was laid upon the nervous system. All the organs, he said, were dominated by the nervous energy. This gave them their tone which, when exaggerated, passed into spasms, and, when enfeebled, manifested itself as atony. Thus in the last analysis all diseases were morbid affections of the "nervous principle," and treatment must primarily be guided by a recognition of that fact.

Kindred in many respects, though markedly divergent in

others, was the "Brunonian system," founded by another Scot, John Brown (1735–1788). Brown was a very remarkable man, at once a genius and a rogue. He entered the medical profession after having been a minister of religion and then a schoolmaster. A heavy drinker, he became deeply burdened with debt, and thereby found his way into prison. Nevertheless his *Elementa medicinae*, published in 1780, caught on. He set out from the doctrines of Cullen, in whose house he had lived for a long time as private tutor. But, as already said, he differed in various respects from his patron. According to Brown's teaching, the decisive factor in bringing about disease was not excess or defect of nervous energy, but the stimulus, the exciting factor, which set nervous energy in motion. No doubt the nerves and the muscles had the quality of irritability, thanks to which vital manifestations occurred. But these responses only arose through the effects of a stimulus. Stimuli might arise from without, from the environment; but they might also arise within the organism. The emotions were among such stimuli. The whole of our life was a condition determined by stimuli and only maintained by stimuli.

In virtue of its irritability, the organism responded to stimuli. If the stimuli acted within a normal range, the reaction of the organism would be normal. Then the individual would be healthy. Certain stimuli, on the other hand, such stimuli as poisons, infective substances, high temperatures, violent emotions, could not fail to lead to disease. Morbific, likewise, were unduly feeble stimuli, inasmuch as stimuli that were above a certain minimum of strength were essential to the maintenance of a healthy life. That was why haemorrhages and unduly low temperatures also led to disease. Thus the generality of illnesses could be dichotomised into two great groups, into plus-diseases and minus-diseases, into those which resulted from unduly strong and unduly weak stimuli, into sthenic and asthenic conditions. An illness began locally, in the organ subjected to excess or defect of stimulus, but could then become generalised.

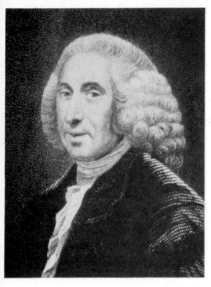 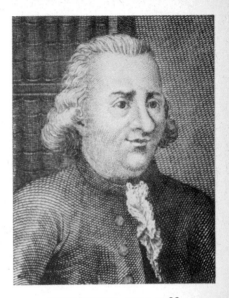

WILLIAM CULLEN, 1710–1790   JOHN BROWN, 1735–1788

In other cases, however, an illness could be general to begin with, and then disclose itself chiefly in local manifestations. According to one type or the other, the treatment should be predominantly local or predominantly general. It must be directed towards counteracting the causes, towards reducing excessive stimulation, as by bleeding, or towards intensifying unduly feeble stimuli by irritants of one sort and another.

Brown's teaching exerted an extraordinary fascination upon many minds. Here there was no longer a question of physics and chemistry, no longer any talk of humoral or solidistic pathology, for the fundamental notions of modern physiology were already broached. The Brunonian system was a genuinely biological theory of disease, and furthermore it gave valuable indications for practice. Unquestionably it was Brown's great merit that he clarified and elaborated the notion of stimulus, which is an essential part of our modern outlook, and that he made it fruitful for pathology. Since he was an innovator, and since the physiological knowledge of his day was elementary, it was natural enough that he overshot his mark, and that he tended to ignore the importance of reaction to a stimulus.

For a considerable period, the Brunonian system secured enthusiastic adherents in all the countries of Europe, and especially in Germany. Curiously enough it was the exposure of a plagiarist which made Brown's doctrine widely known in Germany. A Göttingen physician, Christoph Girtanner by name, who had been in England and had there become acquainted with some of the newer trends, published in 1790 in a French periodical *Deux mémoires sur l'irritabilité considérée comme principe de vie dans la nature organisée*. In these articles he presented Brown's doctrine without making any reference to their originator, who had died two years before. It was not long, however, before the Brunonian source was generally recognised. Thereupon Melchior Adam Weikard, who had been physician-in-ordinary to Catherine the Great and had now returned to Germany, became Brown's apostle upon the continent. In 1795 he translated Brown's *Elementa medicinae*, and, in addition, wrote a number of original works in which he fervently espoused the Brunonian theory and secured for it a great number of disciples. The Romantic Movement was destined to provide an all-too-favourable soil for Brown's teaching.

Let us return to Haller. We left him in Göttingen, occupied in physiological experiments. Since by temperament he was impelled to aim at completion, it was impossible for him to rest content with the fragmentary solution of problems, however fundamental these might be. He could get no rest until he had endeavoured (a bold pioneer) to make a general statement of the principles of physiology. In 1747 his book was published under the title of *Primae lineae physiologiae*, the first of all text-books of physiology. Still he was not satisfied. The *Primae lineae* was no more than a compendium for students and physicians. Its scope was too restricted to allow of a detailed discussion of the various problems of physiology. Yet the foundations for subsequent research could not be laid without a detailed discussion. Haller, therefore, wrote a second book on the topic, *Elementa physiologiae corporis humani*, which appeared in eight bulky volumes between 1757 and 1766. Here all the domains of physiology were treated with the utmost elaboration. Ranging back into antiquity, he critically expounded the views of his predecessors, to end with an account of his own studies. This was a truly monumental work, being concerned, not only with physiology, but also with anatomy and embryology, and with theoretical medicine as well—for in the author's view pathological experience was continually shedding fresh light upon the normal vital processes. Even to-day, after the lapse of nearly two centuries, Haller's great book is a valuable mine to those who desire information concerning the developmental history of any of the problems of medicine.

The publication of the *Elementa* was not begun until after Haller had left Göttingen. In the year 1753 he unexpectedly resigned the post he had filled with so much success at that university to accept a subordinate position in the Swiss State service at Berne. The scientific world was amazed, but he had adequate reasons for the step. Overwork, ill-health, broils with his colleagues, anxiety about the future of his children, to which was probably superadded the homesickness which sooner or later attacks every native of Switzerland who has settled in foreign parts, were the motives which had driven him back to his native soil. The mental strain of the years in Göttingen had been colossal. No relief from that strain was possible so long as he stayed at the university, where, indeed, fresh burdens were continually being heaped upon him. There was only one way out—the way he took.

Haller, then, was at home again. He had set forth seventeen years earlier as an unknown young doctor, but he returned as a scientist with a worldwide reputation. If he had changed in the interval, Berne had changed likewise. As the federal capital, of course, Berne was almost exclusively interested in politics, and took little note of the advances of science. Still, Haller was no longer alone. He remained president of the Göttingen Academy. He carried on an active correspondence with other scientists. The letters he received from them are extant, filling many volumes in the Berne library. Nor did any noted man of learning pass through Switzerland without paying his respects to Haller. Shortly before his death, Emperor Leopold II called on him.

His work went on unceasingly. The lack of the facilities afforded him by the Göttingen Institute made itself felt, but he had an extensive private library and a large amount of notes still requiring elaboration. It was from these that he produced his *Elementa physiologiae*. He also wrote extensive critical bibliographies of botany, anatomy, surgery, and practical medicine. He edited and published editions of the writings of some of the classical physicians. Haller also resumed his botanical studies, republishing his earlier writings on this topic in amplified editions.

From 1758 to 1764 Haller was resident manager of the Bernese Saltworks at Aigle. He lived near by in a rural retreat at Roche. There he had a little kingdom of his own which he studied and which he ruled wisely. At Ferney, close to the other end of the Lake of Geneva, there dwelt during these same years another man towards whom the gaze of Europe was likewise directed—Voltaire. These two, Voltaire and Haller, were both men of the Enlightenment, but were poles asunder. Voltaire was an atheist, a scoffer, a revolutionary, and a man who fought passionately against injustice. Haller was a Protestant, inclining toward pietism, devoid of any sense of humour, and an arch-conservative. His hair bristled at the mere thought of any kind of resistance to constituted authority. He had a profound dislike for Rousseau. Had he survived into the days of the French revolution, that great movement would have filled him with horror, but this affliction he was spared. For Voltaire, philosophy and science had become a unity, of which the famous *Encyclopédie* was the concrete expression. In Haller, just as in many of the German and Dutch scientists, the cleavage of the Baroque epoch persisted. He thought as a rationalist, and he believed as a sincere Christian.

Rumour has it that one day an English ship was seized by pirates who found on board their prize a box of books directed to Haller. Noticing the inscription, the pirate captain hastened to the next port and left the box to be forwarded, feeling that it would be insufferable to rob so famous a man of learning as Herr von Haller.

CHAPTER TWENTY-FIVE

GERHARD VAN SWIETEN (1700-1772)
AND
ANTON DE HAEN (1704-1776)

ALTHOUGH the university of Vienna was not quite so old as that of Prague, which had been founded as the second of German universities in the year 1635, it could, in the eighteenth century, look back to a venerable past. Nevertheless, the history of its medical faculty had been inglorious. It had never taken an active part in the development of the science of healing. The Viennese medical professors stood obstinately upon the old ways. Anatomical teaching in Vienna was pitiable. There was no botanical garden, no clinic, no chemical laboratory. The professors, few in number, were underpaid. No doubt they did not fail to recognise the inadequacies of the institution to which they were attached, but they lacked power to remedy matters.

Then, in 1740, Maria Theresa ascended the throne. She was quick to recognise that a thorough reform of the university of Vienna was essential if it was to remain a university in any sense worthy of the name. The first question was to find the right man for the job.

The Empress's sister Maria Anna was ill in Brussels, far advanced in pregnancy, and her life was in danger. Maria Theresa dispatched her own physician-in-ordinary, Engels, to Brussels, where he called some of his local colleagues in consultation. The Archduchess gave birth to a stillborn child, and her condition grew steadily worse. As a last hope, Gerhard van Swieten, a man of high repute in Leyden, was sent for. Although he did not succeed in saving Maria Anna's life, his assured and tactful ways inspired confidence in the Empress, who invited him to settle in Vienna as her own court physician. She wrote to him in cordial terms as follows:

"I feel it my duty to send you my most sincere thanks for all the trouble you have taken, and to tell you that your conduct has given me the utmost satisfaction. The fact that you are able to put up with Engels' waywardness and to humour him has given me so much respect for your character that my confidence and my friendship have gone out to you apart from your skill in your own chosen province of work. A monarch must ever strive to be surrounded by such persons, and cannot fail to be happy when they are discoverable. I hope you will accept this as sufficient assurance that that tiresome fellow has done you no harm in my estimation. It would be a very great distress to me if I thought that through my action you had been deprived of the delightful calm which you enjoyed, and which is the only happiness we know on earth. All that I am afraid of is what your wife's feelings or prejudices may be, since she is less philosophically minded and more sensitive than you, and therefore more readily open to first impressions. Let me assure you once again that I would rather sacrifice my own interests than do anything to make you unhappy.

"Much as I hope to see you here before long, I leave you perfectly free to come or not to come as you think best, and to refuse my request if you feel disinclined to fulfil it. That would be a distress to me, but it is a pain I would endure rather than sacrifice you and your repose, remaining always inspired with the same feelings towards you. Maria Theresa."

After brief reflection, van Swieten accepted the call, arriving in Vienna during the summer of 1745. The "delightful calm" of which the Empress had deprived him had not been a wholly voluntary one, so that to abandon it was not so difficult as she supposed. Van Swieten was one of Boerhaave's pupils, and perhaps the favourite of them all. No other was so devoted to the master, or on terms of such pleasant intimacy with him. For years the two had lived and worked side by side in the friendliest way, closely linked though there was so much difference between their ages. Van Swieten practised in Leyden, and was a very successful lecturer at the university.

But he was a Roman Catholic, and as such he could not occupy a professorial chair in Leyden. There was no possibility of his becoming Boerhaave's successor. When the latter died, van Swieten had to quit the university. The students rose in rebellion, but without avail. Van Swieten himself had to pacify them, explaining that there was no choice but to obey the law.

Thereafter he had, indeed, "calm" or "repose." Devoting himself to his private practice, he began to write a great commentary on Boerhaave's *Aphorisms*. The master's heritage was to be adequately preserved, and was to bear rich fruit. In fact, the *Aphorisms* were so concise, so curt, as to need elucidation. Van Swieten, if any one, was intimately acquainted with Boerhaave's ideas. Moreover he had quantities of notes which, being a skilful shorthand writer, he had made during the clinical demonstrations.

He was now forty-five years of age. Had it not been for Maria Theresa's summons he would probably have remained for the rest of his life a general practitioner in a small Dutch town. History would have taken little notice of him, regarding him as no more than one among the very large number of Boerhaave's pupils. For, as a physician, he was not endowed with exceptional talent; nor was he inspired with the investigatory impulses of such a man as Haller. But fortune willed it that in early middle age he should be raised to a position in which he could develop to the full his slumbering talent for organisation. The Empress, who had absolute confidence in him, gave him a free hand.

Having come to Vienna as physician-in-ordinary to the Empress, van Swieten soon began to give lectures in the imperial capital, not in the medical faculty of the university but in a lecture-theatre attached to the court library of which he had promptly been appointed director. Here is his own account of the matter: "I am delivering a two years' course of lectures on medicine, devoting the first year to an account of the functions of the human body, to physiology. That is to say, I do my best to make my auditors acquainted with the structure of our body, using anatomical preparations of my own, provided with great labour and at considerable expense, originally for my own instruction and for that of my children should any of them prove themselves inclined to devote themselves to the study of medicine. A few years ago, I should never have dreamed of being able to use these preparations for purposes of public education. Since coming to Vienna, I have enlarged this small collection of mine by a few additional specimens likely to be of use to my students.

"In the second year of my course I discuss pathology, i.e. the doctrine of illnesses, their causes, characteristics, symptoms, together with the suitable remedies and the best way of applying them. This leads me to materia medica, that is to the history of remedies, their doses, their preparation, etc.

"When a pupil has grasped all this, the next point is to expound to him the nature of disease in detail, with references to the best authors who have written upon it and perhaps an elucidation of obscure passages, in order to show what progress has been made in the treatment of the various diseases from the earliest times down to our own day."

There can be no question but that these lectures must have been a great advance upon the medical instruction hitherto given in Vienna. Still, much remained to be done. The faculty and the whole system of medical teaching needed reorganisation from the ground up. Before van Swieten had been four years in Vienna, the Empress asked him to formulate proposals with this end in view. It behoved him, therefore, to establish a genuinely modern faculty. The task was much more difficult in Vienna than in Göttingen, which was an entirely new foundation. The difficulty in Vienna was that the reformer had to

208

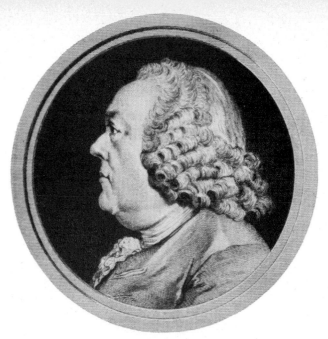

GERHARD VAN SWIETEN, 1700-1772

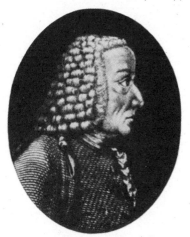

ANTON DE HAEN 1704-1776

reconstruct a venerable and sovereign faculty, one greatly impressed with the importance of its chartered rights. Only a few years earlier, the faculty had petitioned for a confirmation of its privileges. It was soon to become plain that no effective reform would be possible without abrogating these same privileges.

In January 1749, van Swieten submitted a memorial to the Empress. Three weeks later was issued the decree which was to give the Dutch physician's proposals the status of a law.

The most essential feature of the reform was that the university was to be subjected to the State authority. Henceforward the professors would be appointed and also paid, not by the faculty, but by the monarch. The real chief of the faculty was not the dean, inasmuch as a special representative of the government was appointed as principal. This special representative had the last word as regards examinations, the granting of degrees, of licences to practise as an apothecary, and all academic affairs. The whole examination system was reconstructed. Any one who wished to practise medicine within the limits of the monarchy must have taken his degree either at Vienna or in one of the provincial universities; but whereas the Viennese examinations gave a right to practise in all the patrimonial dominions of the empire, those of a provincial university were valid exclusively for the province concerned. The fees payable on taking a degree, which had been enormous, were greatly reduced.

In the same imperial decree, van Swieten was appointed director and president of the faculty.

Naturally enough the faculty, whose traditional privileges and powers were thus annulled, was indignant. It protested against being superseded by van Swieten, a foreigner. Protests were fruitless. The Dutchman carried out his reforms with the strong hand needed for these innovations. The imperial decree had merely smoothed the ground, and had been in accordance with the spirit of the times. In other countries, likewise, the absolutist State had quashed the powers of the universities and had made itself supreme in academic education. What was now needed was that this supremacy should be skilfully used for the training of really efficient doctors, and also for the promotion of research. Such were the new tasks of the university.

Not merely had fresh institutions to be created, for, more important still, men of the new time able to animate them must be recruited. Here Leyden was made the exemplar. A botanical garden and a chemical laboratory were established, Nikolaus Joseph Jacquin, the noted Dutch botanist, being put in charge of them. Great stress was laid upon the study of anatomy. The dissecting-room hitherto available was in a pitiable condition, for its windows were broken and it was unwarmed in winter. The study of anatomy, moreover, needed in addition to a dissecting-room, bodies and collections of specimens. These wants were supplied. It was arranged that not only the corpses of executed criminals, but also the bodies of those who died in certain hospitals, were to be supplied for anatomical study. Dissected specimens were bought, chiefly in Holland. An able anatomist was acquired in Lorenz Gasser, whose name has been preserved in the Gasserian ganglion. Van Swieten wisely separated the chair of anatomy from that of surgery, for the anatomist was apt to be a specialist in the dissection of dead bodies without any experience in operative surgery. Two practising surgeons, Jaus and Leber, were appointed professors.

Next it was essential that Vienna should become famous as a centre of clinical instruction, since this was the field of work upon which the renown of Leyden had above all depended. What could be more natural than to summon one of Boerhaave's pupils, a man who had grown up in the clinical tradition of the Dutch university? In 1754, Anton de Haen, one of van Swieten's fellow students, came to the imperial capital. Following the Leyden precedent, twelve beds in the City

Hospital were set aside for clinical instruction—six beds occupied by men and six occupied by women.

In due time it became plain that Europe indeed possessed a new medical centre. Whereas in 1748 Maria Theresa had found it necessary to ask the faculty why so many Austrian students went to foreign parts to take their degree (which, she said, was a discredit to the university and disadvantageous to the State), things had now changed so much that the Viennese faculty attracted foreign students in increasing numbers. A new medical school had come into being. The old stem from Leyden, carefully nurtured by van Swieten, had put forth fresh shoots.

Van Swieten's activities in the same service were by no means exhausted by the foregoing extensive reforms. He devoted himself to the improvement of the whole province of medical activity over which he presided, seeing to it that there should be improved teaching, under State supervision, of the minor grades of persons engaged in the work of healing— barber-surgeons, midwives, and so on. The house physicians at the hospitals and the district physicians were also appointed by the State. It became, furthermore, part of the policy of the absolutist State to care for the welfare of its subjects by strict measures of sanitary control.

Not restricting his activities exclusively to medical work, van Swieten busied himself in other domains as well. I have already said that he was director of the court library. In addition he became censor. This office had hitherto been exclusively in the hands of the Jesuits, who were omnipotent in Vienna. It was part of van Swieten's policy that no State within the State should be tolerated, that there should be no second power rivalling the governmental authority. Although he did not succeed in fully excluding the Jesuits from the censorial board, he was able to limit their powers to a considerable degree. He took his duties as censor seriously. In the Viennese National Library there is a manuscript volume containing shorthand notes by van Swieten relating to 3,120 works on which he had passed judgment as censor. No less than 595 of these had been refused publication. He came into conflict with the Jesuits in connection with the reform of the other faculties of the university, and there, likewise, he was able to restrict their power.

We have a contemporary description of van Swieten's daily work: "He rose at five and went to court at half-past six. Returning home at eight or nine, he shut himself up in his study and worked there until two o'clock in the afternoon. Then he had his dinner, which occupied an hour. After that he devoted an hour to giving free medical advice to the poor and then went on working in his study until seven in the evening. At this hour he paid a second visit to the court. At nine he ate a frugal supper and went to bed at half-past ten.

"He followed this daily routine very closely, and would only modify it in extremely urgent circumstances. Any one who came to Vienna hoping to see him might just as well start on the return journey next day. Thus he worked twelve hours daily, and even more, for he was never idle, finding some sort of mental occupation when he was out walking or driving. He had a remarkably good memory, and even when well up in years could repeat hundreds of verses from the classical poets. In addition to his native Dutch, he could speak Latin, Greek, French, German, Italian, Spanish, and English—and could even make some headway in Magyar. In conversation he was pleasant and cheerful, especially among intimates, who were however few in number. Strict though he was where his public duties were concerned, he was kind-hearted to the unfortunate. With a liberal hand he helped the needy, often assisting those who came to consult him, not only with money to buy medicines, but with considerable sums to provide the necessaries of life.

"Above all, he had an open purse to aid gifted students of medicine, many of whom were maintained wholly at his cost."

It is easy to understand that a man so overwhelmed with public administrative work had no time for scientific labours. Van Swieten's calling lay in another field than that of pure science. Still, the commentary on Boerhaave's *Aphorisms* begun in Holland was continued and finished in Austria, so that, when published, it became a widely used manual. Posthumously there appeared his *Constitutiones epidemiae et morbi potissimum Lugd Bat. observati*—notes made when he was practising in Leyden from 1727 to 1744—a work which reflects the spirit of Boerhaave.

Throughout the twenty-seven years of his residence in Vienna his relations with Maria Theresa remained most cordial. On the day of his death, June 18, 1772, she wrote to Archduke Ferdinand: "The loss I have sustained this afternoon through van Swieten's death has turned all my joy into sorrow. I must admit that I am inconsolable. Even when he was lying dangerously, hopelessly ill, I still felt that he was with me. He died, or, rather, he ceased to live, without a death-struggle, remaining fully conscious to the last, and continuing to communicate by signs after he had lost the power of speech. He is irreplaceable, especially so far as I am concerned. In many matters I had great confidence in him, and my confidence has always been merited."

A few months later she wrote: "I miss van Swieten more and more." Year after year she bore the day of his death in memory, writing, for instance, in 1778: "J'ai aujourd'hui un grand jour de dévotion, l'anniversaire de van Swieten, qui est pour mon particulier une perte irréparable."

We have learned how the Viennese medical school came into being. If we want to become acquainted with its functioning, we must turn to consider the man who was for many years, as director of the clinic, the motive force of its activities— Anton de Haen.

Like van Swieten, de Haen was a Dutchman, a Catholic,

and one of Boerhaave's pupils. De Haen was only four years younger than van Swieten. They were, however, men of very different types, as is shown plainly enough by their likenesses. Van Swieten's head is that of a self-reliant and distinguished man. The energy of his features is that of one wont to command and accustomed to unconditional obedience. Nevertheless his expression is gentle, kindly, manifestly genial. Persons with a double chin are rarely ill-tempered!

How different is Haen's countenance. In him we see the hard-bitten lineaments, the rigid gaze, of a fanatic. Apart from this portrait, we know that de Haen had an extraordinarily difficult character. He made no friends, was blunt to his associates, arrogant, impatient, a savage controversialist, fiercely adverse to such innovations as the doctrine of irritability, inoculation with the smallpox, and percussion. During old age he became more and more immersed in mystical speculation, writing about magic and about miracles. All the same, he was an untiring worker and a great clinician.

In a word, de Haen's historical significance depends upon the brilliant, the unparalleled success with which he developed clinical methods. Let us recall what this meant. Hospitals, as they came into existence early in the Middle Ages, had been nothing more than gratuitous or semi-gratuitous rest-houses for poor and weary travellers. Only by degrees did they become transformed into places for the care of the sick, into places where, from motives of Christian charity, patients could secure the attention which it was impossible for them to receive at home. Then, towards the close of the Middle Ages, medical treatment was provided in the hospitals, especially in those maintained by the municipalities. Even then, however, the hospital doctor was not officially appointed as such to devote all or most of his time to hospital patients. He was merely the town doctor (in most cases), appointed to give medical aid to the poor, and, for a small addition to his salary, entrusted with the care of the sick in the hospitals. No doubt as early as the sixteenth century in Padua and during the seventeenth century in Leyden, the hospitals were officially turned to account for purposes of clinical instruction and of demonstration—but they did not even then become centres of research. The pathological literature of that era is almost exclusively based upon observations made in private practice.

By slow degrees hospitals were transformed into foci of medical research. By slow degrees was it recognised that the hospital patient, removed from his domestic environment, housed in a place where he can be observed daily or hourly by the doctor, and where all his excretions can be kept for examination, is the ideal subject for the study of disease. Since Sydenham's day, the main interest of pathological observation had been directed towards the study of particular diseases, and here was the best way of studying them. It was not only pathology which could be studied in hospital patients, but also the success or failure of remedial measures. So long as a sick man or woman was at home, it was impossible to know exactly what had been eaten, what medicine had been administered, how far the doctor's directions had been followed. In hospital, on the other hand, the patient was under continuous control.

Boerhaave's clinic worked methodically in this direction, but it was no more than a modest beginning. De Haen made a much greater advance along the same lines with his Viennese clinic. De Haen's literary works consist of eighteen volumes which were published in the year 1758 under the title *Ratio medendi in nosocomio practico*, and which consisted entirely of the annual reports of the clinic, of clinical histories, and clinical lectures. Case reports unexampled in number and wealth of detail were here offered to the medical world. Nowadays a hospital publishes its clinical histories in exceptional cases only. In the middle of the eighteenth century, when the concepts of particular diseases were still in a flux, every precise clinical history was a valuable document.

Now, de Haen's clinical histories were of the most meticulous

215

exactitude. First of all, by appropriate questions, the anamnesis and the subjective symptoms were established. Then the status praesens was considered, the greatest possible care being taken to ascertain the symptoms of which there was objective evidence. For this purpose, inter alia, use was made of the clinical thermometer, which had been occasionally employed by Boerhaave, but was now for the first time used extensively in clinical work. Then the changes in the course of the illness were recorded with the utmost care from day to day, with notes as to the effect of treatment. If a patient died and a post-mortem examination was made, a full report of this was appended to the clinical history; and a critical consideration of the whole case followed.

All this was done, not in order to prove a "system," but in order, soberly and concretely, to depict the course of particular diseases. It was the expression of a scientific empiricism conceived on thoroughly sound lines. Stoll, who continued de Haen's clinical work, stated clearly the object of all these case-histories by saying: "When we have before us several clinical histories of one and the same illness and have been able to compare each with the other, we can deduce guiding principles for practice and formulate didactic aphorisms."

In the therapeutic field, likewise, de Haen exercised a fertilising and purifying influence, showing himself decisively opposed to the fussy over-activity of many physicians of his day; by pointing out that the systematic administration of sudorifics was frequently injurious; and that in many cases the expectant method was the best way of treating acute illnesses, without any interference with their natural course.

The reader will perceive that de Haen's clinical method was that of our own day. We, of course, have far better methods of investigation at our disposal. We can make much more precise examinations, and we have the firm standing-ground of pathological anatomy beneath our feet. Nevertheless, the guiding ideas are the same. Perhaps a fanatic like de Haen was needed, a man who would carry out his principles with the tenacity of a monomaniac.

It was only to be expected that two such strong personalities as van Swieten and de Haen should found a school. Crantz, one of van Swieten's pupils, was sent to Paris to study surgery and midwifery in the French capital. Then, returning to Vienna, he became lector of midwifery there, and gave practical instruction in St. Mark's Hospital. Another pupil, Anton Störck (1731–1803), who succeeded van Swieten not only as teacher but also as physician-in-ordinary to the court, did especially good work in advancing our knowledge of the use of drugs. The attempt of the Viennese clinic to simplify traditional therapeutics necessarily encouraged the search for simpler but more effective remedies. First experimenting on himself and then administering various medicines in the hospitals, Störck studied the effect of hemlock, meadow-saffron, aconite, stramonium, and henbane, writing brief and clear monographs about his experiences. De Haen, be it noted, would have nothing to do with these new drugs.

In his pupil Maximilian Stoll (1742–1788) de Haen had a worthy successor, who not only maintained but increased the prestige of the Viennese clinic. Stoll continued the publication of the annual report, adding to the number of case-histories, and giving a more sharply defined description of various diseases: lead-colic, for instance; and pulmonary tuberculosis, of which he himself eventually died. Following up one of Sydenham's ideas, he tried to grasp the nature of the epidemic morbid constitution, coming to the conclusion that many diseases (for the most part epidemic diseases) were of a gastro-bilious nature, and that the treatment of all these must therefore begin with the use of emetics and purgatives. The view is certainly one-sided, but it contains a kernel of truth.

The reform and the subsequent remarkable progress of the Viennese faculty set an example for the provincial universities.

In Prague, Pavia, and Budapest, changes were instituted after the Viennese model, and by degrees clinical instruction made progress.

Van Swieten died in 1772; de Haen in 1776; and Haller in 1777. Thus the great generation of the disciples of Boerhaave came to an end, but their work lived after them. An admirable new university had come into being at Göttingen, and the Viennese medical faculty was thenceforward an important factor in the progress of European medicine. Vienna, of course, had its ups and downs; but the Austrian capital was again and again to produce great doctors whose thoughts and deeds were to fertilise the healing art.

CHAPTER TWENTY-SIX

JOHN HUNTER
1728–1793

THE scene changes, and we are back in England once more. No one who goes to London should fail to visit the museum of the Royal College of Surgeons. He will find there, in five great halls, thousands upon thousands of preparations and dissections belonging to the domains of human and comparative, of normal and pathological anatomy. But he will see there likewise objects such as are not to be found in ordinary anatomical museums. For instance he will find the skeleton of O'Bryan, the Irish giant, who was seven feet six and a half inches high, and beside it the skeleton of a Sicilian dwarf, a girl who at the age of ten was only one foot eight inches high. He will also find the skeleton of a famous racehorse, and that of a greyhound which belonged to a man of high rank.

At the first glance these curios show us that we are not in a typical modern collection. We become aware of the collector's spirit of the seventeenth and eighteenth centuries, when rarities and whimsicalities vied with classified scientific objects for a place in museums. The museum of the Royal College of Surgeons was, in fact, mainly grounded by the collection of an eighteenth-century surgeon named John Hunter, a Scotsman by birth. After his decease, his collection was bought by the government for £15,000.

Hunter, however, was no mere collector. He occupies a leading place in the history of surgery and of medicine, so that it will repay us to become more closely acquainted with him.

In childhood he was the despair of the elders of his household, and no one ever anticipated for him a great career. He was the youngest of a family of ten, of whom (such mortality was characteristic of the age) three died in childhood, and four in early youth. The father, a petty laird in Lanarkshire, was quite a veteran when John was born, and the mother spoiled her Benjamin, giving way to all his whims. At school he was an unsatisfactory pupil, so that his schooldays were short. Capricious and ill-tempered, when he could not get his own way he would howl for hours in succession. The only things he really liked doing were playing practical jokes or wandering in the woods in search of birds' eggs. He also had a way of asking inconvenient questions. "When I was a boy," he said of himself in later years, "I wanted to know all about the clouds and the grasses and why the leaves changed colour in the autumn. I watched ants, bees, birds, tadpoles, and caddisworms. I pestered people with questions about what nobody knew or cared anything about."

What was to become of him? One of his sisters had married a timber-merchant in Glasgow. Perhaps he could work in the business? But there, too, he made a poor showing. By this time he was twenty, and something must be done. For a youth of his sort it seemed that the only career open would be to enlist. However, before taking this desperate step, he would try another plan. His brother William, the pride of the family, lived in London. William Hunter was about ten years older than John, had studied medicine in Glasgow, was a successful surgeon, and was devoted to anatomical studies. Perhaps William would help him, could find a use for him. John wrote to London, and William agreed to give his young brother a trial.

In 1748, therefore, John Hunter journeyed to London, and became William Hunter's assistant. He arrived at a lucky moment. Since the beginning of the year, William Hunter had been giving private anatomical lectures to operative surgeons, with practical demonstrations. Wonder of wonders, the ne'er-do-well proved his mettle as William's assistant! He worked all day and far on into the night, kept the dissecting-room in good order, and showed himself an adept at securing the requisite bodies. Soon, moreover, he became a skilled dissector.

He had an excellent teacher in Brother William, who was a distinguished anatomist, surgeon, and accoucheur. William Hunter's treatise *On the Human Gravid Uterus*, first published in Latin in the year 1774, a huge folio enriched with thirty-four magnificent copper-plate engravings, has become a classic. William was an enthusiastic collector, not only of anatomical preparations, but also of books, manuscripts, medals, and paintings. His library and his anatomical collection are preserved in the university of Glasgow. The collector's fire is a contagious passion. The younger brother was soon attacked by it, and it persisted for the rest of his life.

Anatomy is not an easy profession for a young man who has had a poor education. As we have seen he had had very little schooling, and had never been at a university. Still, in those days it was possible for him to become a surgeon, so, on William's recommendation, John Hunter entered as surgeon-apprentice at Chelsea Hospital, transferring later to St. Bartholomew's and then to St. George's. In Cheselden and Pott he had excellent teachers, and after a few years he had mastered his craft. William wanted John to make up for the defects of his general education, so he sent the young man to Oxford, but John stayed only a few months, saying when he returned: "They wanted to make an old woman of me, or that I should stuff Latin at the University; but these schemes I cracked like so many vermin as they came before me."

His interests were in a very different field. With the utmost zeal he now devoted himself once more to anatomical studies, realising that one who wishes, not merely to describe but also to understand the organs of the human being must make himself acquainted with the organs of the lower animals as well. He must dissect as many different kinds of animals as possible. Anatomy must be comparative anatomy. Only through a comparison of the organs of men and those of other animals is it possible to understand the general functions of life, whether

221

normal or pathological. To comparative anatomy, therefore, he turned. He was not an anatomist in the ordinary sense. He never wrote a text-book of anatomy. How easy it would have been for him to engage a copper-plate engraver and, getting prints made of his numerous preparations, to produce monumental illustrated works. He had no thought, however, of doing anything of the kind. In fact he wrote very little upon anatomy; no more than a work upon the natural history of the teeth and a few minor essays—parerga. For him, anatomy was not an end in itself, but a means to an end; especially comparative anatomy and embryology. The latter, likewise, could help him to answer the various questions in which he was interested. Was it not true that animals in the early stages of their development exhibited forms which reminded the observer of the structure of other and simpler animals?

While he was thus busily at work, in the year 1761 he had a severe attack of pneumonia. One of his brothers had died of consumption. His life in hospital wards and in the dissecting-room was not one to be recommended to a man with such morbid tendencies. He was advised to be as much in the open air as possible. For a time he became army surgeon, and then naval surgeon. England was at war with France and Spain. Hunter was present at several engagements, and acquired a great deal of experience. His mental outlook was essentially contrasted to that of the ordinary army surgeon. He was a man of science; his mind was keenly occupied with the problems of general pathology; and every injury he had to treat was for him an experiment. It was during this period of active service that were laid the foundations of a book which was to take decades to mature, and was not to be published until after his death. It is accounted his most important work, and it will be considered presently.

In 1763 the war came to an end with the Peace of Paris, by which France ceded Canada to England. The army was disbanded. Hunter returned to London and settled down as a surgeon. At first his practice grew slowly, for he had no hospital, and a surgeon without a hospital is like a captain without a ship. Well, he had all the more time for his studies and his collection.

He bought a country-house at Earl's Court—for Earl's Court was in the country a hundred and seventy years ago. It was a very original country-house, one which no one could pass without standing at gaze. Never before had so many kinds of animals been seen in the grounds of a country mansion. Behind it was a meadow where birds of all sorts were walking about, especially a great number of geese, whose eggs Hunter wanted for his embryological studies; but there were also pigs, goats, hedgehogs, an opossum, buffaloes, a zebra, an ostrich. The more dangerous beasts—leopards, jackals, serpents—were kept in cages. Many of the birds were rare specimens. There was a pond, for the study of fresh-water life. In the house there were dissecting-rooms, rooms for physiological experiments, and rooms for the storage of collections.

Hunter was perpetually on the look-out for rare beasts. If a gipsy passed by with a dancing bear, Hunter would make a bargain with the man to bring the creature for dissection when it died. The Irish giant cost him much labour and a great deal of money. He was absolutely determined to have O'Bryan's skeleton for his collection. When the giant fell sick, Hunter had him kept under observation. But the Irishman scented danger, and, regarding with horror the thought that his body would be cut up, he made his friends promise that when he died they would never lose sight of his corpse until it had been sealed up in a leaden coffin and sunk in the sea. We are told that bribery and corruption to the tune of £500 were needed before Hunter could get his way. The upshot was that the skeleton is in the Royal College of Surgeons' museum, and that O'Bryan's name has become immortal.

Manifestly such studies must have cost a great deal of money. His practice had to supply the necessary funds. Frequently quoted is the anecdote that when on one occasion Hunter was called away from his work to see a patient he said to one of his friends: "Well, Lynn, I must go and earn this damned guinea, or I shall be sure to want it to-morrow." It was a lucky day for him when, in 1768, he was appointed surgeon to St. George's Hospital, where, years before, he had been a student. Thenceforward his practice rapidly increased. In 1775 he was earning a thousand a year, and in 1783 five thousand a year—an enormous sum for those days. Enormous though it may have been, it did not suffice his needs. His household had gradually increased to forty-five persons: children, a tutor, assistants, servants, gardeners, keepers for the animals. Above all, his collection swallowed huge amounts, so that when Hunter died he left nothing but his collection and debts.

Being now a hospital surgeon, he had pupils, some of whom lived with him and were his constant companions. Among them was a young man with whom he became peculiarly intimate, and with whom in subsequent years he kept up a correspondence. This was Edward Jenner.

Just as his brother William had given courses of private lectures on anatomy, so in the autumn of 1773 John Hunter began to give private lectures upon the theory and practice of surgery. The course lasted from October to April, three lectures every week, the fee for the whole being four guineas. Hunter was not a good lecturer. He could only read from his manuscript, and before every lecture he was extremely nervous, so that sometimes he had to take thirty drops of laudanum in order to compose himself. Nevertheless, his lectures were of the utmost interest to those competent to understand them. He conveyed much more information than had been promised in the prospectus. What he discoursed upon was not the theory of operative surgery, but rather that which to-day we call "general surgery," a domain which had not hitherto been segregated. Nor indeed did Hunter call it by that name. It comprised general surgery, and more, namely anatomy, physiology, and

224

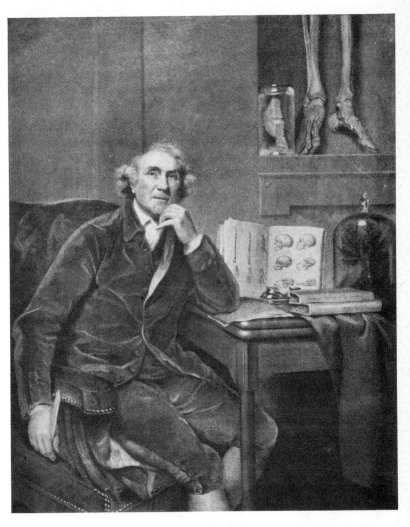

JOHN HUNTER, 1728–1793

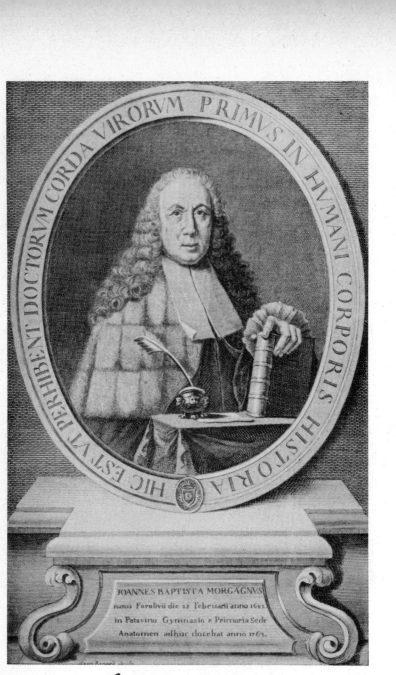

GIOVANNI BATTISTA MORGAGNI, 1682–1771

pathology. In all these fields he put forward original ideas, the result of prolonged observations and experiments. Hunter was not a qualified physician, had not been trained in any academic faculty. He was an empiric in the best sense of the term, and approached the problems of pathology from the practical aspect, in a mood quite free from prejudice.

One of the illnesses which in the eighteenth century was left entirely to the surgeons for treatment was syphilis. Hunter attacked this difficult problem, and wrote a great work upon it, *On the Venereal Disease*, published in 1786, which remained a standard text-book well on into the nineteenth century. Valuable as this treatise is in many respects, it contains serious errors, and errors which are all the more instructive because they were originated by experiment. In his day there was much dispute as to whether gonorrhoea and syphilis were but two manifestations of one disease. Hunter inoculated himself with what he believed to be gonorrhoeal pus, with the result that a chancre formed at the site of inoculation. The identity of gonorrhoea and syphilis seemed to have been proved. Just as in former days people had believed in the infallibility of logical deduction, so now were experimenters inclined to put blind faith in the results of experiment. What we have to learn is that one experiment, taken by itself, proves nothing, and that the correct interpretation of experiment is more important than the experiment itself. [The presumption is that the pus with which Hunter inoculated himself, the pus from a urethral discharge, was derived—in part at least—from an intra-urethral syphilitic chancre.]

The closing years of Hunter's life were years of unceasing toil. He was up before six in the morning, and worked until nine in his dissecting-room. Until noon he saw patients at home, and then went on his rounds. At four in the afternoon he had his principal meal, after which he slept for an hour. Then he gave lectures. After that his secretary took down from his dictation what he had observed during the day. At midnight the family went to bed. The footman brought his master a freshly trimmed lamp, and Hunter remained at work till one, two, or even later in the morning. He quarrelled with his brother William, to whom he had owed so much at the outset of his career. He suffered much and for several years from angina pectoris, which ultimately proved fatal.

In 1794, a year after his death, appeared the ripest fruit of his life-work, *A Treatise on the Blood, Inflammation, and Gunshot Wounds*—a work which is a milestone in the development of general pathology. The theory of inflammation was the wrestling ground of speculation. Each school, every trend, had its own theory. Practice brought a wholesome corrective, holding fast as it did to well-tried methods of treatment, regardless of theory. As late as 1822, C. H. M. Langenbeck, the Göttingen anatomist and surgeon, wrote: "If we compare the theories concerning inflammation with the treatment of this malady, we find the most divergent views in respect of theory, whereas as regards treatment there is unanimity. Writers theorise diversely about inflammation, but genuine practitioners treat the disease in the same way."

Hunter was the first investigator since the days of antiquity to advance the theory of inflammation a stage. By simple observations and lucid experiments he was able to interpret processes of inflammation more clearly than they had ever been interpreted before. He recognised that inflammation is a reaction of the organism to any kind of noxious influence. Determinative of the type and the course of any particular inflammation, he said, were the exciting cause, the constitution of the body, and the peculiarities of the affected part. He was well acquainted with the three main types of inflammation: alterative, secretive, and regenerative. "Inflammation in itself is not to be considered as a disease, but as a salutary operation, consequent either to some violence or some disease. . . . Inflammation is not only occasionally the cause of diseases, but it is often a mode of cure, since it frequently produces a

226

resolution of indurated parts, by changing the diseased action into a salutary one, if capable of resolution." Thus the curative value of inflammation was plainly recognised.

Wherein does Hunter's historical significance lie? He worked at anatomy all his life, and yet his true field of work was not anatomy pure and simple. He was one of the most successful surgeons of his time, but many another surgeon among his contemporaries did more than he to promote the advance of operative surgery. His position in the history of the healing art must be sought elsewhere. In the eighteenth century, medicine and surgery were two distinct provinces. At the university the physician received instruction in surgery, but usually from anatomical specialists not one of whom had ever done so much as lance a boil. No scientific progress in surgery was to be expected from such quarters. The practising surgeon, on the other hand, was as a rule a rather imperfectly educated handicraftsman. Even though surgery was steadily advancing, and such institutions as the Académie Royale de Chirurgie founded in Paris in the year 1731 had had a valuable influence, the interest of surgeons was concentrated upon practice. When a surgeon, here and there, felt impelled to engage in scientific work, his main concern was likely to be to effect an improvement in operative technique. Very rigid limits were imposed upon operative surgery in those days, owing to the impossibility of producing general anaesthesia, and owing to the almost universal prevalence of the various forms of wound infection. Surgeons, therefore, kept their minds fixed upon particular and very narrowly defined groups of maladies. Their thoughts turned in a circle round the diseases due to "external injuries," as they phrased it; and such maladies as stone in the bladder, rupture, fistula, etc., whose treatment they tried to improve.

It seems to me, then, that Hunter's main significance was that he threw open the field of surgical observation and experiment to general medicine, enabling all doctors to turn it to account. He was a working surgeon like the rest of them;

227

but he was also a man of science. For him a wound was something more than a practical problem. He was not content to ask, "How can I best heal this wound?" He inquired: "What does the wound signify to the organism? By what mechanisms does the organism safeguard itself against the effects of the wound, immediate and remote?" In this way, almost imperceptibly, he passed from the domain of surgery into that of pathology. His anatomical and physiological studies safeguarded him against getting lost in a maze of speculation. As a practitioner, he advanced by practical measures, set the organism tasks, made experiments. Not having been trained as a physician, approaching the problems devoid of preconceptions and from without, he saw much which had remained hidden from the doctors.

Along this path he was a pioneer hastening greatly in advance of his time, and he constructed the first bridge between surgery and medicine.

CHAPTER TWENTY-SEVEN

GIOVANNI BATTISTA MORGAGNI
1682–1771

ONCE more there came a voice from Padua, a voice that was to resound throughout the medical world. Again an anatomist of Padua was to bring about a considerable advance in the healing art. Towards 1700, quiet times had befallen this university city of ancient renown. The great days were over. The current of foreign students was no longer flowing southward but northward, was setting steadily towards Leyden. But when in 1711 the Venetian government summoned to Padua a general practitioner of Forli, Giovanni Battista Morgagni by name, it made a lucky hit, for it had discovered a man who was to give new renown to the venerable faculty.

Morgagni was well grounded for his new task. He had studied medicine in Bologna, and had become assistant to his teacher, Antonio Maria Valsalva (1666–1723), who had written an outstanding work upon the ear. Indeed, for a twelve month Morgagni had acted as Valsalva's substitute when the latter had followed a call to Parma, and had at this date published his first anatomical observations. Then, however, just like Haller twenty years later, he settled down in his native city as a general practitioner.

Now came the summons to Padua. He was appointed assistant professor of theoretical medicine. Four years later he became professor of anatomy instead, thus occupying the chair which Vesalius and so many famous anatomists had held before him. He was twenty-nine years of age when he went to Padua. Haller, it will be remembered, was summoned to Göttingen at the age of twenty-eight.

Morgagni's life was uneventful, that of a man of science who lives remote from the world of affairs. His hours were filled with conscientious teaching, indefatigable labours in the dissecting-room, consultations, and an extensive correspondence with his professional colleagues. There did not yet exist an abundance of periodicals eager to publish the most trifling observations, to make the most seemingly inconspicuous ideas widely known. In the eighteenth century, an investigator who believed himself to have discovered something new began its dissemination by communicating with his colleagues, subjecting his observations to their criticisms. A letter of the kind, swelled to the size of a monograph, was read aloud in a friendly circle, was passed from hand to hand, gave rise to discussion and to control-experiments. There was no thought of publication until matters had ripened. The letters exchanged by the scholars of those days are stimulating reading. They give us a lively impression of the workshops of research. People disclose their personality much more freely in letters than in printed publications. If we know the history and biography of learned men of the eighteenth century better than those of their fellows belonging to earlier epochs, this is because of the innumerable letters which have been preserved in MS., and some of them in print.

Morgagni published very little. He was an exceptionally conscientious scientific worker, but he lived a secluded life, and (apart from the before-mentioned letters) his work remained little known to his contemporaries. Half a century rolled by, and he was nigh upon eighty years of age. Then, in 1761, he published *De sedibus et causis morborum per anatomen indagatis libri quinque*—five books concerning the seat and the causes of maladies anatomically studied. What did this mean? It meant that illnesses were localised. The seat of an illness was an organ or several organs. Through the working of morbific factors, anatomical changes were produced in the organs. These changes were not of a haphazard character. They determined the particular disease, decided its nature. They were the cause of the morbid symptoms.

230

Was this outlook upon illness novel? Yes and no. No one who had made post-mortem examinations, no one who had made a close study of human organs, could have failed to come across abnormal anatomical conditions from time to time; for the bodies that were dissected were not only those of executed criminals (a large proportion of whom were young and healthy persons). We have already learned that in the days of antiquity Erasistratus detected pathological changes in the organs, and drew far-reaching inferences from what he saw. After the Renaissance had begun, observations of the kind were multiplied. Nearly all the anatomists of the sixteenth century noted and described pathological changes of this sort. They were especially interested in malformations, which from very early days had stimulated people's imaginations.

Collections were made of gall-stones and vesical calculi. It was obvious that these accretions, and many of the other abnormalities that were noted, must be the product of abnormal tissue change, and that, by a vicious circle, they must, once formed, interfere with normal functioning. In the seventeenth century, observers began to preserve dissections of abnor-malities, and to make extensive observations. The Genevese physician, Théophile Bonet (1620–1689), published in 1679, under the title *Sepulchretum* a comprehensive work comprising all the pathologico-anatomical observations he had been able to shark up. It was a mish-mash in which there were sound nuggets interspersed amid a mass of fables. Bonet was not an anatomist. First and foremost he was an indiscriminate collector, but he recognised to what good uses a collection would be put. The sub-title of his book was *Anatome practica*. It was a work on applied anatomy, written with an eye to the practice of medicine. Such an anatomy seemed to him "pathologiae genuinae tum nosologiae orthdoxae fundatrix"—the foundation of a true doctrine of pathology and of a genuine theory of disease. Thus his outlook was thoroughly sound. If he failed, nevertheless, to draw sound conclusions from his observations, this was not merely because he possessed a second-rate intelligence, but because of the general inadequacy of the knowledge of his day.

If an anatomical change is to be brought into causal relationship with a morbid symptom, the observer must first be acquainted with the normal functioning of the organ concerned. Not until then can he judge how far a symptom is the expression of disordered function. In other words, pathological anatomy presupposes a knowledge, not only of anatomy, but also of an anatomically grounded physiology. Not until well on into the eighteenth century, not until the days of Albrecht von Haller, had the new physiology advanced so far as to enable anatomical concepts to make the next step and to advance into the domain of pathology. Much earlier, indeed, and most characteristically, William Harvey, who clearly recognised the importance of pathologico-anatomical observations, had written that the post-mortem examination of a patient who had died of pulmonary consumption or of some other malady was far more instructive than the cutting-up of a dozen executed criminals.

During the eighteenth century, relevant observations multiplied. In Mantua, Bartoletti studied changes in the lungs; in Turin, the brothers Fantoni investigated changes in the heart, the spleen, and the dura mater. Valsalva was interested in the pathological anatomy of the organ of hearing as well as in its normal anatomy. Morgagni worked along the same lines. He knew and frankly acknowledged the value of his predecessors' work, Bonet's not excepted. Like Bonet, he recorded the observations of others, and was always grateful for information furnished by his correspondents. But, having a critical intelligence, he knew what to accept and what to reject. For the main part, however, throughout his long life he made a mass of personal observations.

It was his imperishable service that he, pioneer in this respect among writers on pathological anatomy, systematically elaborated an enormous number of observations. Before Morgagni's day, nothing more had been done than to assemble observations haphazard, or to elaborate restricted domains. In this respect, Morgagni reminds us of Vesalius, who had likewise turned the work of his forerunners to account. Vesalius, as the outcome of personal observations, wrote the first complete textbook of human anatomy. In like manner Morgagni, an original investigator, wrote the first handbook of the new pathology, of pathological anatomy. The reader must not, indeed, suppose that Morgagni's opus magnum exhibited the precise classification of a modern textbook of pathological anatomy. It was loosely constructed. The separate chapters had been composed as letters to his colleagues. Moreover, the work was not compiled in accordance with anatomical views, but was put together from the clinical standpoint. It described individual symptoms, symptom-complexes, and diseases as observed in living patients, and then endeavoured to explain them in terms of the anatomical changes discovered on post-mortem examination. Morgagni followed the traditional course of description "a capite ad calcem," beginning with maladies of the head, such as headache, apoplexy, etc. He described and discussed particular cases. The whole great work is a collection of cases. We have seen that the Viennese clinic published similar collections, and that post-mortem examinations were made and duly appreciated in Vienna. The idea in both instances is the same. The difference is, however, that in de Haen's writings the main stress is laid upon the clinical histories, whereas in those of Morgagni it is laid upon the reports of the post-mortem examinations; and that Morgagni's cases are not simply arranged chronologically but are classified in accordance with pathological outlooks.

That is what lifts Morgagni's works up to so high a plane; that is what gives their author an epoch-making importance. Although his book is somewhat primitively constructed, it is a magnificent attempt at a synthesis. It covers the whole field of special pathology, considered anatomically. A symptom is no longer something that hangs vaguely in the air. It is tracked down in the organism, is referred to the organs upon whose disordered functioning it depends. Symptoms, symptom-complexes, diseases, are strictly associated with the various organs. Thus the conception of diseases as entities was strongly fortified. Of course there are "species morborum," different kinds of maladies. What determines whether one kind of malady or another manifests itself is, the organ affected, and the anatomical changes that are taking place therein. The disease is recognised by the material changes associated with it.

It is hard for us to-day to realise how great were the difficulties with which the pathological anatomist had to contend in the eighteenth century. Until then, anatomical interest had been almost exclusively directed towards normal anatomy. In the field of normal anatomy there were still numerous matters which remained to be elucidated. But now a new question pressed for solution. What or where were the limits between normal and pathological structure? When is a deviation from the normal a mere variation, and when is it a morbid change? No one could doubt, of course, that a tumour, a growth the size of a man's fist, must be morbid. Morgagni recognised, however, that minute changes in the tissues of the organs could entail serious consequences. These minute changes, indeed, were the most important, and not the salient instances, the curiosities, which had hitherto been exclusively considered.

We must also learn to distinguish between changes that existed during life and those which have only arisen after death. The bodies obtained for post-mortem examinations were not always fresh; and, besides, the examination sometimes lasted for a considerable time.

Here experience was the only possible teacher, and Morgagni was lucky enough to have extraordinarily abundant material at his disposal. Indeed, the supply of bodies from the hospitals was so large that he could not deal with them single-handed.

Many of the post-mortems had to be entrusted to his assistants and students, and he had to content himself in such cases with their reports concerning the pathological conditions they found. It is interesting to note that there could not in Italy at that date have been any general prejudice against being subjected to post-mortem examination. Persons of all classes, including noblemen of high rank and dignitaries of the Church, were subjected to post-mortem examination by Morgagni. We are told that a great many patients uttered a definite wish to have their bodies examined by him after death. Nor were any objections raised to experiments upon animals. The Church never protested against such experiments, recognising the excellent intentions with which they were made. Morgagni experimented freely, endeavouring by artificial means to produce abnormal conditions.

It may seem surprising that Morgagni did not illustrate his book. Illustrations would certainly have enhanced its value, and there could have been no lack of competent draughtsmen. Almost all works on anatomy at that date were illustrated. Still, Morgagni was not writing a textbook of anatomy but a work on special pathology of which anatomy was no more than a part. Besides, his book was not conceived as a textbook, as is manifest from its epistolary form—though it ultimately developed into a textbook. Finally we have to remember that anatomy is static, whereas pathology is dynamic. We can depict the uterus, which, rare abnormalities apart, is practically the same in all women; but a myoma cannot be generalised in this way. There are large myomata and small ones; they vary in shape and in situation. We can describe a myoma, and can select a characteristic myoma as an example. Morgagni could have given illustrations of some of his preparations. But the decision which preparations were especially characteristic was hard to make in those days. We know now that all myomata, whatever their outward form may be, have this much in common, that they consist of muscular tissue, and that it is this which makes them myomata. Morgagni could not as yet know so much. His ideas of general pathology were entirely conventional. His chosen field was that of special pathological anatomy, and, as a matter of course, naked-eye pathological anatomy.

Morgagni did not give medicine a new trend. Developmental forces were effecting a strong urge in that direction. The anatomical idea had long since begun its victorious campaign. Yet it does not suffice that a current should be working in the depths. If the current is to become a broad and effective stream, there is need of an engineer who perceives its existence and digs a channel for it. Though not an innovator, Morgagni was such an engineer, and we are therefore fully justified in regarding him as the founder of pathological anatomy. The year 1761 will always remain an important one in the annals of the healing art.

From every physician we expect tact and moral earnestness, but we expect them from a pathologist in a supreme degree. It is the dead who are brought to the latter, persons whom medical practitioners have been powerless to save. All too often an autopsy demonstrates the insufficiency of human knowledge. In such cases the pathologist must not play the part of judge, but must be a helper and an exhorter. It is well that a man of such high character, a man so profoundly impressed with his mission, should have stood upon the threshold of the developing science of pathological anatomy. Morgagni's delicacy of feeling is shown by his refusal to perform an autopsy upon the body of his colleague Vallisnieri and upon that of a bishop with whom he had been linked in close friendship. A pathfinder in the natural sciences, he was also equipped with classical culture, and he devoted his rare hours of leisure to archaeological studies. He was in his ninetieth year when he died.

CHAPTER TWENTY-EIGHT

LEOPOLD AUENBRUGGER
1722–1809

IT seems to have been the predestined lot of Vienna that at all times there should live in that city physicians of genius who do not form part of the official faculty. To-day, for instance, we think of Sigmund Freud, Steinach, and others. It was the same in the eighteenth century, as regards Leopold Auenbrugger.

The more medical thinkers inclined to adopt anatomical ways of thinking in the study of pathology, the plainer it became that diseases have organic seats and that anatomical changes play a decisive part in bringing about disease—the more strongly must the need have made itself felt to discover a means of perceiving these changes, not only on the post-mortem table, but in the living patient. As far as pure science is concerned, it is of the utmost value that the pathological anatomist should be able to confirm or to correct the diagnosis in the post-mortem room; but as regards the patient, such a revision of the diagnosis comes too late. We have to learn how to interpret symptoms, be guided by them to an understanding, to a recognition, of the anatomical changes which give rise to them. The pulse and the breathing afford valuable indications. There was a crying necessity for additional methods whereby the interior of the organism could be studied. Until recently, no direct method was forthcoming. For that, doctors had to wait until the discovery of the Röntgen rays. Surely there must be indirect ways of "looking into" the organism, of obtaining information regarding its internal condition?

A man who wishes to know whether a barrel is full or empty taps it. Auenbrugger was the son of an innkeeper, and must often have seen his father engaged in this simple operation.

237

Well, the human thorax is in many respects like a wine-barrel. Normally, the lungs are full of air, but in certain diseases the air-cells are filled with morbid secretion. If we tap the breast with the fingers, the resulting tone must, just as in the case of a barrel, depend upon the internal condition. When the barrel is full of wine, the note produced by tapping is low-pitched, "dull"; when the barrel is empty (filled only with air), the note is high-pitched, "resonant." In like manner, if the left hand be laid gently on the chest and one of the fingers be tapped with a finger of the other hand, if the air-cells contain air the note is resonant, but if they are filled with morbid secretion the note is dull. Thus by this peculiar way of tapping the thorax, known as "percussion," it is possible to ascertain whether the thoracic organs are normal or morbidly changed.

Auenbrugger was a pupil of van Swieten, and from 1751 to 1762 was first assistant physician and then physician at the Spanish hospital in Vienna. It was there he began his experiments in tapping, in percussion, doing so directly with the finger-tips of one hand, and not, as above described, through the intermediation of the left hand—the present practice. He distinguished between the normal resonant tone, the "sonus altior," the "sonus obscurior," and the "sonus prope suffocatus" or "percussae carnis." These are to this day regarded as the chief percussion tones, three in number, which we distinguish as normal pulmonary resonance (or a somewhat lower-pitched "tympanitic" resonance produced by percussing over the stomach and intestines), as "dullness on percussion" resulting when the lung is consolidated by morbid secretions or when we percuss the liver, and the much higher-pitched tone produced by percussing the larynx or the shin-bone. The significance of these various tones was disclosed by post-mortem examinations.

Auenbrugger experimented and gathered experience for seven years before he published an account of his method. We can realise how great the difficulties must have been when we recall our own early attempts at percussion in our student days.

We percussed until our fingers were sore, and yet, with the best will in the world, we could not (at any rate those of us with a poor musical ear could not) recognise the differences in percussion tones about which our teachers were talking. Yet how easy are matters made for us nowadays. We know the pathological anatomy of the lungs perfectly well. The tones are demonstrated to us by our seniors, so that our ears may become accustomed to them. Auenbrugger had none of these advantages. He had laboriously to work out the anatomical and diagnostical ideas unaided.

It is a matter of familiar experience in hospital wards that persons with "a good musical ear" learn percussion and auscultation far more speedily than those without musical gifts. The significant point is that Auenbrugger was a great amateur of music, and indeed more than an amateur. Not only were musical performances frequently held in his house, but he himself wrote the libretto to a comic opera by Salieri. It would seem that he did not shine in this domain so much as he did in the field of medicine, since otherwise he would scarcely have taken the trouble to provide a text for what Mozart (writing to his father) described as "a pitiable work."

After seven years, Auenbrugger was ready to make his discovery known to the world. On New Year's Eve 1760 he wrote the preface to his book *Inventum novum ex percussione:*

"I here present the Reader with a new sign which I have discovered for detecting diseases of the chest. This consists in the Percussion of the human thorax, whereby, according to the character of the particular sounds thence elicited, an opinion is formed of the internal state of that cavity. In making public my discoveries respecting this matter, I have been actuated neither by an itch for writing, nor a fondness for speculation, but by the desire of submitting to my brethren the fruits of seven years' observation and reflexion. In doing so, I have not been unconscious of the dangers I must encounter; since it has always been the fate of those who have illustrated or improved the arts and sciences by their discoveries to be beset by envy, malice, hatred, detraction and calumny.

"This, the common lot, I have chosen to undergo; but with the determination of refusing to every one who is actuated by such motives as these, all explanation of my doctrines. What I have written I have proved again and again, by the testimony of my own senses, and amid laborious and tedious exertions;— still guarding, on all occasions, against the seductive influence of self-love.

"And here, lest anyone should imagine that this new sign has been thoroughly investigated, even as far as regards the diseases noticed in my Treatise, I think it necessary candidly to confess, that there still remain many defects to be remedied— and which I expect will be remedied—by careful observation and experience. Perhaps, also, the same observation and experience may lead to the discovery of other truths, in these or other diseases, of like value in the diagnosis, prognosis, and cure of thoracic affections. Owing to this acknowledged imperfection, it will be seen, that, in my difficulties, I have had recourse to the Commentaries of the most illustrious Baron van Swieten, as containing every thing which can be desired by the faithful observer of nature: by which means I have not only avoided the vice of tedious and prolix writing, but have, at the same time, possessed myself of the firmest basis whereon to raise, most securely and creditably, the rudiments of my discovery. In submitting this to the public, I doubt not that I shall be considered, by all those who can justly appreciate medical science, as having thereby rendered a grateful service to our art,—inasmuch as it must be allowed to throw no small degree of light upon the obscurer diseases of the chest, of which a more perfect knowledge has hitherto been much wanted.

"In drawing up my little work I have omitted many things that were doubtful, and not sufficiently digested; to the due perfection of which it will be my endeavour henceforth to apply myself. To conclude, I have not been ambitious of

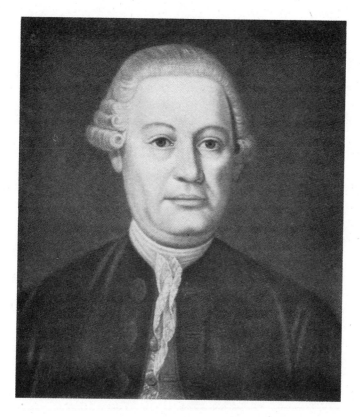

Leopoldus Auenbrugger medicus viennensis.

LEOPOLD AUENBRUGGER, 1722–1809

ornament in my mode or style of writing, being contented if I shall be understood." [Quoted from the English translation of 1824.]

His little book, then, was ready for publication. It could stand on its own feet. Wait a minute, though! The reader must not suppose that Auenbrugger was simply playing with theory. Taking up his pen once more, he appended to the preface a "Monitorium ad omnes medicos"—an exhortation to all doctors:

"Convinced by personal experience, I contend that the sign about which this book treats is of the utmost importance, not only for the diagnosis, but also for the treatment of diseases, so that it ranks in value immediately after the examination of the pulse and the breathing. I contend that an abnormal tone in the thorax is, in every disease, a certain sign of the existence of serious danger."

How was the book to be entitled? The author found it hard to express in any brief phrase the nature of the contents. We have already given it curtailed. In full, the rather cumbrous title ran: *Inventum novum ex percussione thoracis humani, ut signo, abstrusos interni pectoris morbos detegendi*, which being interpreted means "A New Discovery in order, by Percussion of the Human Thorax, to discover Signs for the Recognition of Hidden Diseases of the Chest."

It was in this same year 1761 that Morgagni's great work was published. The two books were expressions of an identical movement, expressions of the advancing anatomical idea. Morgagni laid the foundations of pathological anatomy, and Auenbrugger laid the foundations of anatomical diagnosis.

The expected onslaughts were not lacking. Many doctors paid absolutely no attention to Auenbrugger's discovery. Others declared that it was not a discovery at all, that there was nothing new in what he wrote, since it was to be found in the Hippocratic writings. Yet others regarded percussion as a needless molestation of the sick. Much more distressing to Auenbrugger was de Haen's cold and stubborn silence, for the Dutchman was antagonistic to innovations, took no notice of them, contemptuously ignored them. Nevertheless if there was any place where the new method might have proved fruitful, it was at the Viennese clinic.

Still, the book was widely read, so that in two years a new edition was called for. Many of its readers recognised its importance. Haller declared that percussion was "worthy of close attention, and, it would seem, an entirely new discovery. It is true that proposals of this kind must not be unhesitatingly accepted, but they deserve our respectful attention."

After de Haen's death, when Stoll became chief of the clinic, percussion was more widely practised there, but when Stoll's course was run the method passed for a time into oblivion.

We know to-day how important to medical science was Auenbrugger's discovery. In retrospect it is easy enough to perceive this. Nevertheless, we should be unjust to reproach Auenbrugger's contemporaries for having failed to recognise forthwith the value of percussion. Pathological anatomy was a new science, which had not yet secured general acceptance. The majority of doctors still regarded illnesses as essentially general, and thought that local conditions were subsidiary. Decades had still to elapse before anatomical outlooks secured general acceptance. As we shall see, it was left for French physicians in the beginning of the nineteenth century to realise that percussion was one of the most important methods of examination of the sick, as it has remained unto this day.

In the year 1762, Auenbrugger resigned his post at the Spanish hospital, owing to a dispute with his colleagues. Henceforward he was a busy and favourite practitioner. He took up his pen more than once to write short monographs upon remedies, upon dysentery, and upon influenza. In 1784 the Emperor gave him a patent of nobility.

CHAPTER TWENTY-NINE

JOHANN PETER FRANK
1745–1821

ON August 26, 1766, a young man took his degree as doctor of medicine at Heidelberg. He had had a chequered youth, and a still more adventurous career awaited him. Born at Rodalben near Pirmasens in Baden, he grew up in that borderland between German and French civilisation which was ever and again the seat of sanguinary struggles. His grandfather, a Frenchman, had been a purveyor to the army, and had been killed in the field by marauders. His father, being still a child, had remained with the regiment; then he ran away to seek his fortune, was for a time a petty trader, and at length, settling down as manager of some glass-works, married and had thirteen children. In these circumstances it had been difficult for Johann Peter Frank to take up a life of study, but he managed to get his way. To begin with, he had been educated by the Piarists in Rastatt and by the Jesuits at Bockenheim. Then he had studied philosophy and natural science in Baden, Metz, and Pont-à-Mousson, and had taken his degree as doctor of philosophy. He was, however, attracted to a medical career. His mother was greatly distressed that he refused to enter the Church; and his father was enraged because he wanted to continue his studies instead of taking up a business life. Young Frank, however, got his own way, studying medicine at Heidelberg and at Strasburg.

Now he had become a doctor of medicine. His dissertation upon the dietetics of childhood attracted attention. He showed himself capable of treating a medical problem scientifically. The dean of the medical faculty had a talk with him one day, and urged him to take up some special subject of study. What occurred to him as suitable?

Frank: "A notion has been working in my head. I perceive that doctors are seldom able to obviate those causes of disease which either act in bulk upon the general population or operate independently of the will of individuals (however careful they may be). Yet assuredly many of these causes could be obviated by systematic action on the part of the authorities. Is there any sort of carefully elaborated science dealing with the rules in accordance with which such an end could be achieved?"

The Dean: "There are, doubtless, many specialised institutions aiming at this, but no comprehensive and inter-connected scientific campaign of the kind has hitherto been attempted. Your idea is an excellent one. How would you baptise this child of your mind?"

Frank: "The topic of my inquiry would certainly be *medical*, and, since the carrying into effect of measures likely to promote the general health must be mainly left to a country's *police* [the Germans use this term "police" in a wider sense than the English, to denote public executive authorities and administrative measures of various kinds], the name 'medical police' seems to me appropriate."

Medical police! [The most appropriate modern English equivalent of this term would be "public hygiene." In fact, *Polizei* shades into "policy."] A complete system of medical police measures! This would be an important, and also a strenuous task. To teach rulers how to keep their subjects in good health. Frank was only one-and-twenty when this presented itself clearly to his mind as his life-work. He was seventy-two years of age when the last volume of his *System einer vollständigen medizinischen Polizei* was published (1817). The writing of this work remained the steadfast directive of a life which in other respects was variegated and eventful—even chaotic.

The first requisite, however, was to earn his daily bread, by medical practice. He began at home, but soon took a dislike to the place. Then he tried Rastatt, and here he was forbidden to exercise his profession. Then he went to Bitsch in Lorraine, where one of his brothers was living. Scarcely had he put up his plate, when the authorities interfered, for he had no French diploma. The days when a properly qualified doctor could practise in any land were over. Matters were especially difficult in regions where a few miles' walk involved the entry into the domain of a new sovereign prince. He went back to Pont-à-Mousson, and got a French diploma there, which enabled him to practise in Bitsch. He married a young woman with whom he had been in love for some time, and settled down to his work. But, being restless, he removed two years later to Baden, becoming district medical officer.

He had not forgotten what was to be his opus magnum. This he had now been working at for years, and it had grown into a bulky manuscript. He sent it to a publisher in Carlsruhe, who declined it, for the publishers' expert reader had a poor opinion of it. In a rage, Frank burned his manuscript.

His wife dead of puerperal fever. An epidemic of typhus broke out at Gernsbach. Frank was sent thither, being thus given an opportunity of studying one of these widespread diseases. He sickened of it himself, but recovered. Now he was appointed physician-in-ordinary to the Margrave of Baden-Baden, and became attached to the court in Rastatt. At length our would-be hygienist had a chance of "teaching a ruler how to keep his subjects in good health." Frank set to work energetically. The first essential obviously was that there should be adequate provision of medical aid, for there was a great scarcity in this respect. He drafted a plan for the instruction of midwives and surgeons. At this juncture his patron died, the last margrave of the dynasty. The territory passed to the Baden-Durlach line in Carlsruhe. Frank's appointment was confirmed by the new ruler, and he stayed on in Rastatt as "director of midwives and territorial accoucheur." Over and above the supervision of the training of midwives and the control of their work, it was incumbent upon him "whenever summoned, to give the necessary assistance to poor women in labour without extra fees." He insisted that every midwife under his control should keep accurate notes of her cases, hoping thereby to obtain important statistical data.

Four months later came the offer of a better post. He removed to Bruchsal as urban and rural physician in the service of the Prince-Bishop of Spires, to whom in 1775 he became physician-in-ordinary. Here, too, he continued his work of reform. He saw to it that the midwives were better instructed, with the result that mortality in childbirth fell promptly from 1 in 85 to 1 in 125. He also founded a surgical school where he himself was one of the teachers.

He was no longer a beginner. He had been able to acquire practical experience. The moment had come for taking up his great work once more. In 1776 he wrote a small pamphlet, expounding his aims, and inviting his colleagues to supply him with material. The task was a difficult one, for conditions varied greatly from one State to another. He received only a few answers, but in 1779 appeared the first volume of his *System einer vollständigen medizinischen Polizei.* The motto of the work was "Servandis et augendis civibus." This volume dealt with the topics concerning which Frank was especially well informed: reproduction, marriage, pregnancy, childbirth; the domain which seemed to him supremely important, since he considered that maintenance and increase of population were among the chief duties of the State. He discussed various special problems, considering the position of affairs in foreign States even as far as the East, and quoting examples from history, wherein he disclosed remarkable learning. Then he went on to speak of various measures incumbent upon the authorities, and to make proposals for reforms many of which seem to us thoroughly modern. For instance, he demanded that persons "with exceptionally severe and disadvantageous hereditary maladies" should not be allowed to marry without close medical examination.

The introduction to this first volume breathes the spirit of the Enlightenment. Let me quote the opening paragraphs:

"The internal security of the State is the aim of my general science of police [hygiene]. An important part thereof is the science which will enable us to further the health of human beings living in society and of those animals they need to assist them in their labours and for their entertainment, acting in accordance with definite principles; consequently we must promote the welfare of the population by means which will enable persons cheerfully and for lengthy periods to enjoy the advantages which social life can offer them without suffering unduly from the vicissitudes and the variations to which social life cannot fail to expose them as soon as they have resolved to tame the wildness of nature and to renounce certain advantages which in no department were so overwhelming as under the rude and strenuous conditions of human beings before they became artificialised.

"Medical police [hygiene] therefore, like the science of police [public welfare] in general, is a defensive art, is a doctrine whereby human beings and their animal assistants can be protected against the disadvantageous consequences of crowding too thickly upon the ground; and especially it is an art for the promotion of their bodily weal in such a way that, without suffering from an overplus of physical evils, they may defer to the latest possible term the fate to which, in the end, they must all succumb. How strange it is that this science, which day by day grows more essential to our race, should still be so little cultivated, having received attention here and there only and to a minimal extent, while never, so far as I know, being systematically cultivated. This may be due to the fact that only of late have people begun to realise the value of a human being and to consider the advantage of the population; and because these calculations, as their first effect, have given rise to the philanthropic contemplation of

247

the causes to which many attribute the alleged falling-off [in the quality] of our race."

In an earlier chapter we learned how the Greek spirit and the Roman capacity for organisation generated, in ancient times, a highly developed system of hygiene. Amid the storms of the folk-migrations, classical hygiene fell into decay. The aqueducts and the canals of the Romans crumbled to pieces. To the men of the early Middle Ages, the personal hygiene of the ancients, their numerous baths, their salves, their bodily exercises, all the care they took of the physical frame, seemed a meaningless effeminacy—since the soul was the only thing that mattered. But the body is the vessel, the container of the soul. The body must be preserved in good condition. Hygienic ideas reawakened in the towns of the later Middle Ages. Dietetic rules were observed. Public baths were inaugurated. A vapour bath was found to be not merely healthy, but pleasurable, making one who had taken it feel well and cheerful for the whole of the next week. Pestilences raged across Europe alarming men's minds, and compelling them to attempt counteraction. Doctors and the public authorities joined forces to erect a wall against these plagues, to protect society from their ravages.

Despite this, the state of public health was pitiable; mortality, especially among the young, was terribly high. There was little improvement even during the Renaissance, in the sixteenth and seventeenth centuries. Oriental plague was continually reviving. Smallpox, diphtheria, tuberculosis, measles, puerperal fever, typhoid and typhus (the two were not yet distinguished), and malaria claimed countless victims. In the seventeenth century statistical records were begun. Imperfect though they were, they told a plain tale. People became greatly alarmed. The State was menaced with depopulation. Something had to be done.

In the eighteenth century, therefore, a vigorous movement

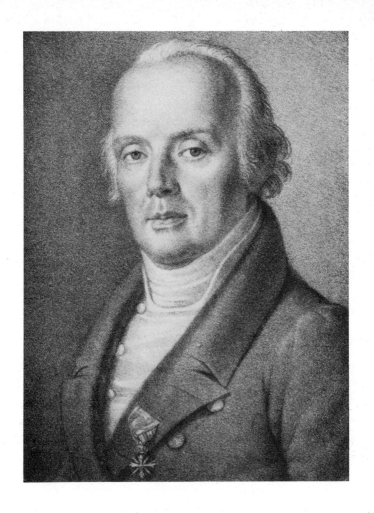

JOHANN PETER FRANK, 1745–1821

for the promotion of public health began. It was sustained by the Enlightenment. Primitive man, whose life was a more "natural" one, was (Frank tells us) strong and healthy: he was also good and happy. Civilisation had worked untold mischief. It had enfeebled man to such a degree that he fell an easy prey to every illness; it had manifestly corrupted him and made him unhappy. "Return to nature," was the call of Jean Jacques Rousseau. Women must prepare themselves for maternity by leading natural lives. It was essential for them to suckle their own children. What had children become? Mere dolls, playthings for grown-ups. From their earliest days they were swaddled in garments which cramped their growth, and they led lives unsuitable to their age. What was the result? They became crippled, both in the mental and in the bodily sense. The child must be set free. Education became a burning question. Rousseau wrote *Emile*.

Doctors were coming to recognise that prevention was better than cure, that the prophylaxis of disease was one of their most important tasks. What was to be the method of preventive medicine? Two ways presented themselves. We may term them the conservative and the revolutionary way, respectively.

The conservatives declared that the populace was like a child, incapable of understanding, or of spontaneously discerning what was good for it. Just as in a family it is the duty of a father to educate his children by means of prohibitions and commands, so in the State it behoves the monarch to educate his subjects—to educate them towards health. Under the advice of his physicians, he will forbid them to do what is injurious and order them to do what is desirable. Thus he will be able to counteract the noxious influences of civilisation, enabling man to enjoy its benefits unhindered. Sanitary regulations always existed, but, as the results showed, these had been inadequate. They must be revised and strengthened.

Those of the other school, the revolutionists, with Rousseau as their leader, took a different view. Nothing worth having could come to the populace from above. Tyranny and corruption held sway. Unnatural ways of living were worse at court than anywhere else. A straightforward simplicity prevailed among the common people; genuine kindliness, childlike innocence, and also sound reason. If the common people were unhappy, that was because they were not sufficiently enlightened. They were sick because they were ignorant. They must be properly instructed concerning health and disease, as well as concerning other matters. A campaign of hygienic popular enlightenment began. A flood of books, pamphlets, and newspapers to inform townsfolk and countryfolk—and especially the latter—about these things issued from the press.

The movement was a part of that which led to the proclamation of the rights of man, and ultimately to the growth of liberalism.

Frank was a typical representative of the conservative trend. His work is the hygienic monument of the absolutist State, of enlightened despotism. His book does not, indeed, spurn the idea of direct popular instruction, but it seemed to him that the safer route was that of "police"—of authoritative measures. Let me give an example to show how far he was inclined to interfere with individual rights. In the chapter entitled "Better Regulation of the Amusement of Dancing," he enlarged upon the dangers of dancing for young girls, and concluded as follows:

"The authorities are therefore justified in prescribing the duration of balls, were it only for reasons of health. They will do well to forbid certain unduly active dances, such as the so-called waltz, and the like. They should forbid parents and other elders to allow young women to indulge without supervision in such violent pleasures or to do so at certain unsuitable times. They must prohibit the dispersal of the dancers until at least half an hour has been passed in repose after the dancing has been finished. Above all they must acquaint every one, and especially young girls, with the probable result of the failure of attending to such regulations."

The book had a wide circulation, for it fulfilled a need, and within a year a new edition was called for. All the same, it brought a good deal of trouble to its author. He had inveighed against the celibacy of the priesthood, and the Church was outraged. This was extremely inconvenient seeing that Frank was in the service of a bishop, who was, moreover, a man of uncertain temper.

Simultaneously with the publication of the second edition of the first volume in the year 1780, there appeared the second volume, which discussed fornication and the hygiene of childhood. Very important questions were considered: prostitution, venereal diseases, abortion, foundling-hospitals. Throughout Europe, venereal diseases were working havoc. Their dissemination was promoted by the moral corruption of the upper classes and by the promiscuity of the lower. Some regarded venereal disease as a punishment for sin; others looked upon it as an unavoidable evil, as the effect of the poisoned arrows of Venus, whose wounds Mercury could heal. Nobody knew how to deal effectively with this pest. Everywhere superstitions and prejudices stood in the way. Here, too, however, Frank took a clear line, demanding the segregation of prostitutes in brothels, the extirpation of clandestine prostitution, the forcible control of prostitutes. Frank, nevertheless, knew perfectly well that it was not prostitutes alone who were responsible for the spread of venereal disease. Logically authoritative, therefore, he insisted "that all persons, whether male or female, ascertained to be infected with venereal disease should be restrained from intercourse until this was known to be safe because they had been completely restored to health." One-and-a-half centuries were to elapse before an effective law for the prevention of venereal diseases was to become possible.

After three years, in 1783, came the third volume, which treated of the hygiene of food, clothing, and habitation. Then there was a longer pause. Not until 1788 was the fourth volume published, for in the interim there had been a great change in Frank's life. He had remained physician-in-ordinary to the Bishop of Spires for nine years, and no longer felt at ease in this post. His scope of activity was unduly narrow. The old unrest seized him. Now he was a man with an established reputation. His books had shown what he was capable of. Almost simultaneously he received three offers, being invited to Mainz as professor of physiology and "medical police"; to Göttingen and to Pavia as professor of practical medicine. Which should he accept? In a non-committal way, he negotiated with the three universities simultaneously. Finally he rejected the offer of Mainz, but was half inclined to go to Pavia. Then he accepted the Göttingen post, though he had been nominated professor in Pavia after already pledging himself to the German university. In the end, therefore, he removed to Göttingen, the famous Protestant university, which had summoned him although he was a Catholic. He began his professorial work there in May 1784, visited the sick attended by a train of students, delivered lectures upon general and special pathology and therapeutics and also upon physiology, and, it need hardly be said, upon hygiene as well.

Hardly had he been a year in Göttingen, when he had had enough of the place. He was overworked, and he found the climate too harsh for him. Besides, he was obviously a square peg in a round hole. His true business was not to teach students but sovereign princes. His preferred field of work was not the narrow one of a university but the wide one of a State. The post in Pavia was still open; the Italians still wanted him. Making up his mind quickly, in the spring of 1785 he travelled south by way of Vienna.

He found he had made a good choice. Here there was an extraordinarily comprehensive region of activity. He was not only clinical teacher and chief of the hospital, but also proto-physicus, that is to say director-general of medical affairs in

Austrian Lombardy and in the duchy of Mantua. At once he began to realise his plan of organisation. As a start, the medical faculty of Pavia was radically reformed. New chairs were established. The students of internal medicine were constrained to attend surgical lectures, and the students of surgery to attend lectures on internal medicine. The medical curriculum was to last five years, and the surgical curriculum four. A separate surgical clinic came into being, and an apothecaries' school was founded. A museum of pathological anatomy was established. Next with his reforms Frank reached out beyond the limits of Pavia. He made a great number of official tours, with the result that, everywhere he went, the hospitals, the work of the apothecaries, and that of the midwives was improved. By degrees Frank came to be regarded as the leading expert in the construction of hospitals. When Genoa wanted to found a clinic, his opinion was invited. On the death of Joseph II he was summoned to Vienna to inspect the General Hospital there, which was in a bad way. In the preface to the fourth volume of the *Medizinische Polizei*, published as already said in 1788, Frank, who had during the last years acquired so much new experience, wrote as follows: "An additional advantage of this work is that I am in a position to carry into effect a large part of my medical proposals, and am therefore able to adjudge their consequences and their difficulties better than can most writers." The volume treated of "Security-Institutions, in so far as they affect Public Health"—that is to say accidents and crimes, their recognition and prevention. Thus the main topic of this volume was what we now classify as forensic medicine.

This same theme was continued in the fifth volume, which also discussed the disposal of the dead. Therewith the circle of human life from birth to death, with all its hazards, had been fully considered, and it would seem that a certain degree of finality had been attained. When the fifth volume appeared, in 1814, Frank was in Vienna, once more in Vienna, at the close of his career, ready to take rest at last. What had transpired between the publication of the fourth volume and that of the fifth? Every reformer has to overcome obstacles. The stronger his hand, the more vigorous will be the opposition. Thus in Italy Frank had encountered much criticism, which went so far that complaints against him were lodged at court. True, he had made good, he had come through with flying colours, and his adversaries had been punished. Still, the perpetual intrigues against him had sickened him with Pavia. In 1795 he was summoned to Vienna to take part in the deliberations of a military sanitary commission. Then he was offered the directorship of the General Hospital, and remained in the Austrian capital.

The General Hospital was perhaps Joseph II's most magnificent creation in the medical field. Frank had been acquainted with it almost from the outset. In 1785, when he passed through Vienna on his way to Italy, he inspected it thoroughly. The Emperor asked him what he thought of the place, whether it pleased him.

Frank: "Admirably, and it has reconciled me to the idea of so large a hospital."

Emperor: "Why were you inclined to object to an institution of this size?"

Frank: "So large a clock seldom keeps good time."

Emperor: "This one does!"

Frank: "Yes, it keeps good time because it has a very heavy weight to drive the wheels."

Frank's perspicacity had not misled him. When the "very heavy weight" was removed, when Joseph II died in 1790, the clock stopped working. Frank had to be summoned to set it a-going once more. Being appointed chief of the General Hospital, he displayed his wonted capacity for organisation, improved the administration, established strict discipline, had a new post-mortem room built, and founded a museum of pathological anatomy. Above all, he devoted himself to the

254

clinic, which had been neglected since Stoll's death. The number of beds available for purposes of clinical instruction was doubled. Frank himself took over the professorship of clinical medicine, and his lectures were greatly esteemed. He had also found time to write a work in several volumes on clinical medicine, and this was widely read.

One might suppose that Frank had satisfied his ambitions. He was in the capital of the empire, and held a high position there. The famous Vienese clinic and one of the largest hospitals in the world were under his charge. But here, too, he encountered adversaries. Stifft, physician-in-ordinary, intrigued against him. The Church had an animus against him, for it had not forgotten what he had written about the celibacy of the clergy. The upshot was that one day Frank set out again on his travels, removing as a clinician to the university of Vilna, accompanied by his son Joseph, who was appointed professor of pathology there. After spending a year in Vilna, he was summoned to St. Petersburg, being given a princely salary as physician-in-ordinary to the Tsar and director of the medico-surgical academy there. He worked for three years in the Russian capital, and then fell sick of dysentery.

He had had enough of Russia, and longed for repose. Besides, his great work was still unfinished, and he had much more to say. He wished to return to some quiet place in Germany where he could continue his literary labours, and he decided upon Freiburg-im-Breisgau. He travelled to Moscow, recovered his health there, and went on to Vienna, arriving in 1809. At this date, Europe was in flames. There was no question, for the moment, of travelling any farther. Napoleon was attacking Vienna for the second time. Frank narrowly escaped his grandfather's fate. A marauder stole his watch, and was even on the point of killing him. Marshal Lannes had both his legs shot through at the battle of Aspern-Essling. Frank was called in consultation, but the case was hopeless. Napoleon himself consulted Frank a few weeks after the battle of Wagram. He wanted Frank to come back with him to Paris. "Your reputation is widely known in my empire. You should settle down in Paris, where you would have an excellent position. We have many first-class men there, who know how to appreciate others' merits." Frank gave the proposal serious consideration, Bitsch, Baden, Rastatt, Bruchsal, Göttingen, Pavia, Vienna, Vilna, St. Petersburg. Should he now go to Paris? There would be much of interest to see there, new institutions, new laws. That which he had been advocating all his life had been realised in the French capital. But he was an old man, and suffered from gout. It had produced a painful impression upon him, painful physically as well as mentally, that the Emperor, who had received him mother-naked in a bath, had kept him standing for a whole hour. Napoleon's physician-in-ordinary, Corvisart, made it plain enough that a competitor would be unwelcome. Frank decided that if the Emperor gave him an express command, he would go to Paris; but that if he were left free choice, he would prefer Freiburg.

The Peace of Vienna was signed. Frank found himself in the much-desired Freiburg. He had a "huge grandfather's chair" and a long table. His coffee, the "drink of the gods," was excellent, and the work on the fifth volume of his great book was making rapid progress. But he found it hard, after such manifold activities, to lead a perfectly quiet life, with no patients, and to play the role of reverend senior. In 1811, when the manuscript of the fifth volume was ready, he wearied of Freiburg and returned to Vienna.

In Vienna he remained until his death, carrying on once more a large practice, and writing his sixth volume. It was the crown of the work, a great fresco, "Concerning the Healing Art in General, and concerning its Influence upon the Welfare of the State" and also "Concerning Institutions for Medical Education."

Frank's death took place six years after the Congress of

Vienna. The restoration had occurred throughout Europe. In the domain of hygiene this took the form of a gloomy reaction. The tide of public health, which had been in full flood during the Enlightenment, had ebbed. The State had lost its absolutist power. The bourgeoisie was growing rich, and had no interest in the public welfare. Beneath the surface, however, the seeds of a new revolution were germinating—the industrial revolution. Fresh dangers threatened the health of the population. Unforeseen problems were emerging and were demanding active solutions. Towards the middle of the nineteenth century, a new hygienic movement began. Experts looked back to the work of Frank, whose treatise was an imposing monument handed down from the eighteenth century.

CHAPTER THIRTY

EDWARD JENNER
1749–1823

IN the days when Frank was director of the General Hospital in Vienna—in the year 1800—there broke out in the imperial capital a severe epidemic of smallpox. This gave an excellent opportunity for the trial of a new material for inoculation which had just arrived from England.

In those days, smallpox was one of the most dreaded and most devastating of the infectious disorders. It is estimated that in Germany alone more than thirty thousand persons died annually of the disease. Many of those who escaped with their lives were horribly disfigured. Nowadays pock-marked faces have almost disappeared. Only those who have travelled in the East are familiar with them. But in the eighteenth-century streets, wherever one went, pock-marked persons abounded.

It is true that even then doctors were not altogether helpless in face of the disease. A peculiar method had been imported from the East as a protection against the pestilence. It was known that those who had had an attack of smallpox were protected against further infection with this disease. Also it had been noticed that epidemics varied in severity, some of them being attended by a very high mortality, and others so mild that there were few deaths. Obviously, then, it was a great advantage to have the smallpox when a mild form of the disease prevailed. Those who had thus suffered were protected for the rest of their lives. It was thanks to these considerations that an attempt was made to induce the disease artificially during a mild epidemic, instead of leaving infection to chance. In Hindustan, in such cases, children were wrapped in the clothing of smallpox patients. In China, the powdered scabs that had fallen from the skin were blown into the nostrils

258

through a tube. It was also noticed that smallpox virus often became less virulent when preserved for a time and allowed to dry. In Central Asia, a mitigated virus of this sort was introduced beneath the healthy skin by needle-pricks. Such methods were used in Africa by slave-traders and slave-raiders, in order to protect their "wares" from decimation by smallpox. The same thing was done in Turkey. There, female slaves from the Caucasus (Circassians) were renowned for their beauty, and commanded high prices. If they fell sick of virulent smallpox, and became pock-marked, they were worth nothing at all. For this reason they were inoculated in early youth, and an inoculated slave-girl commanded a higher price, since the purchaser was guaranteed against her having her face spoiled by the disease.

In Constantinople, at the beginning of the eighteenth century, Lady Mary Wortley Montagu, wife of the British ambassador, became acquainted with this method of inoculation. Being a lady of much energy, and free from prejudice, she took the risk of having her own children inoculated by a Greek physician. The children showed the customary reaction, having no more than a very mild attack of smallpox, recovering quickly, and being thenceforward immune. On her return to England in 1718, she tried to induce her friend the Princess of Wales to follow her own example, and have the royal children inoculated. There was some natural hesitation about risking these "more valuable" lives, so experiments were first made upon persons of no importance, seven criminals and six orphan children being inoculated and subsequently exposed to ordinary smallpox infection. They also proved immune, and at length, in the year 1722, the great venture was taken, and the young princes were inoculated.

The example thus set by the court gave a splendid advertisement to inoculation with smallpox, then termed "variolation." The practice spread rapidly all over England. Variolation centres, at which specialists in inoculation did the work, were established everywhere. From England the method spread to the Continent, though slowly, being first tried at Geneva in the year 1749, by Dr. Tronchin—Geneva having at that date peculiarly close relationships with England. Voltaire was interested in the new practice and did his best to make it generally known.

There can be no doubt that many lives were saved by variolation. Still, smallpox persisted in frequent epidemics, which claimed numerous victims. Although inoculation became more and more general, it was by no means universal. Even in our own day there are plenty of persons who regard the deliberate inoculation of an infective virus as a sinister proceeding. Objections of the kind were probably much commoner in the eighteenth century. The distrust of inoculation felt in many circles was not without justification. Variolation was certainly not free from danger. The substance inoculated was pus derived from a fresh smallpox pustule. The usual practice was to dip a thread in the pus, to dry it, to scarify the patient's skin, and to bandage the pus-impregnated thread upon the scarified surface. Thus what was transmitted was an essentially dangerous disease. Even though the variolators learned to mitigate the virus by preserving it in the dried state for a time, it still sometimes happened that an inoculated person became attacked with severe smallpox, which involved grave risk, not only to himself, but to all who came in contact with him. Furthermore, inoculation was effected from human being to human being. However much care was taken, there always remained a possibility that in addition to smallpox some other illness—especially syphilis—might be transmitted. Variolation, therefore, was not an ideal preventive method, and there was great need of discovering a virus which could immunise patients against smallpox without exposing them to serious danger.

In the closing years of the eighteenth century news came to Vienna that such a virus, an ideal substance for inoculation, had been discovered in England. Von Ferro, the Austrian sanitary authority, took up the matter. "Since it was very difficult to find any other children whose parents would consent to have them inoculated by the new method, and, besides, I wanted to keep the inoculated subjects under close observation, I inoculated my own children." He did this on April 30, 1799. Ten days later, a young physician from Geneva, who had lived in England for a time and had then settled down in Vienna, did the same thing. The results were satisfactory. Next this same Carro inoculated various other children, and by 1801 he was able to report observations upon two hundred cases. He was enthusiastic about the results, devoted himself ardently to the new method, and passionately defended it against its adversaries. For adversaries there were! Stifft, physician-in-ordinary to the Emperor, took a reactionary line as usual, and even succeeded in getting inoculation with the new English virus prohibited, though the prohibition was shortly afterwards withdrawn. In 1800 there was a smallpox epidemic, and it was incumbent upon the experts to adopt a definite attitude for or against the English virus. On November 1, 1801, Johann Peter Frank inoculated two sick children with the new substance at the hospital. Pustules formed at the site of inoculation, dried into scabs, and the scabs fell off. On November 12th, thirteen of the children which had been inoculated with the English virus were inoculated with ordinary smallpox. Not one of them showed any morbid reaction. They had been immunised. Thereupon the government issued a circular in which the new method of inoculation was officially recommended.

What was the virus which gave such remarkably good results?

The discoverer of the new method of inoculation was an English surgeon, Edward Jenner by name. We have heard of him already as one of John Hunter's pupils and for a time an inmate of Hunter's house. The two men had remained closely linked, and Jenner preserved a grateful admiration for Hunter. In 1773, when four-and-twenty years of age, Jenner settled as a general practitioner in his native town of Berkeley, Gloucestershire. His practice flourished, he acquired local renown as a surgeon, and was generally liked. In addition to purely medical and surgical work, he was (as was to be expected in a pupil of Hunter's) much interested in natural history, reporting his observations from time to time to his London teacher.

Round Berkeley, and elsewhere, the cows occasionally suffered from a malady in which pustules closely resembling those of smallpox appeared on the udders and the teats. Jenner called the illness "variolae vaccinae"—cowpox. This malady was transmissible to human beings. The cowherds and milkmaids became infected from time to time with similar pustules, which appeared on their hands and arms. The trouble, however, remained purely local, the attendant general symptoms being of trifling importance, and there being no tendency to the outbreak of a generalised crop of pustules.

There was a widespread belief among the common folk that those who had suffered from what Jenner called cowpox, and had not before this been affected with smallpox, remained immune to the latter disease. In his practice, Jenner had often to undertake variolation. From time to time a landowner would have himself, his family, all the members of his household, and the staff at his farms inoculated with smallpox. Now, again and again Jenner noticed that in some of the cowherds and milkmaids variolation had no effect, and when he inquired into their history he was informed that they had previously suffered from cowpox. This cowpox might have occurred fifty years or more ago.

Was the popular notion sound? Did an attack of cowpox confer immunity to smallpox? If so, there was ready to his hand an ideal virus for inoculation against smallpox, a virus that was effective and innocuous. The idea was thrilling, but

262

Jenner had far too critical an intelligence to jump to a conclusion. He continued his observations for many years. The result confirmed him in his belief, and at length he had recourse to experiments. On a farm not far from Jenner's home cowpox had broken out, and one of the milkmaids became infected. On May 14, 1796, Jenner inoculated a boy of eight, James Phipps by name, with matter taken from one of the milkmaid's pustules. The youngster had a characteristic attack of cowpox, and speedily recovered. Then, on July 1st, he was inoculated with the virus of true smallpox, but no reaction followed, nor yet when the smallpox inoculation was repeated a few months later. Jenner was satisfied. An attack of cowpox rendered the patient immune against true smallpox. Cowpox lymph was the ideal virus for inoculation.

Jenner wrote an account of his observations and sent it to the Royal Society. The members of that learned body shook their heads and returned the country doctor's manuscript. This one experiment, however interesting, did not convince them. It seemed incredible to them that a malady affecting the lower animals could, transmitted to human beings, protect the latter against a properly human epidemic disease.

Undismayed, Jenner continued his experiments, always with the same result. At length, in 1798, he published a booklet consisting of 75 pages and containing 4 plates, entitled *An Inquiry into the Causes and Effects of the Variolae vaccinae*.

The work opens in the style of the Enlightenment:

"The deviation of Man from the state in which he was originally placed by Nature seems to have proved to him a prolific source of diseases. From the love of splendour, from the indulgences of luxury, and from his fondness for amusement, he has familiarised himself with a great number of animals, which may not originally have been intended for his associates.

"The Wolf, disarmed of ferocity, is now pillowed in the lady's lap. The Cat, the little Tyger of our island, whose natural home is the forest, is equally domesticated and caressed. The Cow, the Hog, the Sheep, and the Horse, are all, for a variety of purposes, brought under his care and dominion."

It must not be supposed, however, that the author wasted many of his pages on such tirades. He proceeded to give a concise and clear description of cowpox, a disease which he (erroneously, as we now know) believed to be identical with horsepox. Then came the description of twenty-three cases, from which he drew his conclusions, and he ended by saying: "In the meantime I shall myself continue to prosecute this enquiry, encouraged by the hope of its becoming essentially beneficial to mankind."

The booklet secured, generally speaking, a cool reception. The doctrine it conveyed was too unfamiliar. Others tried to repeat the experiments, and were unable to obtain the same results. Jenner, however, stuck to his guns. In 1799 he published further observations, and he issued yet a third booklet in 1800. In these later essays he explained where his adversaries had gone wrong.

By now the experiences acquired were so extensive that even the most sceptical began to be convinced. Confirmative observations poured in from other lands. We have seen how the discovery was welcomed in Vienna. Ere long the new method of inoculation was being practised everywhere. It became plain that Jenner's discovery was of the utmost importance, and as early as the year 1802 the British parliament showed the nation's gratitude by voting Jenner the sum of £10,000. Five years later a further grant of £20,000 was voted. In such matters the English have always been free-handed. What were £30,000 as compared with the value of Jenner's discovery to the nation?

Enthusiasm cooled when, after a while, it became manifest that the immunity conferred by this method of inoculation did not last throughout life. Further experience showed, how-

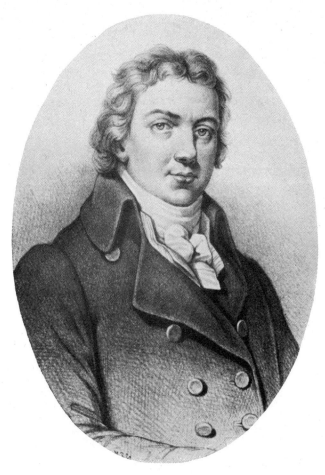

EDWARD JENNER, 1749–1823

ever, that immunity could be renewed by a repetition of the inoculation.

Thus inoculation with smallpox was replaced by inoculation with cowpox. "Vaccination" was substituted for variolation. A means had been discovered thanks to which smallpox became a preventible disease. During the latter half of the nineteenth century, vaccination was made compulsory in most civilised countries, with the result that smallpox is now extremely rare.

CHAPTER THIRTY-ONE

XAVIER BICHAT

1771–1802

WHILE in Italy Frank was reorganising medical matters in Lombardy, and while in England, in rural retirement, Jenner was carrying on his momentous experiments, there were going on in France events of worldwide historical importance which were to leave an imprint upon the progress of medicine. To this matter, we must now turn.

In Paris the old medical faculty persisted like a fossil, its one thought being to stand upon the ancient ways, to maintain its traditional rights. Evolution had passed it by. Leyden, Vienna, and Göttingen were now flourishing centres of medical learning. The clinic had become the main pillar of medical instruction. Enormous advances had been made in anatomy, physiology, and chemistry. Pathological anatomy had come into being. But at the Paris faculty, as of old, "learned doctors" were discussing ancient texts, and were breeding a type of physician which belonged to days long past. No doubt the faculty realised now and again that there was something amiss. In 1778, it sent in a memorial asking for the establishment of a clinical professorship. But the time for this had passed. The ablest physicians (of whom there were plenty in France) had joined other organisations.

In 1776, despite the fierce protests of the faculty, Lassonne and Vic d'Azyr had founded the Société Royale de Médecine, a finer institution than then existed in any other country, an organisation bringing together all the doctors of France for joint work in the furtherance of the medical sciences. A petty practitioner in the most out-of-the-way village could at any time address himself to the Society with questions and suggestions, and could acquaint it with his observations. Far-

266

reaching tasks were contemplated and Vic d'Azyr elaborated a program for the reorganisation of medical education.

French surgeons had since 1731 possessed a similar institution, the Académie Royale de Chirurgie, a body whose most outstanding and influential member was Antoine Louis. Now came the Revolution! The States General assembled at Versailles on May 5, 1789. On July 14th of the same year the Bastille was stormed. On August 27th the Rights of Man were proclaimed. The Revolution became continually more radical. The King tried to escape, but was recaptured. The government declared war against Austria. The Tuileries was stormed. By a decree of August 8, 1792, the medical faculty was unceremoniously dissolved. France became a republic. Louis XVI perished beneath the guillotine. On August 8, 1793, the Convention decided to abolish all the corporations which had been subsidised by the State. This decree applied to the Académie de Chirurgie, the Société de Médecine, and to the provincial medical faculties and surgical schools.

Therewith medical education and medical practice in France were reduced to chaos. There was no longer either instruction or control. Anyone practised who wanted. The lack of properly qualified doctors soon made itself felt, especially in the army. France was at war with half Europe. Six hundred physicians and surgeons had already fallen at the front. The gaps in the army medical service were filled by new recruits, many of them no more than young students.

The Convention had made a clean sweep of the old institutions, and it was necessary to rebuild from the foundations. It commissioned one of its members, Fourcroy, a physician and an able chemist, to draft a plan for reorganisation. He carried out his task as speedily as possible, laid his scheme before the Convention on November 27, 1794. It was adopted amid general approval, and steps for its realisation were promptly begun.

The first requisite, of course, was to provide doctors for

the army. Three Ecoles de Santé were established; in Paris, Montpellier, and Strasburg respectively. The word "medicine" was carefully avoided in the description of these schools. From the first it was to be made plain that medicine and surgery were not, as heretofore, to be two sharply distinguished occupations, carried on by persons who had received a different sort of training in each case, but that there was to be a unique healing art to subserve the needs of the public health. What was to be effected half a century later in Germany at enormous expenditure of ink and paper, namely the unification of medicine and surgery, was achieved in France at one stroke.

To each Ecole de Santé there were affiliated for medical training three hospitals, one for internal disorders, one for surgical diseases, and a third for rare cases and exceptional complications. The teaching body consisted of twelve professors with twelve assistant professors. Laboratories were provided. All the new specialties were represented. The curriculum was thoroughly modern, and teaching was in the vernacular. Each district in the republic could nominate a student who would be trained gratuitously as an "élève de la patrie."

Thus France, whose medical institutions had hitherto been obsolete, acquired betwixt night and morning the most admirable institutions for teaching and research. This was not a mere change of framework; the entire mental attitude of the doctors was modified. They no longer looked backward, but forward. They were eager to scan all the new trends, and they took up their duties with zeal. The Paris school opened with 600 students, and within a few years there were 1,500. The new possibilities of medical instruction attracted young men of talent from all over the country. By the opening of the nineteenth century, French clinical medicine was far in advance of that of other lands, and guided the progress of medical science for several decades.

At the outbreak of the Revolution there can be little question that, in Pierre Joseph Desault, France possessed the most distinguished surgeon in Europe of that day. He was one of the founders of topographical anatomy, and there is scarcely any other domain of surgery which he did not enrich. He was surgeon at the Hôtel-Dieu, where even before the Revolution his work as a surgical teacher had been greatly valued by a large number of students. When the Ecole de Santé was founded, to him was entrusted the directorship of the surgical clinic.

It was the rule at Desault's clinic that every day, before the clinical instruction of that particular day opened, a practitioner should read a detailed report upon the last day's clinical lecture. On one occasion the specified practitioner was not forthcoming. A student sprang into the breach and, extempore, gave so brilliant an address that his auditors were delighted. The student was Xavier Bichat, to whom Desault's attention was thus directed.

Bichat was the son of a country doctor who had studied in Montpellier and Lyons, and had then, like other young men of his age, been called up for military service. Since 1793, he had been in Paris. Desault took a great liking for the modest, shy, and gifted youth. He invited young Bichat to come and live with him, made him editor of the "Journal de Chirurgie," and did all that was possible to promote Xavier's advancement. However, Desault died in 1795.

The old scientific societies had been dissolved, and new ones arose to take their place. Bichat himself, in 1796, founded the Société Médicale d'Emulation de Paris, in which young doctors assembled for debates concerning the problems of general medicine.

For it was general medicine, above all, which interested Bichat. He did not wish to practise as a surgeon. His chosen fields were anatomy, physiology, and general pathology. In 1800, he became physician at the Hôtel-Dieu. He had hoped to be appointed professor of anatomy and physiology, but another candidate received the preference. He therefore gave private lectures and demonstrations, which were well attended. He worked with febrile energy, experimenting, dissecting, and making post-mortem examinations. Indeed, he spent day and night in the post-mortem room, and is said to have made as many as 600 examinations in one year. His health was poor, and he died when only just over thirty years of age.

Though his end was thus premature, he left behind him a number of notable books, of which three may be mentioned: *Traité des membranes*, 1800; *Recherches sur la vie et la mort*, 1800; and *Anatomie générale appliquée à la physiologie et à la médecine*, 1801.

Bichat's trend was that which proceeded from Haller and led by way of the Montpellier school to vitalism. Like Haller, he considered that life has its own laws, that physiological processes are fundamentally different from physical ones. Vital manifestations are determined by "propriétés vitales," by qualities immanent in living substance, which cannot be explained but only observed. Life is the sum of all the functions which resist death. Bichat's vitalism was not a vitalism of the study, but derived, like contemporary vitalism, from the laboratory. His work is permeated with and enlightened by the results of experiments, so that it was regarded with respect even by materialistic physiologists.

Bichat's main service to medical science, however, did not consist in this general vitalist outlook which he shared with many eighteenth-century physicians, but in the importance he ascribed to particular organs in disease. Morgagni had declared that some particular organ was always the seat of a disease. Yet it was observable that when different organs were diseased, the symptoms were sometimes identical. Pinel, with whom we shall become more closely acquainted by and by, had explained this by assuming that in such cases the malady must affect organs which, though differently placed, had like internal structure. There was a good deal in the idea, but it was too generalised.

Bichat took up this notion. What did the organs consist of? Of tissues, which Bichat termed "membranes." Bichat recognised or distinguished simple tissues to the number of twenty-one. We must not forget that the animal cell had not yet been discovered, so that it was still impossible to be aware that the tissues were aggregates of cells of like form and function. Bichat had to classify his "membranes" in accordance with coarser characteristics than those of cellular structure, and that is why there were, as he thought, so many of them.

The organs are built up out of these tissues. The tissues are the sustainers of vital functions, both normal and morbid. Consequently the seat of a disease is not the organ as a whole, but a tissue. Any tissue in any organ could become diseased apart from the other tissues of which the organ is made up. Indeed, that is what usually happens. Well, if like tissues become diseased in the same way in different organs, identical morbid symptoms necessarily arise.

Bichat studied these tissues in detail, studied their structure and above all their qualities: their qualities after death, their elasticity, their behaviour when treated by heat, acids, alkalis, etc.; and also their vital qualities, their reactions under normal and pathological conditions.

In this way Bichat pushed the anatomical way of regarding pathology a stage farther, from the organ to the tissue. When, a few decades later, the animal cell was discovered, an additional advance inevitably followed, and Virchow's cellular pathology came into being.

Bichat stood at the turning-point between two epochs. He reached back into the eighteenth century. He built upon the foundations laid by Haller and Morgagni. All the same, his work embodied the program of the nineteenth century. He pointed out the road along which medical science was to travel: analysis of morbid phenomena with the aid of physiological concepts, and a reference of these same phenomena to their anatomical substrata.

CHAPTER THIRTY-TWO

JEAN NICOLAS CORVISART (1755–1821)
AND
PHILIPPE PINEL (1755–1826)

DESAULT, as we have shown, was the founder of modern clinical study in France so far as surgery was concerned; one of Desault's pupils, Corvisart, did the same work for French clinical medicine. Just as after the extensive reorganisation that took place during the year 1794 Desault became director of the first surgical clinic, so did Corvisart become director of the first medical clinic. Like Desault, moreover, Corvisart had been actively at work as a clinician several years before this. In 1788 he had been appointed physician at the Charité, as successor to his teacher Desbois de Rochefort, organising clinical work there in an exemplary fashion and with an almost military precision.

Corvisart had originally been destined for the legal profession. At school he was not only diligent at his studies, but had distinguished himself by bodily vigour. His father was solicitor to the crown, and took the lad into his own office. Corvisart, however, found the copying of legal documents a tedious affair. Whenever he could, he escaped from this thraldom, made his way into the Latin Quarter, listened to one lecturer or another, visited the Hôtel-Dieu (the largest hospital in Paris), and there gave ear to what Desault had to say. He found this fascinating. At length he broke away from his father's profession, and became a medical student. Having been trained in Desault's hospital, in 1782 he qualified as a doctor, and was appointed parish physician at a minimal salary. Naturally he looked out for a better post. Ere long there was a vacancy at the hospital founded by Madame Necker. He applied for it, and presented himself before the governing body,

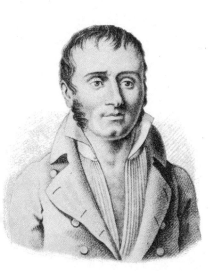

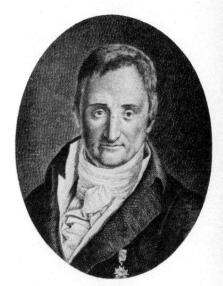

XAVIER BICHAT, 1771–1802   PHILIPPE PINEL, 1755–1826

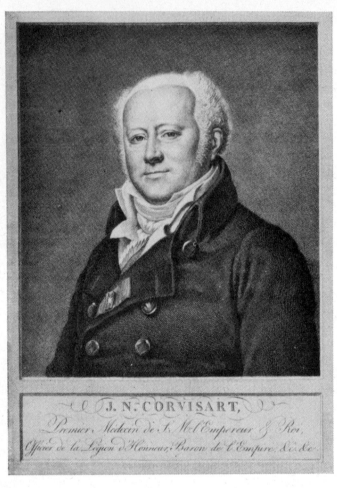

J. N. CORVISART,

Premier Medecin de S. M. l'Empereur & Roi,
Officier de la Légion d'Honneur, Baron de l'Empire, &c &c.

Corvisart

JEAN NICOLAS CORVISART, 1755–1821

which was outraged to find that the young man wore no wig! In other respects his qualifications and recommendations were satisfactory, but it was impossible to appoint him as hospital doctor unless he would wear a wig. Corvisart refused to give way upon this point, and, in his letter declining the post, wrote: "Respect for outward signs must not degenerate into superstition."

Now he devoted himself to anatomy and pathology. During a post-mortem examination, he pricked his finger. In those days before antiseptics had been discovered, this often meant fatal blood-poisoning. With stoical calm, watch in hand, Corvisart awaited the expected rigor, but was lucky enough to escape. Faced with the choice of devoting himself to surgery or to internal medicine, he decided in favour of the latter, and worked at the Charité, of which, a few years later, as we have learned, he became medical director.

Now he was a clinician, but there was no clinical tradition in France. He therefore determined to get into touch with the Viennese school, since the Vienna clinic had set an example to the world. Of the three books he wrote, two were translations of those by Viennese physicians. He studied Stoll's writings, and in 1797 translated the latter's *Aphorisms*. Here he learned of percussion, a method of which he had never heard in Paris. "Percussion made a strong impression upon me, and I think that since then I have practised it unceasingly, whether in obscure diseases of the chest or in those that were simple and easily understood. It never led me astray if the condition of the patient was such as to allow me to make full use of it. On the other hand, I must frankly admit that I have known of many grave errors in diagnosis on the part of those who knew nothing of percussion or neglected it." For twenty years Corvisart practised percussion and developed its use. Since then it has formed an inseparable part of a clinical examination.

A French translation of Auenbrugger's *Inventum novum* had appeared in 1770. The translation was a bad one. The translator had never practised percussion, and did not even believe in the method, which did not seem new to him for he supposed it to have been mentioned in the Hippocratic writings. In 1808, therefore, Corvisart made a fresh translation, enriched with an elaborate commentary. Auenbrugger's booklet was entirely renovated, and was expanded from 95 to 440 pages. This made it possible for the new method to bear rich fruit. Clinical medicine had advanced so far that the great majority of practitioners were thinking anatomically, and were trying in every case of illness to refer the symptoms to changes in the bodily organs.

In the year 1797, Corvisart was appointed to a second academic post, becoming professor of practical medicine in the Collège de France. Here he shone as a teacher. A great number of physicians were trained by him. In the morning he went his round at the Charité, accompanied by a train of students as he moved from bed to bed, examining each patient with the utmost care. "The medical training of the senses" was his watchword and his program. Students must learn to use their sense-organs. Everything depended upon accurate observation. By the bedside of the sick, theory was silent, for the only thing that mattered was to see and to hear. Corvisart was himself a marvellously keen observer. We are told that one day, looking at a portrait, he said: "If this picture is a faithful one, I cannot doubt that the original must have died of heart disease." Inquiry showed that such had been the case.

When a patient died in the clinic, a careful examination of the intact body was first made. Then came the autopsy, and immense was the delight of the doctor and his pupils if this confirmed the diagnosis. Still more instructive, however, were instances in which discrepancies arose. They gave Corvisart an opportunity of showing in masterly fashion how and why he had erred, and, of explaining what was to be learned from these new observations. In the evenings he delivered theoretical addresses at the Collège de France, speaking extempore as a

274

rule, and discussing cases which had been treated in the morning.

Thus in the Paris clinic the road entered upon by Morgagni was systematically followed. Patients were examined with the utmost thoroughness; if they died, their bodies were subjected to post-mortem examination; then the clinical history and the report of the autopsy were mutually confronted. For the time being, so Corvisart thought, theory was of minor importance. The first essential was, in the then state of medical knowledge, to collect an abundance of accurate observations, to make precise pictures of diseases. Still, the outlook was not one-sidedly anatomical. Physiology, too, was given due weight. "The physician who fails to combine pathological physiology with his anatomy will never be anything more than a more or less adroit, diligent, and patient prosector. In practice he will be vacillating, unstable—especially as far as the treatment of organic lesions is concerned."

What loomed before Corvisart as destined to be his opus magnum was a work which, following Morgagni's example, *projected* he would call *De sedibus et causis morborum per signa diagnostica investigatis et per anatomen confirmatis*—that is to say "Concerning the Seats and Causes of Diseases, as studied in accordance with Diagnostic Signs and confirmed by Anatomy." But for this a new Morgagni would have been needed! Corvisart felt unequal to so mighty an undertaking, which would, moreover, have been premature. There had not as yet been collected a sufficiency of material. The book, therefore, would have been a mere fragment. Corvisart devoted himself to and finished a portion of the task; an extremely *concrete* important part, namely that of diseases of the heart. In 1806 he published his *Essai sur les maladies et les lésions organiques du coeur et des gros vaisseaux*. Hitherto, doctors had been unable to cope with diseases of the heart. Corvisart, applying his method to their study, achieved notable results. First of all he was able to show how common are organic diseases of the heart. He also insisted upon the need for distinguishing functional from organic heart diseases. With the help of percussion he tried to form a clinical picture of the particular diseases of the heart. He was further able to distinguish between hypertrophy and dilatation of the heart, and made a thorough study of the course of cardiac insufficiency or, as we now call it, failure of compensation.

Thus Corvisart's clinic served, not only to train more competent physicians, but also to advance research by a long stride. His study of heart diseases showed what the new method could effect.

In 1807, Corvisart became physician-in-ordinary to Napoleon, and his new duties tended more and more to withdraw him from his work as a clinical teacher. His practice increased from day to day, and his social obligations became more comprehensive. Napoleon was a difficult and exacting patient, but Corvisart got on with him very well. It is recorded that the Emperor once said he had no faith in medicine, but he had faith in Corvisart.

After the fall of the Empire in 1815, Corvisart likewise vanished from the stage. He had been paralysed by an apoplectic seizure, and retired to his country estate. He was not the founder of a school, but he had trained many distinguished pupils, among them such men as Laennec, Bayle, Dupuytren, and Bretonneau, who worked along his lines, and continued his labours.

A contemporary and associate of Corvisart was Pinel. Corvisart was medical director of the Charité, Pinel that of the Salpêtrière, where women suffering from mental and nervous disorders were cared for. Corvisart was professor of practical medicine at the Collège de France, and Pinel was professor of hygiene and subsequently of internal pathology at the Ecole de Médecine. Though belonging to the same epoch, and indeed born in the same year, the two men were radically different. Look at their portraits. Corvisart has the aspect of a self-confident man of the world, and we know that he was not afraid to express his views to Napoleon frankly. Pinel's countenance betrays his character, shows him to have been retiring, reserved, timid. Fundamentally different, likewise, were Corvisart and Pinel in their medical outlook and in their whole way of thinking. [Extrovert and introvert, pyknic and asthenic, respectively!]

Pinel had entered the medical profession by a devious route. The son of a country practitioner in poor circumstances, he had begun his career as a divinity student, but subsequently transferred from this branch of study to philosophy, upon which topic his doctrines were akin to those of the sensualists, the followers of Condillac. For a while he was engaged in the pursuit of natural science, and did not begin his medical studies until he was thirty years of age. Having worked at Toulouse, Montpellier, and Paris, in 1798 he published his opus magnum, *Nosographie philosophique, ou la méthode de l'analyse appliquée à la médecine*. In two decades the book ran through six editions, and secured for Pinel a large following.

Pinel was both philosopher and scientist, but especially the latter. For him medicine was one branch of the natural sciences, and must be studied in exactly the same way as botany, zoology, or mineralogy. Diseases were entities, just like the species of plants and animals. Every illness had its natural course, with which it behoved the doctor to become acquainted. Pinel, like Corvisart, greatly esteemed the Viennese school, more especially because the clinical teachers in the Austrian capital had studied the course of so many diseases. A doctor, when consulted by a patient, should first decide the true nature of the malady, and thereafter must pigeon-hole it in its proper place in a natural system. Pinel's work revolved round this attempt to formulate a natural system of diseases.

We see that Pinel worked along the lines which had come down from Sydenham. One who holds that there are "species morborum" will necessarily endeavour to classify these species systematically, just as a botanist classifies plants and a zoologist classifies animals. Linnaeus (a qualified medical man as well as a botanist) had written a work entitled *Genera morborum.* One of his contemporaries, the French physician and botanist Boissier de Sauvages, had in the middle of the eighteenth century penned a *Nosologia methodica,* and in the subtitle of this classification of diseases he declared that his works were conceived in the spirit of Sydenham and constructed in accordance with the method employed in botanical science. He distinguished one from another 2,700 types of disease, which he arranged in species, orders, and families. The Linnaean system exercised a contagious influence, so that many doctors of that date were convinced of the need for a tabular classification of maladies resembling the tabular classification of plants.

Pinel's book was an expression of this trend, though he worked with different instruments. He knew the writings of his forerunners well enough, but regarded their systems as erroneous, as unduly artificial and too complicated. Their mistake had been that they were ready to regard mere symptom-complexes and complications as distinct diseases. That is why they had established such a multiplicity of species, which did not correspond to anything actually existing in nature. A particular disease must be analysed until its essential form came to light, and this must be the basis of classification. The lines of classification must be determined (herein we recognise the gulf between Pinel and his precursors) by physiological and anatomical considerations. Pinel was continually regarding anatomical fundamentals. How, for instance, were inflammations to be classified? In accordance with the tissues affected by it. There were, for instance, inflammations of the skin, of the mucous membranes, of the serous membranes, of the parenchyma or functional elements of the various organs, of the muscular tissue, and so on.

It is easy to understand why Pinel's books had so striking

278

a success. He wanted, as practical-minded doctors had again and again wanted before his day, to extricate medical science from uncertainty, so that it should no longer grope in the dark. His contemporary Corvisart had revived the old saying that medicine was an "ars conjecturalis," an art guided by guesses. For Pinel, however, medicine was one of the natural sciences, and must be made as exact a science as botany or mineralogy. A doctor at the bedside of his patient must observe all that was going on as accurately as Hippocrates (whom Pinel greatly esteemed) had observed. Then, proceeding analytically, he must decide the true character of the malady with which he had to deal and ascertain its place in the classificatory system. That was the purpose of diagnosis. In fact, the doctor's duty was almost finished when he had made an accurate diagnosis. Who could be bold enough to maintain that he had ever really cured a disease?

Attractive though Pinel's *Nosographie* was, it was a premature and fallacious attempt. In his day the knowledge of pathological anatomy was not sufficiently far advanced to warrant such far-reaching inferences. Nay more, it was to become manifest in the sequel that no such system as he aimed at establishing is possible. The strength of our contemporary theories of disease lies in the fact that we have renounced any idea of complete systematisation and are content to define as best we may certain groups of illnesses.

Clinicians of Corvisart's type worked causally. They tried to discover the pathogenesis of a disease, to throw light upon the causal chain, link by link, from the first appearance of a morbific cause until the disappearance of the last symptom. It was a long and tedious road they had to tread. Much remained obscure, much was still inexplicable. But it is the road along which we are still advancing to-day. Moreover, it is the road whose goal is treatment, is the cure of the patient. Pinel's method, on the other hand, was descriptive. Just as, for Condillac, the understanding was nothing more than the capacity for speech, nothing more than the power of expressing sensation in linguistic symbols, so, likewise, for Pinel, the only thing that it behoved the doctor to do was to discover a suitable denomination for the disease with which he was confronted. The manifest outcome of such views was his therapeutic nihilism.

All the same, there were various fields of medicine in which the descriptive and analytic method proved extremely fruitful, especially where no clear images of disease had hitherto existed and where pathological anatomy was still at fault. These two reservations applied, in particular, to psychiatry and dermatology. For thousands of years, diseases of the skin had been regarded as disturbances of the body-juices; as "eruptions," as outbreaks, of peccant humours. Very little attention had been paid to typical forms, colours, and changes in these eruptions, since such matters were regarded as of secondary importance. It was time, and more than time, for doctors to undertake precise descriptions of specific eruptions, just as a botanist describes plants. In the year 1806, one of Pinel's pupils, Jean Louis Alibert, began the publication of a great work, enriched by magnificent coloured plates, on morbid manifestations in the skin, and attempting to construct a natural system of skin diseases classified in families, orders, and species. A classification of such diseases from the pathologico-anatomical outlook was not yet possible, owing to the lack of sufficient knowledge of the local changes. It was not until 1845 that the famous Viennese dermatologist Ferdinand Hebra was able to attempt this.

In psychiatry, too, all that was practicable was a purely descriptive account of the various disorders of the mind, since their pathologico-anatomical explanation was not yet possible —and, indeed, as regards many types of mental disorders, is still impossible to-day. It was, doubtless, known that bodily conditions, various kinds of intoxication, infectious disorders, and diseases of the brain could give rise to mental disorders.

In 1793 an Italian physician, Vincenzo Chiarugi by name, published at Florence a book containing sixty-two reports of post-mortem examinations made on patients who had died of mental disorders. Speaking generally, however, the autopsy on one who had perished while suffering from mental disorder rarely disclosed any changes in the brain, and it was therefore a long stride in advance when the descriptive method was applied to reduce the symptomatology of diseases of the mind to some sort of order.

Here Pinel himself led the way. He was superintendent of an asylum, and had a vast amount of material under observation. He wrote a book on mental disorders. But his greatest service in the domain, perhaps the most important outcome of his life-work, was that he alleviated the unhappy lot of the insane. Personal experience had made him a psychiatrist. One of his friends had gone mad, had run away into the woods, and had been devoured by wolves. In 1792, Pinel was appointed superintendent at Bicêtre. The conditions there were horrible. The patients were kept in chains, were treated worse than wild beasts. In 1788, Mirabeau had written a pamphlet describing the horrors that went on at Bicêtre. The sick, he said, had not even a doctor to look after them. "The new inmates are heedlessly flung into this wild rabble of lunatics, and any ragamuffin who comes along with a few sous in his pocket can be gratified by the sight of the menagerie." When the Revolution came, it brought freedom of a kind even for the insane. They, too, were entitled to the "Rights of Man." But the change for the better did not come of itself. Pinel had to work hard for his reforms. He went in person to the Convention, was able to make the deputies agree that the chains should be removed, and that henceforward the insane should be regarded and treated as ordinary invalids. He worked for many years to improve things, first at Bicêtre and subsequently at the Salpêtrière. What had been penitentiaries were transformed into hospitals.

In 1822 anti-clerical disturbances broke out at the Ecole de Médecine, which had once more become a faculty and was affiliated to the university of Paris. For a few months the faculty was closed. When it was reopened, some of the members of the professorial staff failed to secure reappointment. One of these was Pinel.

CHAPTER THIRTY-THREE

RENE THEOPHILE HYACINTHE LAENNEC
1781–1826

FRANÇOIS JOSEPH VICTOR BROUSSAIS
1772–1838

CORVISART'S work had made plain to every doctor the value of percussion in the recognition of diseases of the chest. It produced tones which threw much light upon the anatomical changes which were going on within the thorax. A doctor could "hear" the condition of this important region of the body. But were there not other sounds in the thorax, sounds spontaneously produced, and not artificially evoked as were percussion tones? If a man is suffering from severe bronchitis, we hear even at a distance the whistling made by the breath as it passes into and out of the bronchial tubes. By laying his ear against the chest, the doctor can hear a good deal more. The Hippocratists had long ago pointed out that certain sick people had strange noises going on in their chests. "It bubbles like boiling vinegar," and "It creaks like a new leather strap," they had said. Still, little use could be made of these perfectly accurate observations until doctors began to think anatomically. At length, in the nineteenth century, when on all hands efforts were being made to "see" into the interior of the living body in order to discern the anatomical changes that were going on when it was sick, such sounds acquired a new value. The doctor who applies his ear to the front of the chest hears the heart-sounds. In many illnesses, these heart-sounds were modified.

Laennec, one of Corvisart's pupils, was a pioneer in insisting upon the importance of listening to the heart-sounds. In 1816 he had been appointed physician-in-chief to the Hôpital Necker (hospital physicians needed no longer to wear a wig!); and, like his teacher, he was especially interested in diseases of the chest. He found, however, that there were great difficulties in direct auscultation. Among hospital patients, before they had been thoroughly cleaned up, it was apt to be very disagreeable to the doctor; and in obese women it gave unsatisfactory results. Laennec had under his care an exceedingly stout woman suffering from heart disease. Listen as he might, he could not hear the heart-sounds clearly. On his way to visit this patient, Laennec was passing through the courtyard of the Louvre. A heap of old timber was lying in one corner, and some children were playing there. They had discovered a new game. One of the pieces of wood was a long beam. A youngster had his ear at one end of it, and another was signalling by tapping the other end. This gave Laennec an idea. He quickened his steps, and, when he reached his patient asked for a quire of letter-paper. Having rolled this paper into a cylinder, he applied one end of it to the site of the cardiac impulse and listened at the other end. The result was marvellous. He could heart the heart-sounds much better, much more plainly, than with his ear on the chest. Moving his paper cylinder from place to place, he listened to the sounds that were forthcoming all over the heart. Then he listened to the breath-sounds. They were so loud that they startled him. The stethoscope had been discovered, the auditory tube which was to become symbolical of latter-day physicians as the urine-glass was of the medieval doctor. Indirect auscultation had replaced the direct method. A new process of physical examination had been revealed, a new means of access to the interior of the organism.

The next thing was to develop this new method. The doctor must ascertain the nature of the various sounds to be heard through the stethoscope, and what they respectively signified. The route was that which had been taken by Auenbrugger and Corvisart in the case of percussion: meticulous observation of living patients and checking of the results by autopsy. For three years Laennec worked strenuously, and at length, in 1819, published in two thick volumes his *Traité de l'auscultation médiate et des maladies des poumons et du cœur.* By now he was tired out, for he had never been robust. Relinquishing his labours for a time, he returned to his native province of Brittany, where he led a retired life for two years, reading classical authors and studying the Celtic tongues.

Laennec had the closest ties with Brittany. He was a pious Catholic and a fervent royalist. Born at Quimper, he grew to manhood in Nantes, living with an uncle who was a doctor. It was natural enough that young Laennec should enter the medical profession. Revolution and counter-revolution were raging in this part of the world. His uncle was called up for service, the lad went with him, and studied the elements of medicine and surgery practically, in the field. Then, in 1800, he went to Paris for formal instruction, was a distinguished student, and took his degree in 1804. The whole medical school was devoted to research, for the Revolution had made scientific investigation a part of professorial duty. The law which had called the Ecole de Santé into being demanded of the professors, "that they shall unceasingly endeavour by thorough investigations to perfect all the sciences which can contribute to the progress of the healing art." For the better attainment of this end there was established the Société de l'Ecole de Médecine de Paris, to which the teaching faculty and the more energetic among the younger men belonged. In 1820, this society was transformed into the Académie de Médecine. Laennec had from the first played an active part in the work of the society, especially in the fields of pathological anatomy and parasitology. In 1812 he was given a post at the Hôpital Beaujon; and two years later one at the Salpêtrière; until finally, as we have seen, he became physician-in-chief at the Hôpital Necker.

After his breakdown in health, Laennec stayed two years in Brittany, and by 1822 was sufficiently restored to come back to Paris. This same year he was appointed professor of practical medicine at the Collège de France, and a year later became clinical professor at the faculty. His book had secured a dubious reception. Many doctors failed to recognise the advantages of the new method; and there were not a few who dreaded that these physical methods of examination would lead to a mechanisation of the healing art, whereby true physicianship would be stifled. They failed to realise that what they were opposed to was no more than a modest beginning, that the century then opening was to create an arsenal of apparatus and instruments, with the result that morbid manifestations would come to be considered more and more objectively and would to an increasing degree be quantitatively recorded. Still, approving voices soon made themselves heard, and became increasingly frequent. Those who had grasped the value of percussion, could hardly fail to recognise that of auscultation. From all over the world doctors made their way to Paris to study the new method in the Charité under Laennec's guidance. No more than a few years, however, were vouchsafed to him in which to give this instruction. In 1826, just after publishing a second and enlarged edition of his book, he fell ill once more. He returned to Brittany, but this time the change of air worked no benefit, and ere long he died of pulmonary consumption, one of the diseases he had so carefully studied.

Laennec was something much more than the discoverer of auscultation. He was a distinguished anatomist and a great clinician. The invention of the stethoscope was remarkable, but even more remarkable was what he himself did with the instrument. His book is a milestone in the history of diseases of the chest, both those of the heart and those of the lungs. A new domain of special pathology had been opened. New conceptions of various maladies had been established, both clinically and anatomically. His book contained brilliant descriptions of diseases of the bronchial glands, of bronchiectasis, of emphysema, of pulmonary infarcts, of both gangrene and

286

oedema of the lungs, of the various stages of pneumonia, and of pulmonary consumption. The more closely doctors became acquainted with particular diseases and the more comprehensive the grasp of their mechanism, the more purposive, as the years went by, did treatment become. Obviously, the new pathological ideas could not take immediate effect in therapeutics, but Laennec always remained fully aware that the doctor's first duty is to promote the welfare of the patient, and he tried to do this by making use of the means which experience had shown to be the most effective.

Like Auenbrugger, Laennec had musical gifts. He was an instrumentalist as well as an amateur, being, we are told, an excellent performer on the flute.

Just as Pinel stands beside Corvisart, so does Broussais stand beside Laennec. These men formed complementary and contrasted pairs. The world of medicine in Paris was cloven in sunder in the second decade of the nineteenth century as well as in the first. Laennec and Broussais differed from one another even more noticeably than did Corvisart and Pinel. They derived from the same region of France, being both of them Bretons. Yet two men of more divergent type are hardly conceivable, were it only in externals. Laennec was of slender build, a man of phthinoid constitution; Broussais was a thick-set man of great stature. Laennec had a gentle utterance, and spoke very much to the point. Broussais was rhetorical, often thunderous. Laennec, as previously said, was a Catholic and a royalist. Broussais was a hard-shelled atheist, a son of the Revolution, a supporter of the Emperor, and an enemy of kings.

His education was rough and sketchy. When his father, a country practitioner, returned from his rounds, the youngster had to mount a horse and deliver the medicines. Becoming involved in the whirlpool of the Revolution, in 1792 he went to the front. After that, he studied medicine in the hospitals at St. Malo and Brest, and then served as naval surgeon against the English, sometimes in government vessels and sometimes in privateers. Returning home after one of these voyages, he found that both his parents had been killed by the royalists. A year earlier than Laennec, he went to Paris, working under Bichat, Corvisart, and more especially Pinel, whose adherent he became—to develop into a savage adversary in due course. Having taken his degree, he was appointed army surgeon, and played an enthusiastic part in the Napoleonic campaigns. These campaigns gave him plenty of experience. After the fall of Napoleon, he returned to Paris, and was appointed assistant professor at the military hospital of Val-de-Grâce.

His first book was published in 1808—a large work entitled *Histoire des phlegmasies ou inflammations chroniques*, in which he put forward some very original views. From 1816 onwards he produced a number of writings, under various titles, expounded the same doctrine (a pathology peculiar to himself), and carried on an active polemic against the dominant medical ideas. He was fiercely opposed to the conception of disease which had tended to become ever more firmly established since the seventeenth century, to the notion that it is a sharply characterised entity. Inasmuch as this same notion was being most clearly and energetically fathered by Pinel, it was natural that Pinel should be his chief target. Yet not Pinel alone, but also Corvisart, and all doctors of those days, were doing their utmost to differentiate and to describe diseases set apart one from another by their clinical course and their anatomical seats. "There are no such diseases," said Broussais bluntly. "They are but the products of a disordered imagination." There was no essential distinction between one malady and another. What determined the difference between particular diseases was nothing but the degree of excitation, stimulation, or irritation.

Of course there were pathological changes in the organs. In the opening decades of the nineteenth century, no one

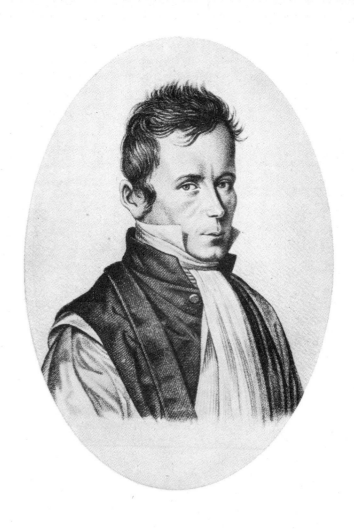

R. TH. H. LAENNEC, 1781–1826

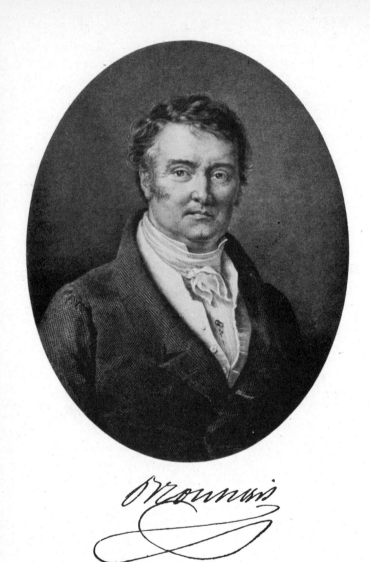

FRANÇOIS JOSEPH VICTOR BROUSSAIS, 1772–1838

could possibly deny that—Broussais least of all, since he had made a very large number of post-mortem examinations. The real question, however, was: Which is cause and which effect, which primary and which secondary? Tubercular and cancerous changes were only products of an inflammation. This inflammation was almost always the primary disease. Irritation gave rise to inflammation. It was local to begin with, but by "sympathy" the most widely separated organs could become affected. If, however, we made a sufficiently careful investigation to discover the original, the primitive seat of the inflammation, we should almost always find it in the gastro-intestinal canal. The disease of diseases was inflammation of the gastro-intestinal canal, gastro-enteritis, caused by irritation. All other maladies were subvarieties of this. In every case, therefore, treatment must be directed towards the stomach and the intestines. The remedies to be applied were diet and bleeding—leeches being especially useful. Since Broussais had a great number of disciples, the consumption of leeches increased so inordinately that within a few years the French sources were exhausted, and leeches had to be imported from abroad, chiefly from Bohemia and Hungary. In 1824, the number of leeches imported was 100,000; in 1827, it had increased to 33,000,000, to decline in 1828 to 25,000,000. Blood flowed forth in abundant streams. Broussais' opponents said that vampyrism had got control of the healing art.

Broussais propagated his doctrine under the designation of "physiological medicine." It need hardly be said that it was not accepted without a fight. Pinel was old, and was therefore little inclined for controversy. Laennec, however, in his lectures, crusaded against "the so-called physiological medicine." But Laennec's lectures were poorly attended. He was not a good speaker; and, being an invalid, he could speak only at long intervals. The students flocked by preference to hear Broussais, and to laugh at his sarcasms directed against the ontologists. During the struggle, there were some tragical incidents. A student, wishing to confirm the soundness of Broussais' doctrine that the syphilitic virus was a fable, inoculated himself in the arm with the fresh discharge from a syphilitic sore and acquired a typical hard chancre. Thereupon he was treated, in due accordance with Broussais' method, by remedies directed towards the gastro-intestinal canal, since the chancre, which was "no more than a local irritation," ought thereby to be dispelled. However, the expected result was not forthcoming, and the student had a severe attack of generalised syphilis. Shaken in his faith, and reduced to despair, he committed suicide.

In 1830, after the July revolution, Broussais was appointed professor of general pathology at the Academy of Medicine in Paris. But by now his popularity was on the wane. The views of Laennec, elaborated by able pupils of the inventor of the stethoscope, were continually gaining headway.

CHAPTER THIRTY-FOUR

KARL ROKITANSKY AND JOSEPH SKODA
1804–1878   1805–1881

THE work of Corvisart, Laennec, and their pupils had made the Parisian clinic world-famous. Everyone who wanted to study the new methods of clinical examination, everyone who wanted to learn the last achievements in pathological anatomy, hastened to Paris. "Thither came almost all the youth of the medical world. Nowhere are conditions more splendid, more multifarious than in Paris," wrote as early as 1841 Carl August Wunderlich, a young instructor in Tübingen. Twice he had visited Paris. But he had also been in Vienna, and had met able young scientists there. It was his impression that new life was blossoming in the Viennese faculty, for he wrote: "I believe I am entitled to regard as a new school this fresh trend of research in German medicine which, though originated by one man, has found zealous helpers, and which is impressive, not perhaps because of the number of its representatives, but because of their quality and the momentous character of their production. And I believe that I do wrong to no one when I style by the name of the young Viennese school the peculiarities of these able investigators, who, though each of them works in his own original way, display a quality which is unmistakably common to them all."

The old Viennese school, inaugurated by van Swieten's activities, had decayed by the turn of the century. Frank had departed in 1804. Stifft, the physician-in-ordinary to the court, was all-powerful. The importance of the faculty was continually on the decline. Joseph II had abolished Latin as the medium of instruction, but now it was re-introduced. The professors were subjected to a rigid censorship. It would have been futile to look for useful talent in Vienna. No doubt there were a few able men there, such as Kern, the surgeon who introduced the open treatment of wounds; or Boër the accoucheur; or Beer the ophthalmologist. Vienna was the first German-speaking university to establish a separate ophthalmic clinic, this being done in the year 1812. In 1818, the first professor of ophthalmics was appointed, and instruction in ophthalmics was declared obligatory. In 1805, when Frank's influence had not wholly evaporated, a special chair in medical jurisprudence and "medical police" had been founded. Still, as a school of medicine Vienna was, for the time being, outworn, and France unquestionably led the world in medical matters.

Now, however, in 1840, Wunderlich found a new school in course of formation at Vienna. Its creator was the pathological anatomist Karl Rokitansky. Let me quote once more from Wunderlich, who wrote when his impressions were recent: "It is only a few years since the extraordinary professor of pathological anatomy, Dr. Karl Rokitansky, began to publish occasional papers in the Austrian medical annals—essays contrasting strongly, not only in respect of form, trend, and contents, with most of those among which they appeared, but likewise with all others to which we have grown accustomed in Germany. With each new essay it became clearer that it was not merely the important observations which deserved attention (for these might have been made by any one who had had similar opportunities), but that a peculiar and logically consistent spirit breathed through these apparently dry articles, animating them, and lifting them far above the level of ordinary post-mortem reports. The essays followed one another in brief succession; they ran counter to many of the doctrines current at the time in Germany; and they were couched in an impressively original style which gave them convincing force. Setting forth from observations made at autopsies, they expanded to discuss general and pathological topics, and threw valuable light upon the indications for treatment. They did not remain isolated, being followed up by papers and books penned by other Viennese physicians, such as Kolletschka, Skoda, Helm, Schuh, and various younger authorities, who, writing in the same or in a similar sense and setting out from the same principles, dealt with the most diversified domains of medicine and achieved results such as had not been paralleled since the days of Laennec. Manifestly these writings proceeded from one source. However independent of one another the individual authors seemed, the reader could not fail to recognise in them an intellectual trend which must have been the outcome of their following a single example.

"In the Institute of Pathological Anatomy new life had been instilled since Rokitansky had come to work there. Doctors from foreign parts assembled year by year in greater numbers. Once more there was something to be learned in Vienna; once more there were things to be seen in Vienna which would be vainly sought elsewhere."

Rokitansky was born in Königsgratz in the year 1804; he studied in Prague and in Vienna; then, in the latter city, he had become Wagner's assistant in the Pathological Institute, and had in due course been appointed Wagner's successor. In 1844 he was made ordinary professor of pathological anatomy. Thanks to his work, the Pathological Institute became the centre of the faculty. Again I will quote Wunderlich: "Thither were sent the corpses of those who had died in the various wards of the General Hospital. . . . The post-mortem examinations were made . . . by the professor of pathological anatomy, to whom no more had been communicated than the diagnosis and a brief sketch of the clinical history. It might seem as if this arrangement would be undesirable, and in certain circumstances it doubtless would have been so. In the case we are now considering, it was almost exclusively for the best. . . . Whereas previously the work had been done too analytically, an endeavour being made to regard the series and groups of symptoms in their interconnection as a general picture and

293

to deduce their relationships with the actual findings, it had been forgotten that there was no secure or stable starting-point, but only fugitive, manifold, diversely interpretable phenomena. Instead of this, Rokitansky followed the opposite course. He made his post-mortem, recorded the results, and then worked backwards, asking himself: 'How could what I found have been brought about? What different physical and physiological possibilities could have produced the alterations which the body displays?' Inasmuch as he weighed these possibilities against one another, he was able in the end to arrive at a probability—and that is what we always have to content ourselves with in the art and science of medicine. . . . Many conditions were requisite if this method were to prove successful; and if in previous attempts such success had been lacking, no doubt the reason was because the requisite conditions were wanting. Widespread experience in the field of pathological anatomy must be the foundation, unless the whole procedure is to eventuate in deception. The Viennese Pathological Institute no longer numbers its post-mortem examinations by the hundred, and Rokitansky can refer to the records of thousands of autopsies in the case of many of the particular diseases. I do not believe that any other pathological institute in the world can vie with Vienna in respect of these numbers. But numbers alone would count for nothing were it not for the comprehensive views, the inborn and well-trained faculties of the observer. We have but to read one of Rokitansky's post-mortem reports in order to be filled with respect for the way in which he regards matters. This plastic, descriptive language; this definiteness of expression; the vividness of all his words—these things guarantee the accuracy of his statements. . . . The application of mechanical and physiological laws demands still higher faculties, unless it is to be utterly vain and futile. . . . The most important condition, however, is that the investigator should be able to formulate the problems of pathology and therapeutics accurately and

294

clearly, and should approach them from the clinical outlook. Now, there are numerous indications in Rokitansky's writings to disclose his mastery in this respect, although we have to admit that much is still to be expected from the future. All the same, the road has been opened up, the method has been disclosed, its practicability has been proved, and the importance and soundness of the results hitherto achieved is incontestable."

Let us inquire into the causes of the advance which the Viennese school made upon that of Paris, and wherein lies the main difference in the working methods of the two. In France, pathological anatomy was mainly carried on by the clinicians themselves. Corvisart, Laennec, and the rest of them, either did the post-mortem examinations with their own hands or had them performed by their assistants. The material available to any one of them was restricted. In the Hôpital Necker there were one hundred beds, and in the Charité no more than forty. In Vienna, on the other hand, there had taken place a division of labour between the clinicians and the pathological anatomists. Pathological anatomy had become an independent discipline. Centralisation came to be regarded as of enormous importance. The bodies of all those who died in the huge General Hospital at Vienna passed through Rokitansky's hands. He had command of an unparalleled amount of material for pathological study. The specialisation of research, which was in due time to become so characteristic of German-speaking medicine and was to yield such a rich harvest, began in Vienna.

Rokitansky elaborated his observations for publication in a three-volume work, which appeared during the years 1842–1846. Morgagni's book had been compiled exclusively from a clinical standpoint. It was natural, too, that French works of the kind, written for the most part by clinicians, should take a mainly or exclusively clinical view. Not until 1829 did a Strasburg pathologist, Lobstein by name, the first professor of pathological anatomy in France, publishing his *Traité d'anatomie pathologique*, adopt, as pioneer, a classification of his material from anatomical outlooks. Rokitansky followed this example. His *Handbuch der pathologischen Anatomie* attracted widespread attention. Virchow, who was not in most respects kindly in his attitude towards Rokitansky, wrote at the close of the nineteenth century that the latter's *Handbuch* had from the outset shown itself the best of all manuals on this topic, and had served as the true foundation of practical medicine. "We may without circumlocution describe it as the finest blossom of 'organicism,' not only because of the masterly achievements of descriptive natural science side by side with the vividness and precision of the description of the diseases of the individual organs, but also because of the abundance and accuracy of the personal observations it contains. Down to the present day it has remained unrivalled."

Rokitansky, however, did not limit himself to the description of what he actually saw, for he transcended the limits of anatomy. In a great many diseases the anatomical conditions found on post-mortem examination were so trivial that they failed to explain the severity of the illness. Obviously, then, in addition to localised maladies of the organs, there must be generalised diseases. Rokitansky was too much the anatomist not to seek a local habitat for these diseases. Their habitat must be the blood, the only tissue which is universally present in the body—a tissue just as much as muscular tissue or nervous tissue, although the intercellular substance of the blood is fluid. Thus Rokitansky was brought back into the domain of the old humoral pathology, and he tried, by means of his doctrine of "crasis," to combine the teachings of humoral pathology with anatomical views. He called in chemistry to his aid. The blood contains fibrin and albumin. Morbid changes in these, caused especially by oxidation, gave rise to a crasis, a pathological condition. But a general disease had a tendency to localise itself. Thus diseases of the organs resulted from a dyscrasia. Nevertheless, the converse was possible. An organ

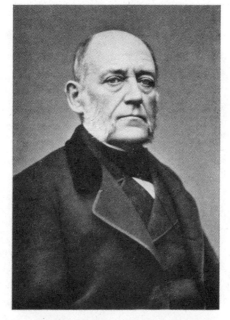

KARL ROKITANSKY, 1804–1878

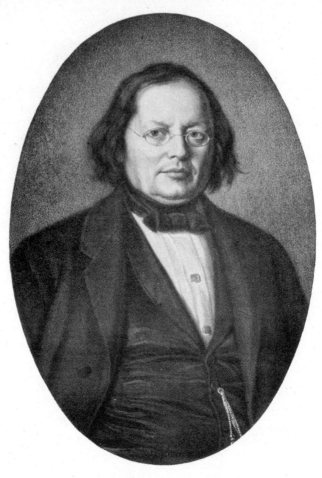

JOSEPH SKODA, 1805–1881

might be primarily diseased, and, as a sequel, a generalised malady might arise.

The doctrine of crasis was erroneous and could not be maintained because its chemical presuppositions were unsound. Here Rokitansky had left the field of observation and had wandered off into speculation. Virchow, who greatly admired those parts of the *Handbuch* which dealt with Rokitansky's direct observations, subjected the doctrine of crasis to ruthless criticism.

In 1875, Rokitansky retired from active work. Let me quote a passage from his farewell address: "Actuated by one of the most urgent needs of the day, I devoted myself to pathological anatomy as a branch of investigation likely to prove fruitful to clinical medicine, and was able, on German soil, to give it so much importance that it became possible to describe it as the true foundation of a pathological physiology and as the fundamental method of natural research in the domain of medicine."

Virchow's *Cellularpathologie* had been published in 1858. Rokitansky's star had paled before the rising sun of Virchow. Still, we must never forget that we owe to Rokitansky a large proportion of our present pathologico-anatomical knowledge. The observations he made speedily became general property, and were no longer labelled with his name. Furthermore his doctrine of crasis, erroneous though it was in many respects, contained a kernel of truth, as latter-day chemistry and serology have shown.

Next to Rokitansky, Joseph Skoda was the centre of attraction of the new Viennese school. Among Skoda's audience, writes Wunderlich, were "professors, imperial councillors, and practitioners of long standing, animated with an eager determination to learn the mysteries of auscultation and percussion." Skoda found it difficult to rise to eminence in his profession. He was born in poor circumstances, his father being a locksmith at Pilsen. One of his brothers also became a locksmith, taking over the paternal workshop, and developing it into one of the largest industrial undertakings in Austria, the Skoda Works. Another brother became a doctor; and young Joseph, likewise, wished to enter the medical profession. At this time, however, the family was very short of money, so that he nearly took the monastic habit. Then, when some one was found kind enough to advance a little money, Skoda went on foot to Vienna and began his medical studies there. He eked out a livelihood by giving private lessons, acquiring in the process a mastery of mathematics and physics, for which he had a talent, so that his chiefs strongly advised him to specialise in these subjects. However, he stuck to his preference, took his degree in 1831, went to Bohemia to help in the fight against cholera, and then returned to Vienna to work as unsalaried assistant physician at the General Hospital.

Skoda was acquainted with the recent medical literature of France, and had read much about percussion and auscultation. There was no one in Vienna who could give him practical instruction in these subjects, so he was self-taught in the new methods of investigation. The reader will readily understand that he had to cope with enormous difficulties. The timbre of the various percussion tones and that of the sounds heard on auscultation can scarcely be described in words. But it was these very difficulties which gave an impetus to Skoda's work. They compelled him to study the wide domains of percussion and auscultation from the first elements. He had to follow anew the long road which had been travelled since the days of Auenbrugger. He percussed, he auscultated, and then went to watch Rokitansky's post-mortem examinations. Being a skilled physicist, he tried to reproduce percussion tones and auscultation sounds experimentally, outside the body, with the aid of apparatus. The French had worked empirically. They had heard a great deal, and had with the utmost conscientiousness recorded the sounds associated with particular diseases. Skoda, on the other hand, inquired into the physical causes of every sound. The French had used similes to describe much of what they heard, speaking of a "cracked-pot" sound (bruit de pot fêlé), of a "purring" sound, and so on—vividly descriptive, no doubt, but not altogether scientific. Skoda's endeavour was to discover lucid physical terms.

In this way he was enabled to plumb the depths of physical diagnosis, and to render it far more objective. Before his day, auscultation and percussion had been methods that were only at the disposal of those capable of a considerable measure of imaginative insight. When Skoda had made the physical causes of the phenomena clear, however, it was much easier both to teach and to learn the new methods. A clarified terminology promoted clearer understanding.

Laennec's interest had been centred upon diseases of the lungs. Skoda, on the other hand, devoted himself above all to auscultation of the heart. He made a thorough study of the cardiac impulse, and of the origin of the heart-sounds, striving to localise them with anatomical precision, and distinguishing sharply between a normal heart-sound and a murmur or bruit.

Additional difficulties arose in his path. The patients complained of the doctor who worried them so much with percussion and auscultation, who was continually "mauling them about," so, one fine day, Skoda was transferred to the department for mental disorders. However, he continued his experimental work in the mental ward, and, on the quiet, was also allowed to pursue his investigations concerning diseases of the chest. At length, in 1839, appeared his monograph, his opus magnum, *Abhandlung über Perkussion und Auskultation*, which ran through numerous editions, and constitutes the foundation of modern physical diagnosis.

Once more, however, there happened in this case what we have seen so often before, namely that an epoch-making book was at first misunderstood, nay ridiculed. Hildebrand, Skoda's chief, who regarded himself as endowed with musical talent, declared that he had never been able to hear a pneumonia play the fiddle!

Meanwhile Skoda had been engaged in general practice, and, in the year of the publication of his great work, had accepted a position as parish doctor. His merits, however, were attracting wider attention, and he was becoming renowned for his successful diagnoses. The upshot was that in 1840 he was put in charge of one of the wards for diseases of the chest at the General Hospital, that he might have more extensive opportunities for studying the diagnosis and treatment of these maladies. A year later, he became physician to the hospital, being thus enabled to continue his scientific investigations upon a broader basis, and being likewise provided with extensive opportunities for imparting instruction. In fact, however, far more of those who came to learn from him were physicians already established in practice than young students. Wunderlich gives a vivid account of the contrast between the enthusiasm of the French students for their teachers and the indifference of the Viennese students to the splendid achievements that were going on under their eyes. "Apart from a few exceptions, we note everywhere in Vienna a phlegmatic coldness, a dull schoolboy-like acceptance, a clinging to the letter and a forgetfulness of the spirit, a trust in the traditional. Especially disagreeable in this respect is the impression produced by the lukewarmness of the assistant physicians at the hospitals."

In 1846, Skoda was appointed professor of clinical medicine.

As regards treatment, Skoda was extremely sceptical. His gorge rose against the stimulant or irritant treatment of the apostles of the Brunonian system, which still had a considerable vogue, and against the ferocious leechings of Broussais and his followers. Besides, investigators of Skoda's stamp, whose attempt always is to attain precision, are necessarily at a loss as far as treatment is concerned, since treatment can never be exact. Their therapeutics, naturally, were expectant; that is to say they inclined to let illness run its course, being content to put their patients under the best possible conditions as regards repose, diet, etc. There is justification for the reproach of therapeutic nihilism which has been levelled against the Viennese school. Throughout, Skoda was mainly interested in diagnosis, and Wunderlich characterises the man aptly when he writes: "Skoda's method, in each concrete case, of unriddling and trying to interpret the physical signs left nothing to be desired. His exceptionally wide knowledge of pathological anatomy and his profound acquaintance with physics were the most valuable aids to his insight, . . . and it was by the method of exclusion and by a calculus of probabilities that he arrived at his definitive diagnosis."

Anatomical concepts, scientific medicine, had found a fostering site in Vienna as never before on German soil. Rokitansky and Skoda were attended by a phalanx of men who collaborated with them in full acceptance of their outlooks. In 1841, Franz Schuh was put in charge of the second surgical clinic. He applied the new methods of physical diagnosis to surgery, thus becoming enabled to determine the seat of exudations, abscesses, internal tumours, etc. He was the first to aspirate the pericardium; and in 1847 was the first German surgeon to anaesthetise a patient with ether. Another of Skoda's pupils, Ferdinand Hebra, was the founder of pathologico-anatomical dermatology. Unlike Skoda, however, he was by no means a therapeutic nihilist, but did marvels in improving the treatment of diseases of the skin. I may also mention Oppolzer, the clinician; Hyrtl, the brilliant anatomist, whose *Text-book of Anatomy* ran through two-and-twenty editions; Brücke, the physiologist; Mauthner, the specialist in diseases of children; Türck, the neurologist; and Ernst von Feuchtersleben, dean of the medical faculty in Vienna, who, though he died at the age of forty-three, was renowned as statesman, poet, and philosopher as well as physician. Thus in the middle decades of the nineteenth century there was a widespread feeling that no European doctor's education was complete unless he had spent a considerable period of study in Vienna.

CHAPTER THIRTY-FIVE

JOHANNES MÜLLER (1801–1858)
AND
JOHANN LUKAS SCHÖNLEIN (1793–1864)

IN France the Enlightenment led to the Revolution. Reason had been deified. Napoleon, as banner-bearer of the Revolution, tried to conquer the world. Although, after Napoleon's fall, there were relapses, on the whole the French intelligentsia kept its intelligence riveted upon the real. In 1830, Auguste Comte began the publication of his *Cours de philosophie positive*.

Very different were conditions in Germany. Doubtless in the eighteenth century the influence of French thought upon Germany had been considerable, but this same century also witnessed the blossoming of German classical literature. The Napoleonic era brought distress and poverty, and in 1807, with the Peace of Tilsit, profound humiliation. On December 5, 1811, Jerome, King of Westphalia, wrote to Emperor Napoleon: "Should war break out, all the territories between the Rhine and the Oder will become the scene of a widespread and energetic rising. The main cause of this dangerous movement is something more than hatred of the French and embitterment on account of a foreign yoke; it lies, rather, in the unhappy circumstances of the time, in the utter ruin of all classes, in the enormous pressure of taxation, in military expenditure, the cost of maintaining armies, in the marching to and fro of troops, and repeated, long-lasting vexations of every possible kind. . . . In Hanover, Magdeburg, and the chief towns of my own kingdom of Westphalia, house-owners are abandoning their houses and are vainly trying to sell them at a ruinous sacrifice. . . . Everywhere families are in poverty; capital is exhausted; nobles, peasants and townsmen are

303

heavily burdened with debt and in actual want. . . . What we have to dread is the despair of those who have no more to lose because everything has been taken from them."

In this time of extreme poverty, a wave of idealism swept across the population. The university of Berlin was founded in the year 1810. The foreign yoke was shaken off during the Wars of Liberation. The Germans freed themselves from French influence, and concentrated their attention upon their own people and their own path. *Des Knaben Wunderhorn* was published in the year 1806. People turned away from the materialism of the Enlightenment, fleeing from the actualities of life to the realm of imagination, discovering beauties where they had hitherto been unsuspected. Gothic architecture, the Middle Ages in general, were regarded in a new light, and aroused fresh admiration. The East was discovered. Schlegel found the key to unlock the literature of Hindustan. Baron vom Stein founded the society for the production of the splendid edifice known as the *Monumenta Germaniae Historica*. Romanticism was the order of the day.

The Romantic Movement was not exclusively an affair of the poets or other imaginative writers. It was to an even greater extent a movement of men of learning, among whom physicians and naturalists played a decisive part. The motive force came from Schelling, whose *Ideen zu einer Philosophie der Natur* had been published in 1797. Spirit and matter were one. The real and the ideal were identical, were the conjoint foundation of being. Spirit and nature were two aspects, two stages. Nature was the antecedent phase to spirit. Issuing from matter, the real perfected itself in the human organism; and proceeding from the ego, the ideal perfected itself in artistic production. Mind and matter were identical. This being so, the laws of nature must be capable of direct demonstration in consciousness, and consciousness in its turn must manifest itself in objective nature as natural law. The phenomena of nature and the laws of nature could therefore be discovered

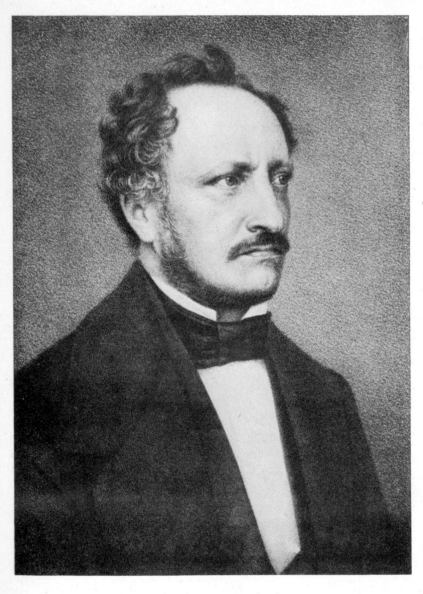

JOHANNES MÜLLER

speculatively by means of rational considerations. Matter had three dimensions. Corresponding with these there were in nature three fundamental energies, electrical, magnetic, and chemical; and in the organism there were to be discerned irritability, sensibility, and the urge to reproduction. Illness was nothing other than a lower developmental phase of life.

Manifestly under such auspices the healing art would necessarily undergo a different course of development in Germany from that which it had taken in France. Whereas in France most investigators, renouncing any attempt at completeness, were satisfied with the gathering of empirical knowledge, in Germany, at the same date, the aim was always at the whole, at totality. Numberless books were written and numberless systems were sought out. They originated, not at the bedside of the sick, but in the study. They purposed to explain everything. Although many of them were ingenious, and some of them contained valuable intimations, their use to medical science was, in the end, small.

Every possible fashion and trend found a suitable soil in Germany. There was not one scientific discovery of prime importance which did not lead to the formation of a system or of systems—electricity, for instance, magnetism, oxygen. The Brunonian system, the theory of excitation, found numberless adherents, and dominated therapeutics for a long time. It was carried a stage farther by Röschlaub, who insisted upon the part played by the vital reactions as against stimuli from without, and who formulated his doctrine in thirty theses. In the domain of medicine as in others, the Germans looked back into their own past, and discovered Paracelsus. A Rhenish doctor, Rademacher, elaborated Paracelsus' teaching into a system which he called "experiential medicine." In 1808 was published the *Organon der rationellen Heilkunde*, by Samuel Hahnemann, the founder of homoeopathy. Hahnemann regarded disease as a disorder of the vital force, which he contemplated as purely spiritual. A doctor, he said, should not concern himself about the nature of illness, but only about its cure. Maladies would be cured by administering in minute or infinitesimal doses those substances which in large doses were capable of provoking similar symptoms. Naturally, too, Franz Joseph Gall's craniological views secured extensive support. Their underlying idea was that which we now term cerebral localisation. Human qualities, said Gall, were localised in different parts of the brain, and this localisation must be manifest in the formation of the skull. Thus originated the doctrine of phrenology, associated with the names of Gall and Spurzheim.

In every one of these multifarious systems there was a kernel of truth. They all contained fruitful ideas. The trouble with them was that their founders, generalising to excess, overshot the mark. The result was that during the first decade of the nineteenth century German medicine was in a hopelessly confused state. There were men of talent in various parts of the country, writing brilliant books concerning God, nature, and human beings; but they and their works did little to promote a knowledge of disease and its cure. Above all the methodology of these writers was defective. They were trying to solve the problems of the healing art, not by observation and experiment, but by speculation. Useful as it is from time to time to elaborate intellectually the mass of isolated observations, necessary as it is again and again to reconsider fundamentals, indispensable as it it in medicine no less than in other departments of knowledge to permeate or environ the data of observation with a philosophical atmosphere—grave dangers obviously arise when a whole generation does nothing else than this. While the French were formulating anatomical conceptions of disease and were developing the methods of physical diagnosis, German doctors were speculating about general topics.

Yet even in Germany a day came when thinkers and observers turned away from natural philosophy to natural science, from the idealist contemplation of nature to the mechanist explanation of nature. As far as medicine is concerned, two men, above all, must be regarded as the originators of this movement: Johannes Müller upon the theoretical plane; and Johann Lukas Schönlein upon the practical. Both of them in youth were immersed in abstract natural philosophy, but they both found a way out of the maze, thus becoming of noteworthy importance to the development of German medicine.

In a commemorative address on Johannes Müller, Virchow said: "Thus he himself became, as he had remarked of his great predecessors, a priest of nature. The cult which he served bound his pupils to him in close ties, as if by a religious bond; and the serious, priestly fashion of his speech and movements completed the veneration with which everyone regarded him. His mouth, with its tightly compressed lips conveyed a notion of severity; around eyes and forehead played an expression of profound thought; every furrow in his face stimulated the idea of a perfectly finished work—thus did this man stand before the altar of nature, freed by his own energy from the fetters of education and tradition, a living witness to personal independence!" The reader need only look at his portrait to gain confirmation of Virchow's striking description.

Johannes Müller was an exceedingly voluminous writer, and his works were widely diversified. He was no less interested in zoology, comparative anatomy, palaeontology, and embryology than in physiology and pathology. He did not make original discoveries of primary importance in any of these fields, but whatever subject he touched was given by him an added depth. Even though the better part of his achievements belong to the domain of pure science, he finds a place among great doctors, not only on account of his *Handbuch der Physiologie des Menschen*, but also because of the influence he exerted upon scientific medicine throughout Germany. It was he more than any other who trained German doctors to think in terms of natural science. His methods were the example they followed, and his Institute was the originating centre for a brilliant period in German medicine. Schwann, the founder of the cell-theory, was trained in his laboratory. There, likewise, Henle received decisive impressions. Müller's physical trend found noted representatives in his pupils Helmholtz, Du Bois-Reymond, and Brücke; his pathological trend in Mekel, Traube, and pre-eminently in Virchow.

Johannes Müller was a Rhinelander. The son of a Coblenz shoemaker, he was born when that town was invested by the French. He hesitated for a long time whether to become a priest or a doctor. It is not unlikely that his decision in favour of a medical career may have been influenced by Goethe, whose writings he read with great enthusiasm, and which perpetually directed him towards concrete nature and away from abstract thought. In 1819 he entered as a medical student in Bonn. He became a member of the Burschenschaft (the German Students' Association, which had been founded in 1815 for patriotic purposes), but he had scant interest in politics, and restricted his activities more and more to scientific fields. He was especially attracted by anatomy. "What does not come under the knife, counts for nothing." Natural philosophy rather than natural science was dominant at Bonn in his student days, and had there an outstanding representative in Nees van Esenbeck. Müller, like the rest, fell under the sway of Schelling's ideas, but he also studied Aristotle. As anatomy fettered his interest more and more, this extremely concrete and practical science formed a counterpoise to idealism, and kept his feet planted upon the solid earth despite the longing of his intelligence to soar into the depths of space. In 1823, Müller wrote a prize essay upon the respiration of the foetus. Having taken his degree at Bonn, he removed to Berlin in order to pass his State examination there. In Berlin he made the acquaintance of Rudolphi the physiologist, who influenced him strongly. Rudolphi was a sceptic who had scant respect for natural philosophy [the reader must remember that this term is used in the German sense, as opposed to natural science], and was continually insisting that anatomy was the prime foundation of medicine. Returning to Bonn in the year 1824, Müller gradually climbed the academic ladder, becoming in 1830 an ordinary professor there, and three years later succeeding Rudolphi in Berlin. He lectured on anatomy, physiology, and pathology, all three subjects being still combined. Not till after Müller's death were separate chairs established. While in Bonn, Müller had made a thorough study of the nervous system and the sense organs. He published a comparative physiology of vision, a work in which he discussed the mechanism of sensation and its relation to mental activity. Bell's doctrine, according to which the anterior roots of the spinal nerves consist of centrifugal fibres and the posterior roots of centripetal fibres, was so thoroughly confirmed by his experiments that thenceforward it secured universal recognition. The doctrine of reflex action was further unfolded by him, and he studied the intimate structure and the development of the glands. Embryological investigations occupied a great deal of Müller's time. His treatise upon the embryology of the genital organs has become a classic.

In 1833 appeared the first volume of his *Manual of Human Physiology*, a work under which several generations of students were trained in that science. It incorporated the important advances made in this domain since Haller's *Elementa physiologiae*. In the interim, anatomy, physics, and chemistry had made enormous strides forward. Oxygen had been discovered. Lavoisier had recognised the nature of oxidation, and had lifted chemistry from the ranks of a purely qualitative to that of a quantitative science. Necessarily these advances took effect upon physiology. More especially, however, was the new handbook distinguished by its method. As far as Germany was concerned, it denoted a turning away from natural philosophy and towards observation and experiment.

Müller also did original work in the field of pathological anatomy. His importance here lay, not so much in the field of actual achievement, as in this, that he was one of the first to insist upon the need for the use of the microscope in pathological study. Bichat had worked without a microscope, and his classification of the tissues had been based upon naked-eye appearances. Obviously we can see far more deeply into the structure of the tissues with the aid of the microscope. Müller tried in this way to formulate a new histological classification of tumours. He described unfamiliar forms of tumours in the cartilages and bones. His researches in this field, however, were soon to be superseded by those of Virchow.

In the domain of chemistry, Müller's investigations concerning the composition of the blood and his discovery of chondrin deserve special mention. One of the finest of his physiological achievements during his days at Berlin was his study of the way in which the tones of the voice are produced in the larynx. In the later years of his life, Johannes Müller was mainly interested in comparative anatomy. Almost every year he went to the seaside, not merely for change of air, but to study marine animals. It was thanks to him that amphioxus became the paradigmatic creature which it remains for youthful students of biology to-day. Müller researches concerning starfish, sea-cucumbers, concerning fishes in general and sharks in particular, and concerning the alternation of generations in the animal world, occupied an outstanding place in the history of zoology and comparative anatomy.

Two events threw a cloud over his declining years. The first of these was the revolution of 1848, which took place when he was rector of the university of Berlin. Müller was entirely unsympathetic towards this movement. By tradition he was a conservative, and he had no interest in politics. The disturbances and the ensuing changes disturbed him at his studies, and compelled him to take a side. He suffered both mentally and physically, and needed a long while to recover. Then, in the year 1855, he went to Norway in pursuit of his researches. On the return journey, his ship was sunk in a collision. His assistant, who was travelling with him, was drowned, and Müller himself was only rescued with great difficulty. By this tragedy his health was greatly affected for the worse, and he grew melancholy. Two or three years afterwards, he died suddenly.

Du Bois-Reymond, calculating Johannes Müller's literary output, declared that it amounted to over 15,000 printed pages and about 350 plates drawn by his own hand—so that, during seven-and-thirty years of his active life, Müller produced every seven weeks matter amounting to 35 printed pages and 0·83 plates. Johann Lukas Schönlein penned, over and above his dissertations, only two works, one of which extended to three pages and the other to one page. None the less he exerted a far-reaching influence, dependent, like that of Johannes Müller, upon his method.

Like Johannes Müller, Schönlein sprang from a Roman Catholic working-class family. His father was a master rope-maker, and the first idea in the family was that Johann Lukas should follow his father's trade. In the end it was decided to allow him to become a student, and in 1811 he was sent to Landshut, then an acropolis of natural philosophy. [Let us emphasise once more that this term is used in the German sense, as contrasted with natural science.] In 1800, under stress of the Napoleonic wars, the university of Ingolstädt had been removed to Landshut. In 1802, Röschlaub was summoned to Landshut, and presided thenceforward over the curriculum. Schelling had been made doctor "honoris causae" at Landshut. It was there that Schönlein received the decisive impressions of youth. Besides the natural philosophers, Tiedemann, summoned from Würzburg in 1805, was working at Landshut, a man of science round whom the current of natural philosophy flowed without influencing him, as a river flows round a rock.

Schönlein attended Tiedemann's lectures as well as those of the disciples of Schelling, and was moulded by Tiedemann hardly less than by the others.

Then, in 1813, Schönlein removed to Würzburg where exceptionally good opportunities of medical education were offered by the Julius Hospital. There, likewise, "natural philosophy" was dominant, Schelling himself having been a professor at the place. Still, at Würzburg there were some of the professors—for instance Döllinger, the anatomist and physiologist—who had escaped this mystical trend. Döllinger had distinguished pupils: Karl Ernst von Baer, the embryologist and discoverer of the human ovum; Pander, the anatomist, who likewise made important embryological discoveries; and Johann Lukas Schönlein.

Taking his degree in 1816 with a dissertation upon the metamorphoses of the brain, in the following year Schönlein was appointed instructor at Würzburg, and three years afterwards was provisionally made chief of the clinic, while in 1824 his appointment became definitive in conjunction with the ordinary professorship of special pathology and therapeutics. He had notable colleagues in the Würzburg faculty, of whom I need mention only two: Textor, who was surgeon at the hospital, and d'Outrepont, who was accoucheur.

Schönlein's claim to historical significance lies in the fact that he was the first to establish in Germany (at Würzburg) a clinic in the new sense; a clinic at which the new diagnostic methods of auscultation and percussion were practised; one where the bodies of deceased patients were subjected to postmortem examination, and where the diagnosis was checked by the result of the autopsy.

Political happenings drove Schönlein from Würzburg. In contrast with Johannes Müller, he was a liberal. Although he never took any very active part in politics, his opinions were generally known. In 1832, two years after the July revolution, he was dismissed from his professorial position, and

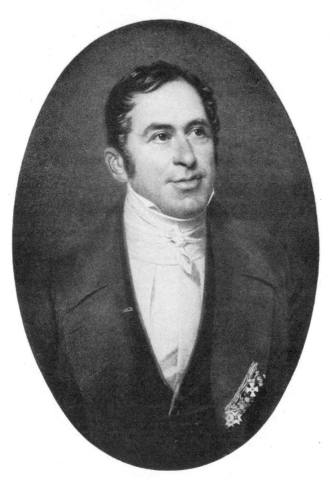

JOHANN LUKAS SCHÖNLEIN, 1793–1864

was offered the post of district doctor at Passau. He preferred to retire from the public service. Political conditions grew more aggravated. After the abortive rising in Frankfort-on-the-Main he was arrested with other liberals. Then a summons to the recently established medical faculty at Zurich opened to him a new field of activity. He felt happy "to breathe the free air of the Alps," saying: "What can be compared with this pleasure?" He wrote: "The hospital is large and well supplied with funds, but stands in need of more extensive changes rendered possible by the political reformation. All parties are agreed upon this matter, so that I do not expect to encounter any serious obstacles. The signs of respect and confidence received from persons of all shades of political opinion are most encouraging, and form a marked contrast to the brutality with which I was treated in Bavaria."

In Zurich, Schönlein was able to carry on his clinical instruction with great success. Pupils flocked to him from near and from far. It was here, too, that he wrote his only two scientific papers, one of which dealt with typhoid crystals, while the other announced an equally important scientific discovery. An Italian observer, Agostino Bassi, had discovered that the silkworm disease known as muscardine was caused by a filiform vegetable parasite which grew in the tissues of the caterpillar. Was it not possible that certain human maladies were caused by similar parasites? Schönlein studied a human skin disease, favus, a malady affecting the hairy scalp, and found that this was indeed caused by a filiform parasite, belonging to the order now known as hyphomycetes—an organism subsequently named, after its discoverer, Achorion Schönleinii. We shall learn in a subsequent chapter how enormous was the importance of this discovery for our conception of the infectious diseases.

Schönlein's practice in Zurich was also extremely gratifying. He wrote about it in a letter: "Furthermore, Zurich is the veritable Golconda of the physician. Day after day, at home or in the Falcon Hotel, I am consulted by foreigners of all nations and by travellers of princely rank, so that my wife is again and again astonished when, at night, I show her the gold pieces with which my pockets are stuffed!" Schönlein's intelligence and wit, which latter was at times a trifle coarse, made him well liked, and served as spice to his lectures. Even to-day, after the lapse of a hundred years, many anecdotes about him are current in Zurich. To give one example, a pupil relates how Schönlein at the clinic said: "You see here a patient who provides sugar, and there another who provides milk. We only want one to furnish us with coffee, and we could start a coffee-house in the clinic!"

His professional reputation increased from year to year. He was invited to become professor at Berne, and was also offered a position as physician-in-ordinary at the court of Brussels. He rejected both invitations. When, however, Prussia sent him a call, asking him to become head of the Berlin clinic, he agreed. The fact was he had always regarded himself as a foreigner in the Swiss environment. He began his work in Berlin at Easter 1840, lecturing in German, though hitherto instruction in the clinic had still been given in Latin. It was he who introduced auscultation, percussion, the use of the microscope, and laboratory methods at the Berlin clinic, and his teaching activities there were extremely fruitful. Even now he wrote nothing. Many of his clinical lectures were published, but these had been recorded by his students.

Schönlein spoke of his school, as contrasted with the natural-philosophical school, as the natural-historical. "We return to those foundations, to those pillars, from which medicine started. Our aim is to read the book of nature, to exemplify a natural-historical trend. The natural sciences are to serve as our guides, and to show how observations must be made in order to gather experience and to elaborate this into facts." Thus he regarded method as of fundamental importance.

Method was what counted. Here was a modest beginning.

Schönlein's clinic was not one out of which vastly important new knowledge could derive, as had been the clinics of Corvisart, Laennec, and Skoda. Only a method was practised and taught; but it was a sound method, the method which was to lead even German clinical medicine away from natural philosophy to natural science, and was thus to enable the Germans, ere long, to overtake and outstrip the investigators of other lands.

In Berlin, no less than elsewhere, Schönlein had to suffer under occasional onslaughts. The ultramontanes of Munich attacked him. Wunderlich criticised his scientific views. He became affected with a goitre, which interfered with his speech, so that in 1859, a year after Johannes Müller's death, he retired to spend his last days in his native town of Bamberg.

Johannes Müller and Schönlein laid the foundations upon which the Berlinese school was to be upbuilded. After their almost simultaneous departure, a new generation rose to the leading position. We shall soon study these men at their work.

CHAPTER THIRTY-SIX

CLAUDE BERNARD
1813–1878

I⊤ is the fate of medical books to age quickly, but there are exceptions. If in contemporary Paris we examine the book-sellers' windows in the neighbourhood of the École de Médecine we shall find exposed for sale a work whose first edition was published in the year 1865. This is Claude Bernard's *Intro-duction à l'étude de la médecine expérimentale.* "Never," wrote Pasteur a year after it was issued, "has anything clearer, more complete, more profound been written about the true principles of the difficult art of experiment. The book is as yet little known because it stands at a level which is so far attain-able only by a few." In due course, however, it became widely known. It has been reprinted again and ever again; it is bought and eagerly studied down to our own day.

When the *Introduction* appeared, Claude Bernard was at the climax of his career. He was professor of physiology at the university of Paris, where a chair for him had been specially established. Simultaneously he was professor at the Collège de France as successor to his teacher Magendie. The aforesaid book opened for him the doors of the Académie Française, so that he received the highest honours obtainable by a French man of learning.

Claude Bernard was a Burgundian, the son of a vine-grower. He was sent in early youth to Lyons as an apothecary's appren-tice. There he began to write plays: a comedy, which had a fair success in a small theatre; and then a tragedy, with which he wanted to try his fortune in Paris. Provided with letters of introduction, he made his way to the capital. Certain art critics read his piece, and advised him to study medicine in preference to becoming a playwright. The upshot was that the apothecary's apprentice became, not a famous imaginative writer, but, to begin with, a student of medicine. Magendie took Bernard as assistant at the Hôtel-Dieu and soon afterwards as demonstrator at the Collège de France.

Until the rise of Magendie, French physiology had been entirely dominated by the views of Bichat, and had thus become strongly vitalistic. Magendie initiated a trend towards positivism. There was, he declared, no such thing as vital force. The aim of physiology must be to discover the laws of what were called vital manifestations, and these laws were identical with those which can be observed in the inorganic world. The only possible method of investigation was experiment. So much did Magendie dread speculation, that he was often afraid of elaborating the results of his own experiments.

It was in this rigidly experimental school that Claude Bernard grew up. He took his degree in the year 1843, when already thirty years of age, with a thesis upon the gastric juice and the part it played in digestion. The ensuing years were devoted to unceasing labour amid the most unfavourable conditions possible to imagine. One who wishes to undertake experimental work to-day will often find veritable palaces at his disposal, laboratories in which the latest acquirements of technique are placed at his service. Claude Bernard had to work in a damp and gloomy hole in the Collège de France. The apparatus he used were constructed by himself, amid great difficulties. Experiments on animals attracted the unfavourable attention of the police. By ill-luck, one day, a dog with a silver cannula protruding from its belly-wall escaped from the laboratory. Bernard was prosecuted, and it transpired that the animal in question had belonged to the commissary of police and had been stolen from him! Then Bernard explained the circumstances, and secured a respectful hearing. Indeed, the commissary of police became his protector, and invited Bernard to remove the laboratory into his own district, where these important physiological investigations could be carried on without molestation.

Every Monday evening a small circle of friends foregathered in Claude Bernard's laboratory, to hear the experimental physiologist's account of his work. They were not all of them doctors, for they included Berthelot the chemist, Paul Janet and Ernest Renan the philosophers. No doubt, in Bernard's hands, physiology had become a pure natural science—but every physiological problem led down to the roots of life, and led therefore, in the last analysis, to philosophy.

A man who should wish to attempt a thorough description of Claude Bernard's life work would have to discuss a large proportion of contemporary physiology, inasmuch as Bernard's discoveries have become a sort of general heritage, and many of his experiments are parts of everyday instruction in the physiological laboratory. I must content myself, therefore, with explaining briefly in which domain his work proved most fruitful. First, come the problems of digestion, to which he primarily devoted his attention. By now chemistry had advanced far enough to enable these problems to be effectively approached. Already in the eighteenth century Lavoisier had shown that organic matter contains carbon and hydrogen, which, when they undergo combustion, form carbon dioxide and water respectively. In 1828, Wöhler, heating ammonium cyanate, had produced a substance which disclosed itself to be urea. Thus from a purely inorganic material, by purely physical factors, a chemical product had been obtained which hitherto had only been known to exist as the terminal product of "vital" changes—of changes that went on within the animal body. This was the first synthesis of an organic substance. The fundamental importance of the discovery was not recognised until subsequent investigators found it possible to produce other organic substances, such as acetic acid and fats. The barriers between inorganic and organic chemistry were thus broken down. What had been called "organic chemistry"

318

became the chemistry of the carbon compounds. It was plain that the chemical changes which occur in living organisms are fundamentally of the same kind as those that take place under artificial conditions in chemical laboratories. At length it had become possible with some prospect of success to study the course taken by the nutritive materials introduced into the organism, to learn how at the outset they were decomposed and underwent combustion, how subsequently they were built up into living substance, to break down again into the terminal products that appear in the evacuations and the secretions. As far as Germany was concerned, the lead was given by Justus Liebig who, in his laboratory at Giessen, elaborated the methodology of organic chemistry. In France, Claude Bernard was attacking the physiological side of the same problem.

A red thread runs through all the work of Claude Bernard. He began, as aforesaid, with the study of the gastric juice and the part it plays in digestion. Then he passed to consider the other digestive juices, studying the effect of the saliva, and the influence of the pancreatic secretion in the digestion of fats. He was especially interested in the fate of the carbohydrates in the organism. He was able to demonstrate that sugar is always present in the blood, and that the sugar of the animal organism is mainly stored in the liver, and partly in the muscles—not however as a sugar, but as glycogen. In 1849, he made the important discovery that when a particular spot in the medulla oblongata is punctured with a needle the blood becomes overloaded with sugar, with the immediate result that sugar appears in the urine. Thus an artificial diabetes mellitus could be produced. It was shown that this puncture of the medulla led to a stimulation of the sympathetic system. Thus was first recognised the importance of the sympathetic nervous system in the regulation of tissue-change or metabolism. By this route, Claude Bernard was led into a new field of research, and began to study the effect of the sympathetic system upon other organs, especially upon the blood-vessels. In a series of papers, he discussed the working of the vasomotor nerves.

It was Claude Bernard's custom to begin his course of lectures with the explanation that there is only one physiology, whose domain is the study of normal and pathological functions. In actual fact, his work was almost as much concerned with pathological physiology as with normal physiology. Extremely important were his investigations concerning the effect of the Indian arrow-poison known as curare, and he succeeded in showing that it paralyses the motor nerves. Following up this line of research he discovered that poisons, speaking generally, do not act upon the organism at large, as had hitherto been almost universally assumed, but that each poison has its own localised region of attack. For instance, carbon monoxide is poisonous because it enters into so firm a combination with the haemoglobin of the red blood corpuscles that they can no longer absorb oxygen in the lungs and convey it to the tissues. Other poisons were examined along similar lines. Then it appeared that what was true of poisons was also, almost as a matter of course, true of remedies. Each of these has its localised influence. Once the locale on which a remedy works is known, it is no longer used blindly in therapeutics, but is administered purposively. In this way pharmacology, likewise, became an experimental science. Thenceforward its aim was, by means of experiments on animals, to show to what degree the bodily functions could be modified by a chemical substance. Having investigated the action of a drug, a chemical compound, upon healthy tissues, it went on to study the action upon the morbidly modified organism. It worked, in fact, along physiological lines, with the reservation that the conditions under which the vital processes were being studied were abnormal. Thus pharmacology entered into the closest relationships with experimental pathology, whose aim, likewise, is the comprehension of vital processes

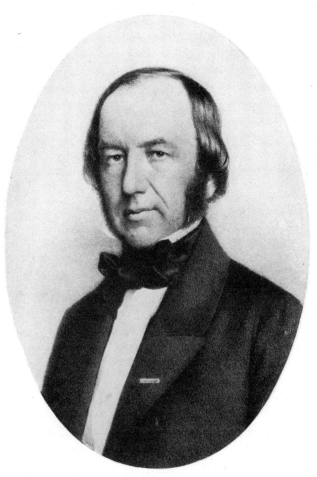

CLAUDE BERNARD, 1813–1878

under abnormal, under pathological conditions. Before all it was a German investigator, Oswald Schmiedeberg of Strasburg, who was to carry experimental pharmacology to unanticipated heights.

Johannes Müller's method, too, had been that of observation and experiment; but Müller had trusted far more to the former than to the latter, in contrast with Claude Bernard, who spent his life in the laboratory experimenting on animals, who in his *Introduction* elaborated the philosophical significance of the experimental method in all domains of scientific medicine, proceeding then to consider practical applications. Johannes Müller wrote in an extremely crabbed style, penning his thoughts as quickly as possible, his only desire being to make his observations speedily known. Claude Bernard's works, on the other hand, eighteen volumes of them, are composed in an extremely clear and cultured language.

The rise of Pasteur to fame, which was soon to follow, was to thrust Claude Bernard's name into the background. This was an injustice. Although Bernard's discoveries were less striking in some respects than those of Pasteur, they were quite as important to scientific medicine.

CHAPTER THIRTY-SEVEN

HERMANN LUDWIG FERDINAND VON HELMHOLTZ

1821–1894

HELMHOLTZ's original aim was to become a physicist, and this indeed he did become. In 1871 he was appointed professor of physics at the university of Berlin; in 1888, a few years before his death, he resigned his post, and became president of the Physico-Technical Imperial Institute. But only through a detour did he become a physicist, and it will always remain an advantage to the healing art that he had to take this detour. Lacking means for the study of physics, he entered as a pupil in the Medico-Chirurgical Friedrich-Wilhelm Institute in Berlin, where young men were trained gratuitously if they pledged themselves, when qualified, to act as army surgeons. Johannes Müller was the most influential among Helmholtz's teachers. Helmholtz took his medical degree in 1842 with a thesis upon the structure of the nervous system of the invertebrata, was appointed assistant surgeon at the Charité, and then army surgeon in Potsdam. While army surgeon, he continued his studies, devoting himself by preference to mathematics and physics. In 1847 appeared his treatise, *Ueber die Erhaltung der Kraft* (The Conservation of Energy).

In his studies on combustion Lavoisier had been able to prove that metals increase in weight when burned, this signifying that, in conflict with the prevailing views, burning resulted in a gain of substance; and he proved that this substance was derived from the air, which lost weight to a corresponding extent. He showed that it was the oxygen in the air which combined with the metal in the process of combustion. Thereby the nature of oxidation had been elucidated; but at the same time a much more important item of knowledge

322

had been won, namely that the sum of the weight was constant —that matter, though it can change its outward aspect and internal structure, remains unchangeable in quantity.

In 1840 Robert Mayer, a doctor from Heilbronn, voyaged to Java as ship surgeon. Following the custom of the day, he practised venesection, and was struck by the fact that the blood he drew from his patients' veins was lighter in colour than he had been wont to see it in Europe. How was this? Obviously the difference must depend upon a change in the thermal economy of the body. By his observations Mayer was led to direct his attention towards the relationships between the development of heat and the oxidized material. As a result of his reflections, he came to the conclusion that not only matter, but also energy, must be constant in quantity. Force or energy, like matter, must be indestructible. No doubt the different forms of energy could be changed one into another, but their sum was a constant. In 1842 Mayer's first paper on this subject appeared in Wöhler and Liebig's "Annalen der Chimie."

Brilliant though Mayer's discovery was, he was not an able enough mathematician to demonstrate it effectively. This demonstration was left for Helmholtz, who had independently arrived at the same conclusion as Mayer, and now, in the before-mentioned work, established the law of the conservation of energy. This was of the utmost importance to physiology, since it was the notion of the conservation of energy which first rendered possible a quantitative consideration of the processes of metabolism.

In 1848, Helmholtz became teacher of anatomy at the Kunstakademie in Berlin and assistant at the Anatomical Museum. Next year he accepted a call to Königsberg as professor of physiology and general pathology. In 1855, he removed to Bonn as professor of anatomy and physiology; in 1858, to Heidelberg as professor of physiology; and finally, as we have already learned, he returned to Berlin as professor of physics. It was a sign of the times that at each remove the scope of his teaching grew narrower. Those were the years in which the trend towards specialisation was becoming marked.

Helmholtz was a physiologist, though his chief interest was physics. It is easy to understand, therefore, why, as far as physiology was concerned, he devoted himself mainly to the physical aspect of that science. He made observations upon the velocity of nervous conduction and of reflex processes, these being of considerable importance to psychology. Out of physiology there was to develop a physiological psychology, working also with experimental methods, endeavouring to bring mental phenomena into rigid relationship with physical laws. This domain received the name of "psychophysics." Its chief founder was Wilhelm Wundt, who in 1857 became professor of physiology at Heidelberg (a year before Helmholtz's arrival), and was ultimately to become professor in Leipzig.

Above all, however, Helmholtz devoted himself to the study of the physiology of the sense organs. His *Handbuch der physiologischen Optik* was published between the years 1856 and 1866, and recorded an enormous wealth of observations and experiments. In 1862 he published his *Lehre von den Tonempfindungen*. Both these works remain of fundamental importance to-day, and a large part of their teaching has been incorporated into the general body of scientific knowledge, although some of the theories put forward—as was only to be expected in the case of such difficult problems—have been invalidated by subsequent criticism in respect of certain details.

In 1851, Helmholtz made a discovery of the utmost importance to practical medicine. We know that in general the pupil of the eye is black, and yet all of us have had occasion now and again of nights to observe a remarkable green sheen in the eyes of a cat. Various theories had been propounded regarding this luminosity of the pupil, but they had hitherto been unsatisfactory. Helmholtz devoted himself with keen interest to the question. He discovered that the human eye, too, has a sheen, though a red one, when the source of illumination is in the observer's direct line of vision, so that these red rays are reflected back into the observer's pupil. If, then, he could succeed in making the observer's eye the source of light, would it not be possible to see the fundus oculi of the observed person? This was rendered possible by a simple apparatus, a concave mirror with a small hole in the middle through which the observer looked as he reflected light into the eye of the patient. The ophthalmoscope had been discovered.

With this instrument, the fundus of the eye could be examined, and—a matter of great importance to the ophthalmologist—morbid changes in the eye could be directly examined. Therewith ophthalmology received a powerful impetus. Whereas hitherto the study of the deeper maladies of the eye had only been possible, in a very unsatisfactory way, on the post-mortem table, the morbid changes could now be directly observed in the living eye. A diagnostic adjuvant of the first importance had been provided.

Helmholtz describes the history of his discovery in the following terms: "I had to explain to my pupils the theory of the retinal reflex, which originated with Brücke. Brücke only just failed to discover the ophthalmoscope. He failed because he had not asked himself to what optical image the rays reflected from the illuminated eye belong. For his purposes at the time, this question was superfluous. Had he asked it, he would have found it just as easy as I did to answer it, and the ophthalmoscope would have come into existence earlier than it did. I turned the problem over and over in my mind, in order to see how I could most simply present it to my auditors, and it was in this way that I hit upon the fundamental question. My medical studies had made me well acquainted with the difficulty ophthalmic surgeons experience in diagnosing the true nature of amaurosis (blindness due to diseases of the optic nerve or of the retina), and I had little trouble in constructing an elementary ophthalmoscope with which to examine the fundus of the eye. At first I found it difficult to use. Had it not been for my firm theoretical conviction that it would be possible to see the fundus, I might not have persevered. But after about a week I was the first who ever succeeded in getting a clear view of the living human retina."

The discovery of the ophthalmoscope affords a striking demonstration of the practical importance of theoretical studies in the field of medicine. Helmholtz was not an ophthalmologist, but a physicist and a physiologist. He made his discovery along purely theoretical lines. It is expedient to refer again and again to such facts as the discovery of the ophthalmoscope inasmuch as to-day we often encounter attempts to degrade the medical faculties to the pursuit of purely "practical" aims.

The development of the new ophthalmology is especially associated with the name of Albrecht von Graefe, who seized on the ophthalmoscope, improved it, and, with its aid, placed the whole science of ophthalmology upon a fresh foundation. His "Archiv für Ophthalmologie," which, in association with Arlt and Donders, he published from the year 1854 onwards, became the focus of the new ophthalmological research.

The discovery of the ophthalmoscope was a big and very important step along the road of anatomical diagnosis. Auscultation and percussion had been indirect methods for the perception of anatomical changes. With the ophthalmoscope, the physician could see directly into the interior of one of the bodily organs, could observe morbid changes more effectively than the pathologist could observe them on the post-mortem table. It was natural, therefore, that an increasing number of attempts should be made to open other internal organs to direct vision. For a long time endeavours had been made to look into the larynx. In 1854, a teacher of singing in London, Manuel Garcia by name, was able to see into the interior of his own larynx with the aid of a little mirror something like a dental mirror. Once more it was a physiologist, Johann Nepomuk Czermak, who seized upon the new invention and developed laryngoscopy, with the result that this method of examination became generally diffused from the year 1858 onward.

In subsequent decades apparatus of various sorts were made for the examination of the internal organs—the urethra, the urinary bladder, the oesophagus, the stomach, and the rectum. Armed with lamps and mirrors, the observer's eye was able to obtain direct information concerning morbid processes in these internal parts. The greatest triumph of diagnosis in this direction followed upon the discovery of the Röntgen rays in the year 1895. Originally applied to the diagnosis of injuries and diseases of the bones, the domain of skiagraphy has been more and more widely extended through the application of contrast substances (bismuth, etc.) which make the gastro-intestinal canal and other organs visible. The Röntgen rays or X-rays have given us an ideal method of studying pathological anatomy in the living body.

There is no need here for discussing the achievements of Helmholtz in the domain of pure physics. It was a rare stroke of luck for medical science that a man with such eminent physical and mathematical gifts should be forced by circumstances to devote a considerable part of his life to medical science. Just as Claude Bernard did so much to develop the chemical aspect of physiology, so did Helmholtz enrich our knowledge of the physical aspect of physiology. In various orations, Helmholtz expounded his attitude towards basic questions of method. No doubt the natural-philosophical wave had ebbed, but Helmholtz's own work had played a notable part in promoting this ebb. All the same, there still existed medical notabilities of a speculative turn of mind who were ready to propound wild hypotheses. As late as 1877, in a speech upon *Thought in Medicine*, Helmholtz said: "But you must not believe, Gentlemen, that the struggle is finished. So long as there exist persons sufficiently arrogant to fancy that by lightning flashes of speculation they will be able to achieve what the human race can only hope to achieve by strenuous labour, there will also continue to exist hypotheses which, put forward as dogmas, promise to solve all riddles at once. So long, moreover, as there are persons uncritical enough to believe whatever they wish to believe, just so long will the hypotheses of persons of the before-mentioned type continue to find credence. Neither of these classes of human beings is likely to die out, and the majority of the human race will always belong to the latter."

Helmholtz recognised yet another danger. In the same discourse he said: "Our generation has continued to suffer from the thraldom of spiritualist metaphysics. The younger generation will doubtless have to protect itself against the thraldom of materialist metaphysics."

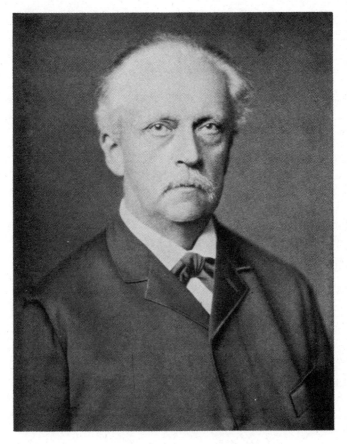

HERMANN VON HELMHOLTZ, 1821–1894

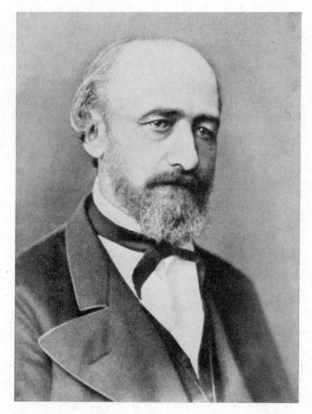

CARL AUGUST WUNDERLICH, 1815–1877

CHAPTER THIRTY-EIGHT

CARL AUGUST WUNDERLICH
1815–1877

ANYONE who to-day enters a hospital and walks up to one of the beds will, if he be a student or a physician, look first of all at the chart which hangs above the patient's head. He will see a curve recording the temperature throughout the illness. When this curve is rising, the illness is on the increase. If it has been high, and has since then been low for several days, we know that the disease has passed its climax, and that the patient is on the way towards recovery. In many cases the curve is extremely characteristic. Crests and hollows alternate with extreme regularity. In such cases, a glance at the temperature chart will often enable us to be practically sure of the diagnosis. Thus in many diseases the temperature curve, the resultant of the morbid processes in the body, gives us standardised information as to the course of the malady.

We have to thank the clinician Carl August Wunderlich for the recognition of these facts. He did not discover the use of the clinical thermometer. We have already seen how, long ago, Santorio, with a primitive instrument, made measurements of bodily temperature; how Boerhaave occasionally and de Haen frequently used the thermometer in their respective clinics. But it was Wunderlich who taught us to read and to understand the curves of fever. He showed that the course of fever is not determined by chance, but reflects the essential nature of the disease; that each of the specific infectious disorders is sharply characterised by the temperature chart. It was mainly through his instrumentality that the clinical thermometer was adopted for daily use by general practitioners, whereas up till then the instrument had been used only in hospitals. Nay more, it made its way into family life. The

329

lay public is nowadays sufficiently instructed to use the clinical thermometer. When any member of a family feels ill, the temperature is taken, and by its indications a decision is made whether it is desirable to go to bed and to send for a doctor.

Wunderlich was the son of a physician. His mother belonged to a family of French refugees. Born at Sulz on the Neckar, he attended the high school in Stuttgart, and subsequently, from 1833 onwards, studied at the university of Tübingen. The Tübingen faculty was, so to say, bred in and in. Almost all the professors had been students at Tübingen, so that little fresh blood was introduced from elsewhere. The teaching was mainly theoretical, and ran along the old lines; but there was an exception in the case of a young instructor, F. A. Schill, who had studied in England and in France, and had learned the new methods. Wunderlich and his friends Roser and Griesinger were in close touch with Schill. When, in 1837, Wunderlich had passed his examination, he felt it essential to go to Paris. He was filled by enthusiasm by what he saw there, studying in one hospital after another. Returning to Tübingen, he became assistant at St Catherine's Hospital, where he turned to practical account what he had learned in Paris, percussing and auscultating the patients. His chief made no objection. In 1839 he paid another visit to Paris, and, after his return, became instructor in Tübingen. Then he journeyed to Vienna, and the outcome of these three journeys was the little book entitled *Wien und Paris, ein Beitrag zur Geschichte und Beurteilung der gegenwärtigen Heilkunde in Deutschland und Frankreich*, from which I have already made copious quotations. This was designed as a guide to young practitioners, as a handbook which would enable them to turn to better advantage travels undertaken with a view to completing their education. It manifested, however, so profound an insight into the problems that were then pressing for solution, it showed so ripe a judgment, that it attracted widespread attention, and people found it difficult to believe that it had been penned by a man only five-and-twenty years of age. In 1841, Wunderlich became assistant at the Tübingen clinic, and, since his chief Hermann was often ailing, he had plenty of opportunities for independent work. The next year, 1842, in conjunction with Roser, he founded a new periodical, entitled "Archiv für physiologische Heilkunde." It was not designed to treat of physiological medicine in Broussais' sense, but was intended to carry on a polemic on behalf of medicine regarded as a branch of natural science and not as a branch of natural philosophy. In the preliminary announcement Wunderlich wrote: "We are here inaugurating an organ to further the knowledge of physiological medicine. This phrase gives a full description of our trend. To establish pathology upon a physiological foundation must be the endeavour of all enlightened minds, for upon that depends the future of the healing art." A little later: "Medicine must be studied as a part of nature. It is fundamentally a branch of natural research. One who should try to study medicine exclusively out of books, instead of at the bedside of the sick, would be committing as gross an absurdity as one who should try to become acquainted with pictures and statues from written descriptions." It was a bold venture on the part of two young men to found a periodical of their own. They regarded none of the traditions as sacred. Germany was to have a scientific medicine based upon the study of nature, just as Paris had or Vienna. They found even Schönlein out of date, and criticised him vigorously when his clinical lectures were published.

Still, mere criticism, mere destruction, achieves nothing creative. Soon a heavier responsibility was imposed upon Wunderlich. As early as 1843 he became provisional chief of the Tübingen clinic, and the appointment was made definitive in 1846. The same year he was appointed ordinary professor. Now it was incumbent on him to show himself a master builder. He enlarged the clinic, though even then there were no more than thirty beds, and if some especially interesting case applied for admission and the beds were full, he would put two of the milder cases into the same bed. He opened an out-patient department, and he took his students with him to visit patients in their homes. Then he entered upon a great task, the writing of a *Handbuch der speziellen Pathologie,* which was published during the years 1846 to 1850.

In 1850 he was offered the headship of the Leipzig Medical Clinic, which had been vacated by the transfer of Oppolzer to Vienna. Wunderlich accepted the appointment, and remained in Leipzig until his death. His inaugural lecture was entitled, *A Scheme for the Firmer Foundation of Therapeutic Experiences.* Recognising clearly that medical treatment had not kept pace with the development of the other medical disciplines, he said: "In former days there doubtless existed various medical schools and sects contemporaneously and successively. They engaged in mutual controversies as regards their theoretical views and their therapeutic principles; but within each school strict rules were enforced, so that the choice among methods of cure was not left to the decision of individuals. To-day, on the other hand, instead of this doctrinaire rigidity, we find that there is complete therapeutic anarchy." In an earlier paragraph of his lecture he had mooted the question: "Has therapeutics, which is the essential social duty of the physician, shared in the before-mentioned advances? Many doubt it; many deny it. As regards treatment, what we need to-day is to expound aims and methods." He insisted that therapeutics, no less than pathology, should be made an exact science. It was true that in this field a sound method was harder to elaborate than in other domains.

It was at Leipzig, too, that he began regular thermometric observations. He published twenty papers on the subject, and finally, in 1868, there appeared his book *Ueber das Verhalten der Eigenwärme in Krankheiten.* For a time he had left the issue of the "Archives" to his friends Roser and Griesinger, but in 1860 he resumed active editorship. His old lust for battle persisted. To attack "natural philosophy," as contrasted with natural science, would, indeed, have been to flog a dead horse; but he became embroiled with Virchow, whose cellular pathology seemed to him open to question. Virchow, however, was publishing "Archives" of his own, and the lightnings flashed back and forth from one periodical to the other.

The cholera epidemic of 1866, and subsequently the Franco-German war, imposed upon Wunderlich extensive organisational tasks. Apart from these activities, he was an admirable clinical teacher. His presence at Leipzig, in conjunction with that of Thiersch the surgeon and Ludwig the physiologist, gave the Leipzig faculty a renown it had never before possessed. The critical inclinations which Wunderlich had early displayed in his work on *Vienna and Paris* led him again and again to discuss matters concerned with the history of medicine. He gave lectures on the topic, and they were printed. The concluding paragraph of this book contained a confession of faith:

"Latter-day medicine recognises its tasks and its duties as part of the immeasurably extensive and sublime science of nature. It has become clear to up-to-date practitioners of the healing art that medicine can only be founded upon facts, and that the understanding of these facts, in so far as it is attainable, can be achieved only through a combination of the facts among themselves. We know, in addition, that genuine facts, trustworthy data, are solely attainable by means of the strictest attention to the methods of investigation and through continually bearing in mind the possible sources of fallacy. The mind is no longer regarded as an outlaw because it is compelled to work in accordance with methods and to subject its impressions to the rigid control of a disciplined logic. No more do we attempt to impose a system upon nature, but strive to disclose being and happening in the utmost possible purity, as they are and wherever they are.

333

"The present rejects one-sidedness in pathological anatomy; it realises that we can know nothing about the conditions which determine organic changes so long as we lack an intimate acquaintance with these changes; it refuses to espouse without qualification either a humoral or a solidist pathology, being aware that both the humours and the solid tissues are part of the organism; it does not expect to arrive at valid conclusions by the use of chemical conjectures, but it insists upon the need for studying and explaining how the chemical substances of the body are combined and decomposed in the sick as well as in the hale; it does not delude itself with the belief that the enigmas of life will all be solved by an advance to the uttermost limits of the visible; but it gives due value to every fact, whether relating to the bulkier masses or to the minutest particles of the body. It regards the sick human being as an organism whose relationships cannot be investigated too thoroughly or studied from too multifarious aspects in the endeavour to explain them; and present-day medicine, in so far as it tries to be neither more nor less than a doctrine of the nature of the sick human being in all the modifications of illness, is entitled to style itself 'physiological.'"

CHAPTER THIRTY-NINE

RUDOLF VIRCHOW
(1821–1902)

WE have already encountered Virchow several times in the present work. We heard of him as a student in Johannes Müller's Institute; there was mention of his severe criticism of Rokitansky's doctrine of crasis, and of his controversies with Wunderlich. Obviously, then, he must have been of a pugnacious disposition. When Virchow attacked Rokitansky, he was five-and-twenty years of age. A year later he founded a periodical of his own, "Archiv für pathologische Anatomie und Physiologie und für klinische Medizin," which was to exercise a far-reaching influence upon the development of medical science throughout the nineteenth century. At that date new periodicals were sprouting up everywhere like mushrooms. The doctors who held to the tenets of natural philosophy had had a great many such periodicals, but their day was done; their organs ceased publication, and the men of the new trend were creating fresh periodicals, nearly all of which are still being published to-day, and which bear the names of their founders, although, naturally, in many respects their characteristics have been modified.

What was Virchow's aim in his "Archiv"? His programme was stated clearly: "The standpoint we propose to adopt and which is already manifested in this first issue is simply that of natural science. Practical medicine as applied theoretical medicine, and theoretical medicine as an embodiment of pathological physiology, are the ideals towards which we shall strive so far as lies within the scope of our powers. Pathological anatomy and clinical work, although we fully recognize their justification and their independence, are both mainly regarded as the sources of new problems whose answers must be supplied by pathological physiology. Since, however, these problems must for the most part be formulated by means of a laborious and comprehensive study of detailed phenomena in the sick and upon the post-mortem table, we maintain that a precise and purposive development of anatomical and clinical experiences is the first and most important requisite of the day. Through an empiricism of this sort there will gradually be brought into being a genuine theory of medicine, a pathological physiology."

Virchow had thus expressed his aims in plain terms, and we see how erroneous it is to regard him as nothing more than an anatomist, although the mistake is still current to-day.

His life is divided into three periods of very unequal duration. The first extends down to the year 1849, being the era of his scientific beginnings, when he was seeking his path, finding it, and defending it. Above all it was an era of social and political activity. Next comes the second period, the Würzburg phase between 1849 and 1856, which was wholly devoted to science, and which led to the propounding of his theory of cellular pathology. The third and last period, which continued for almost half a century, extended from 1856 to his death in 1902. During these decades Virchow lived in Berlin as professor of pathological anatomy and director of the Pathological Institute—the first independent institute of the kind. He had founded a school; he reigned as pope of German medicine, supreme though not without adversaries. Throughout this epoch, his researches were mainly concerned with anthropology.

Born at Schievelbein in Pomerania, as son of the town treasurer, Virchow went to Berlin in 1839 to become a pupil at the army medical school. Johannes Müller and Schönlein were his principal teachers. He took his degree in 1843 and became assistant to Prosector Froriep at the Charité, succeeding him in this post three years later. When Virchow arrived at Berlin, one of the most important discoveries ever made at Johannes Müller's laboratory had just been announced,

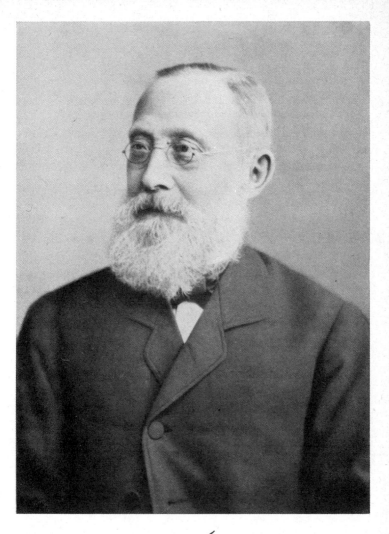

RUDOLPH VIRCHOW, 1821–1902

that of the animal cell. Vegetable cells had been discovered much earlier, as far back as the seventeenth century. An English botanist, Robert Hooke [botany was only one of Hooke's subsidiary activities, for he was mainly a physicist, a mathematician, and what was then called in England a natural philosopher]. Examining a thin slice or section of cork under a powerful magnifying glass, he had detected a structure which reminded him of a honeycomb. But it was not until the compound microscope had been perfected that it became possible to study the minute structure of organisms. In 1833, Robert Brown detected the nuclei in the cells of orchids, and also in those of other plants. It was known, therefore, that plants consisted of nucleated cells, and that the cells were the basic element of plants. Schwann's discovery that the animal organism likewise consisted of nucleated cells was of great importance. In the first place it made manifest the unity of the organic world, since there was an essential similarity in animal and in vegetable structure. But, more than this, the vital functions could now be followed much farther into the depths of the organism. If the cell is the ultimate morphological unit of life, if the cell is the elemental type of organism, then the basic functions of life can be studied in the cell. The tissues, which Bichat spoke of as "membranes," must be aggregates of cells. Although, mainly thanks to Rokitansky's labours, important knowledge had been acquired in the domain of special pathological anatomy, investigators were still groping in the dark when general pathological questions were broached. In the field of general pathology, the door was open to all kinds of vague speculations, for no such thing as a scientific general pathology was as yet possible. In the opening of the nineteenth century, French investigators were still humoral pathologists of the traditional type, except in so far as they preferred to ignore general problems. Rokitansky had tried to bring about a unification of humoral pathology and anatomical conceptions, but the endeavour had miscarried. Now, when

337

animal cells had been discovered, it at length became possible to make a scientific study of the elemental phenomena of disease.

At the outset, however, an error had to be cleared out of the way. What was the origin of the cells? Schwann believed that they were developed out of a rudimentary, undifferentiated, homogeneous substance. He spoke of this as "blastema." The blastema was even thought of as not being alive. For instance, when an inflammatory exudation became "organised," that is to say when it acquired a cellular structure, it was supposed that cells were formed out of the dead substance of the fluid exudation. Virchow was able to refute this theory, and to prove that cells invariably arise out of cells. "Omnis cellula e cellula." Life was continued in no other way than by "a legitimate succession of cell-formations."

The first important piece of work to which Virchow devoted himself was the study of inflammation of the veins, or phlebitis, to which his chief Froriep had directed his attention. This investigation had two extremely valuable outcomes. It threw a clear light upon the previously obscure problems of thrombosis and embolism; and it led to the formulation of a new morbid concept, that of leukaemia.

While still engaged in these studies, Virchow was diverted into other channels by political events, which aroused his passionate interest. In the summer of 1847 there had broken out in Upper Silesia an epidemic which was spoken of as famine fever ("Hungertyphus," now known as relapsing fever). The local authorities did nothing to stay the progress of the plague. At length, when the press gave tongue, the central government in Berlin was forced to take action. In February 1848 a commission, of which Virchow was a member, was sent to investigate. Virchow quickly recognised that the causes of the epidemic were social quite as much as or more than medical. His report took the form of a fierce attack upon the extant regime. Nothing but prosperity, culture, and freedom could bring about an improvement, and these could only be achieved upon the basis of "complete and unrestricted democracy." The report closed with the following words: "All the world knows that the proletariat of our day has been mainly brought into existence by the introduction and improvement of machinery; that in proportion as agriculture, manufacture, navigation, and land transport have, through the perfectionment of apparatus, acquired an unprecedented extension, man-power has completely lost its autonomy, and human beings have become incorporated as mere cog-wheels in machine enterprise—living cog-wheels, indeed, but treated as of no more value than dead matter. The human instruments are regarded as mere 'hands'! Is that to be the ultimate significance of machinery in the history of civilisation? Are the triumphs of human genius to lead only to this, that the human race shall become more miserable? Unquestionably not. Our century has opened what is spoken of as the social age, and the object of its activities must be to reduce to the utmost the purely mechanical parts of human activity, those which fetter men and women most to the soil, to the coarsely material, and withdraw them from the more refined movements of matter. Man should only work as much as is needful to wrest from the soil, from coarse matter, whatever is indispensable to provide a comfortable life for the whole race; but he should not waste his best energies in producing capital. Capital is a title to enjoyment; but why should this title be increased to a degree beyond all reason? Let us increase the possibilities of enjoyment, certainly, but not mere dead and cold possibilities of such enjoyment, which, moreover, when compared with the accumulation of capital, are not a stable possibility, but a perpetually vacillating and uncertain one. The French republic has already recognised this principle in its motto of fraternity; and it would seem inclined, despite the strength of the old-established bourgeoisie, to devote itself to realising the same principle through the power of association. In fact, the association of propertyless labour with the capital of the State or with that of the plutocracy, or with that of the numerous petty possessors, is the only way of improving social conditions. At least, capital and labour power must have equal rights, and living energies must no longer be subordinated to dead capital."

The events of March summoned Virchow back to the metropolis. Although he did not actually lend a hand in the building of barricades, he played an active part in the movement, being above all fascinated by the idea of a thorough-going reform of the whole medical system. The German medical profession was deeply stirred. General practitioners were eager to play a responsible part and to advise in matters relating to public health. They, too, were demanding a reconstruction of the medical system, and self-government for the various professions. They were opposed to State tutelage. A desire for a general medical congress, for a sort of parliament of doctors, secured louder and louder expression. Everywhere medical societies were being formed, and protests were being uttered against "duplicity in the medical profession"—this meaning against a severance of medicine from surgery. The mouthpiece of the movement was a periodical issued by Virchow and one of his friends during the years 1848 and 1849 under the title "Die medizinische Reform." He demanded the foundation of a separate ministry of health and a reorganisation of medical instruction. Appointments to professorial chairs were to be made, as in France, as the outcome of competitive examination. Medical students were to be trained at State cost. He also demanded a legal restriction of the working day for manual operatives. It was, he insisted, the natural right of the impecunious worker to be cared for gratuitously by the State whenever disabled by illness.

A period of reaction followed, and Virchow had to suffer for his advanced political views. He was not positively dismissed from the Charité, but—which amounted to the same thing—his salary was cut off, and he was given notice to quit the room which had been assigned to him as medical officer. Then, in May 1849, came the call to Würzburg. His attempts at social and medical reform had been fruitless, so he devoted himself with redoubled energy to the reform of medical science. The years spent at Würzburg were a time of unresting activity. He had a chance of collecting abundant material and of developing his ideas. He published a number of monographs, and when, in 1856, he was recalled to Berlin, his work was so far advanced that only two years later he was able to deliver to post-graduates a course of lectures which were published in the same year as a book under the title *Die Cellularpathologie in ihrer Begründung auf physiologische und pathologische Gewebelehre.*

In this work, Virchow passed from analysis to synthesis. Pathology, thereby, had become more consciously dominated by anatomical concepts. Morgagni regarded the organ as the seat of disease; Bichat, the tissue (membrane). For Virchow it was the cell. The cell was the sustainer of life. Illness was life no less than was health, life under modified conditions. The cell, therefore, likewise, was the sustainer of disease. Disease, taught Virchow, is the reaction of the cell to abnormal stimuli. When Virchow began his work, a great deal of detailed knowledge had doubtless been collected in the field of the new medicine, of medicine based upon the study of natural science, but a systematic foundation was lacking. The "natural philosophers" had had systems, but the natural scientists had jettisoned these. Virchow, with his cellular pathology, did not try to found a system, and indeed expressly renounced the attempt; but he furnished a principle which was extraordinarily fertile in promoting development, and was competent to render a certain amount of systematisation possible. Before his day, diseases were regarded as entities, this notion being so crudely held in many cases that doctors were apt to regard particular diseases much as if they had been parasitic creatures which held human beings in their clutch. Virchow was strongly opposed to ontology of this sort. Disease, he taught, was life, though life under abnormal conditions, different from those which promoted health. Pathology was physiology, but physiology contending with obstacles. How did disease arise? Through the working of abnormal stimuli upon the organism. These stimuli acted upon the living element, the cell. They gave rise to a lesion, to a disturbance, or to a paralysis of the cell. In other cases, the cell, owing to the changes induced by the stimulus, passed into an irritable condition which—varying in accordance with the strength of the stimulus—manifested itself as functional, nutritive, or formative activities. When the stimulus was exceptionally strong, the cell died.

This cellular pathology was the climax of a development which had begun during the Renaissance. Virchow compelled pathologists to use microscopes, and he placed general pathology no less than special pathology upon the foundation of natural science. The whole edifice of contemporary pathology is upborne on his shoulders. Of course in the seventy-five years that have elapsed since the publication of his book science has not stood still. Many of Virchow's views have been superseded, in respect of certain details; but they have been superseded thanks to the working out of his principles.

Only in one respect can it be said that a fundamental change has taken place in our views during this three-quarters of a century. Virchow's cellular pathology is emphatically localist. His doctrine directed attention to parts of the organism, and these, in his view, formed a community rather than a unity. "The organism," he wrote, "is not a unified but a social apparatus." It is "not a circumscribed unity." Subsequent investigations, however, have turned our thoughts in the contrary direction. Bacteriological research has supplied us with data which in many respects transcend the limits of cellular pathology. We have come to regard the intercellular substances as likewise living, even though their life is of a somewhat different kind from that of the cells. But if they have a normal

342

life, they can also have a morbid one.—Nevertheless, these advances are no more than developments of Virchow's teaching, which still remains the essential foundation of our outlook on disease.

Cellular pathology had a profound influence upon every domain of medicine; especially marked was its effect upon treatment. We have seen how Claude Bernard tried to discover the points of onslaught of remedies in the organism. It was Virchow's work which enabled doctors to realise that the points of onslaught are not the organs in general but the cells. We now know that there are peculiar affinities between particular cells and particular chemical substances. Thanks to the recognition of this, both pharmacological and dietetic treatment have become far more purposive.

Virchow, who survived into the twentieth century, lived through the bacteriological era. He was hesitant in his acceptance of the results of bacteriological investigation, protesting, for instance, against the view that the presence of the tubercle bacillus in an organism was equivalent to tuberculosis. Again and again he insisted upon the part played by the cells, even in the pathogenesis of the infectious disorders. What constituted tuberculosis, he said, was not the tubercle bacillus, but the reaction of the organism, that is to say of the cells, to the bacillus. Since the cells react variously in different individuals, different individuals will sicken from tuberculosis in various ways.

During the latter half of his long life, Virchow continued to be a prolific writer, publishing a treatise in many volumes on tumours, numerous monographs in his "Archiv" upon the multifarious problems of medicine, and an increasing number of anthropological studies. As a member of the Prussian Landtag and as a municipal councillor he belonged always to the left wing, to the opposition, and did excellent service, especially in the matter of educational reform. Though no longer the militant of the 'forties, his attitude even in the days of the empire remained radical, and as late as 1879 he had his essays on medical reform reprinted.

Virchow's authority was far-reaching. It is no exaggeration to say that for half a century he guided the progress of German medicine. But, more than this, his influence extended over the world, and his eightieth birthday was the occasion of a demonstration of international homage such as has rarely been paid to any man of science. At numerous congresses, and especially at the meetings of the German Society for the Promotion of Scientific Research, Virchow, as if from a watch-tower, delivered lectures upon the general problems of natural science, medicine, and life in general—addresses which are still worth reading to-day. He was fully aware of his own position in the history of medicine, having, indeed, a historical sense rare in doctors—for, speaking generally, those only can have it whose own life and work is of great historical significance. Numerous papers, introductions to other writers' works, and speeches, bear witness to this historical sense of the founder of cellular pathology, and among these his masterly biographical sketches of his teachers Johannes Müller and Schönlein deserve special mention.

Virchow was the main prop of the Berlinese school which flourished after Johannes Müller's death and was to outdo the splendours of Vienna and Paris. Johannes Müller's professorial chair was partitioned. Even during Müller's lifetime, the professoriate of pathological anatomy was detached, being assigned to Virchow. Now Reichert, an able embryologist and favourite teacher, became professor of anatomy; and Du Bois-Reymond, whose main field of work was the physiology of nerves and muscles, was appointed professor of physiology.

Clinical work found outstanding representatives in Frerichs and Traube. They were men of very different types, and did not get on well together. Frerichs was of cold temperament, and a sceptic in therapeutic matters. He came from Breslau, where he had worked at pathological anatomy. His main fields of research were diseases of the gastro-intestinal tract, disorders of metabolism, and diabetes. Naunyn was the most noted amongst his pupils. Traube had been a pupil of Schönlein, and was a Jew, so that he could not take his degree until 1848, when the disabilities of the Jews were abolished. He was well read in the French literature of medicine, was an expert in physical diagnosis, and was, above all, an extremely able experimental pathologist.

Surgery, likewise, flourished in Berlin. In 1847, Bernhard Langenbeck became director of the Surgical Clinic as Dieffenbach's successor. He was a noted army surgeon, and, like his predecessor, acquired a special renown for plastic operations. In 1868, ophthalmology was detached from surgery, and, as we have already learned, Albrecht von Graefe made Berlin a noted centre for this new specialty.

In the eighteenth century, medicine was still an international, a European science. Everywhere doctors wrote and talked in the same tongue. Even though the course of development was quicker in some countries and slower in others, even though now one city and now another was a more flourishing centre of medical progress, doctors were advancing everywhere along the same paths, were thinking the same thoughts, were treating their patients in accordance with the same principles. The nineteenth century, on the other hand, was characterised by a separate national development in all branches of science. There no longer existed—there does not now exist—a European medicine, but instead French, English, Italian, German medicine. Of course the great discoveries speedily make their way across the frontiers, becoming a general apanage of cosmopolitan medicine. Nevertheless, clinical work, and especially the activities of general practitioners, have in each country a distinct national stamp. In France since the days of the Revolution there has been a steady and tranquil progress, with the clinic always in the centre of things. Characteristic of German development seems to be the fact that it has tended to pass with a violent swing from one extreme to another. In the opening of the nineteenth century Romanticism was dominant, in medicine as well as in other fields; wild speculation; "natural philosophy." Towards the middle of the century there came a powerful reaction, a trend towards the exact sciences, and this, like all such reactions, may have gone too far. The pathological institute became the centre of medicine instead of the clinic. The laboratory became the symbol, rather than the bedside of the sick. All the same, in this very lack of moderation, now in one direction and now in the other, has lain the peculiar force of German medicine, the energy which, embodied in Virchow and his contemporaries, resulted in such remarkable achievements.

CHAPTER FORTY

JAKOB HENLE
1809–1885

LOOKING backward, it seems to us that the nineteenth century was the period in which greater successes than ever before were achieved in the campaign against epidemic diseases. As far as the healing art is concerned, it is the discovery of the causes of contagious illness which has given the latter half of that century its peculiar imprint. Since then, prophylaxis has been the most important task of medicine. In collaboration with governmental authorities and with the educators of youth, the doctor tries to protect society from infections and other menaces to health, and to fortify the individual that he may become able to cope with unfavourable variations in the environment. Along these lines, remarkable successes were achieved within a brief space of time. Many of the infectious diseases disappeared, and others became comparatively rare. There was a marked decline in mortality, and the mean duration of life increased to an almost incredible extent. In this book, therefore, it has now become incumbent upon us to study the lives and the activities of the doctors thanks to whom these achievements were made possible.

It need hardly be said that from earliest times epidemic diseases had attracted peculiar attention. Whereas other maladies could be more or less plausibly explained as the outcome of chills, errors in diet, and so on, pestilence seemed like a natural catastrophe, a malady that was the outcome of Heaven's wrath, affecting vast numbers of persons simultaneously, and spreading like a conflagration. The causes were sought in nature; in influences to which not individuals merely but whole sections of society were exposed; above all, therefore, in the constitution of the soil, in that of the atmosphere; and

347

also in the influence of the stars. Indeed, as already indicated, people were prone to think of suprasensuous causes, of the anger of the gods. In early days, man felt helpless, was helpless, in face of pestilence. It began unexpectedly, and, after a time, it vanished as enigmatically as it had come. Attempts were made to purify the air by huge bonfires. People were afraid of the proximity of marshes, the vapours (often evil-smelling) arising from these were looked upon as the determinants of many epidemics. Malaria, in especial, was regarded as a "marsh fever." Long, long ago there were vague intimations of a belief that minute living organisms might play a part in the origination of such diseases. In the first century before Christ, Varro, in his agricultural treatise *De re rustica* wrote: "In damp places there grow tiny creatures, too small for us to see, which make their way into our bodies through mouth and nose and give rise to grave illnesses."

In the East, of old, people had become aware that certain morbid conditions were transferred from one person to another by contact. He who touched an unclean human being became himself unclean. The supreme form of uncleanness was the disease zara'ath. Anyone who had thus been rendered unclean became an outcast from society. His mere proximity brought with it a danger of infection. In the Middle Ages, the authorities, in their attempts to check the spread of leprosy, followed the principles laid down in *Leviticus* (Chapters XIII and XIV). Thus we see that the idea of contagion was extremely vivid. It had become plain to the men of the Middle Ages that pestilences did not arise solely from environmental influences, but that they were diffused by contact between one individual and another. Furthermore, the study of the oriental plague or Black Death had made it plain that there must be some other means by which the malady was communicated over and above direct contact. It appeared, in the case both of this and of other disorders of the kind, that infection was also communicated by intermediate articles which had belonged to or come into contact with the patient; by what were called "fomites," this meaning literally by porous substances absorbing contagium; by articles of clothing, for instance. It followed from such considerations that the contagion must be a material substance of some kind. A "contagium" must be transmitted from the sick to the healthy, in part by direct contact, and in part indirectly by articles to which the contagium clung. This contagious material, this virus, must be of a very subtle nature, since it was invisible. It was perhaps so subtle that it could be transmitted through the air. Practical conclusions were drawn from these arguments. The campaign against pestilences became a campaign against the contagium, which must be kept away from the healthy and must be destroyed. For this reason, the sick were isolated; their clothing was burned; all articles which had come into contact with them were cleansed as thoroughly as possible. The huge bonfires that were set a-burning in times of pestilence were intended to destroy the contagium in the air. We find these views clearly expressed in the writings of Fracastoro.

In early days the contagium was a hypothetical substance; but the hypothesis of its existence was an extremely fruitful one, and did good service in concrete attempts to arrest the spread of epidemics. Of course investigators were trying to discover the nature of the contagium. The better acquainted they became with it, the more effective would be the measures undertaken to hinder its spread. In the seventeenth century, the Dutch microscopist and naturalist Leeuwenhoek perceived extremely minute living creatures invisible to the naked eye. He was the first to see the infusoria; and he also detected bacteria, minute rod-shaped organisms, in scrapings from his own tongue. There were not as yet any grounds for the belief that these minute organisms, these microbes as we now call them, could be causes of disease, but the mere knowledge that they existed was of great importance.

Likewise before the close of the seventeenth century the Jesuit father Athanasius Kircher examined under the microscope pus and blood from plague patients, and saw in them (so he believed) tiny worms. This led him to suppose that the contagium of oriental plague was a "contagium animatim" or "contagium vivum"; and also that, as Varro had assumed in the first century B.C., minute living organisms must exist in the exhalations from marshes. We now know Kircher's observations to have been erroneous, for the "tiny worms" he fancied himself to have seen were blood corpuscles, present in the healthy no less than in the sick. Still, thanks to him the idea of a contagium vivum became more firmly established.

The problem belonged to the domain of natural science, and could not be solved until greatly improved scientific instruments were at the disposal of investigators. That was why the definitive establishment of the notion of a living contagion was postponed until the nineteenth century, being first effected by Jakob Henle.

Henle was a pupil of Johannes Müller, one of the first, for he had worked under Müller in Bonn. Subsequently, when Müller removed to Berlin, he was appointed the latter's prosector. Becoming suspect to the authorities as a member of the Burschenschaft, he was prosecuted, and was sentenced to six years' detention in a fortress, but was amnestied, and in 1840 went to Zurich as professor of anatomy. There he got into touch with Schönlein who, however, that same year, transferred from Zurich to Berlin. In 1839, Schönlein had published his discovery of the exciting cause of favus. In 1840, appeared Henle's *Pathologische Untersuchungen,* which had been written before leaving Berlin, and which marked a new stage in the doctrine of infectious disorders.

The starting-point of Henle's researches were studies which

had been made concerning fermentation. A French physicist, Cagniard de la Tour, had shown that alcoholic fermentation was always associated with the presence of yeast, and that yeast was a lowly organism reproducing itself by budding or by spore-formation. A few years later, these investigations were amply confirmed by Schwann. It had become plain that such tiny organisms could effect extensive chemical changes. Observers had also discovered that these micro-organisms multiplied enormously in decomposing organic substances. Previously yeast had been regarded as a crystalline ferment, but now it was seen to be a fungus, a living organism. How natural, then, to compare the working of such a ferment with that of the hypothetical contagium vivum. Presumably the virus which was instrumental in spreading epidemics must, like yeast, consist of living organisms.

It was from this point that Henle's studies set out. The first section of his *Pathologische Untersuchungen* was a discussion "Of Miasmata and Contagia and of the Miasmatic-Contagious Diseases." He used the term "miasma" to denote the infective substance which invades human organisms and produces disease. A miasma was the virus of an epidemic or endemic infective disorder. The prototype of miasmatic diseases was malaria, which was not conveyed by direct infection from human being to human being, but was due exclusively to environmental influences. A "contagium," as contrasted with a "miasma," was an infective material which passed from one sick individual to another. The classical instance of such a contagious disease was syphilis, which was not produced by environmental influences, but was always acquired through direct infection from person to person. Most of the other "infectious disorders" were believed to be miasmatic-contagious, this meaning that they were sometimes acquired through contagion from one human being to another and were sometimes produced by environmental influences. If, however, miasma and contagium could cause the same illness, they must

351

be identical. This was Henle's first inference. Well now, of what nature could this infective virus be? Obviously it must consist of a material which, though introduced in very small quantities, could give rise to great biological transformations; must consist of something which grew, which multiplied, in the organism of the sick, increasing (manifestly) through the assimilation of substances foreign to itself. But the only things that could behave in this way were living organisms, subsisting as distinct individuals. The irrefragable inference was that the contagium must be a contagium animatum or contagium vivum. The infective virus of epidemic disorders must consist of living beings, akin to yeast, akin to the minute fungi which Bassi and Schönlein had discovered.

Henle's inferences were cogent. His book was a work of genius. Nevertheless it secured little recognition. The reasons for this failure are obvious enough. However convincing the author's logic, he was unable to demonstrate by actual observations the existence of the living organisms he assumed to exist. The yeast plant could be seen under the microscope, and people were willing to believe the evidence of their own eyes. But they were weary of speculation. After all, Henle's theory of the contagium animatum was no more than a speculation.

The before-mentioned pathological studies formed only a small part of Henle's work. Primarily he was an anatomist, and he did yeoman's service in this field. He was the discoverer of epithelium, was the founder of histology, the science of the minute structure of the tissues. He wrote both a *General Anatomy* and a *Systematic Anatomy*, and these attracted wide attention thanks to their illustrations. While still professor at Zurich he wrote a *Handbuch der rationellen Pathologie*, and founded a "Zeitschrift für rationelle Medizin." Like the investigators in Tübingen and like those in Berlin, he wanted to inaugurate a scientific pathology. Each of these groups had its own journal, and they were at daggers drawn one with

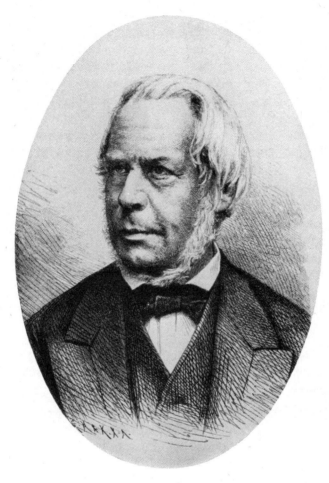

JAKOB HENLE, 1809–1885

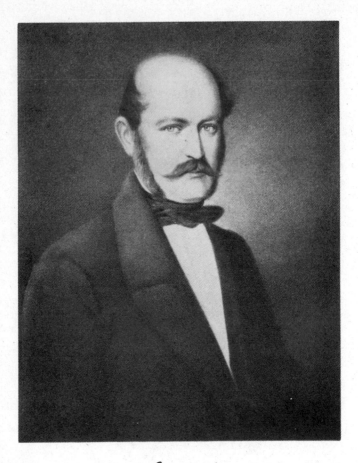

IGNAZ PHILIPP SEMMELWEIS, 1818–1865

another. Fundamentally, however, they were all striving to reach the same goal.

In 1844, Henle had a call to Heidelberg, and in 1852 he removed to Göttingen, where, until his death more than thirty years later, he was busied in fruitful work as a teacher and investigator.

CHAPTER FORTY-ONE

IGNAZ PHILIPP SEMMELWEIS
1818–1865

Now for an interlude, concerning Semmelweis and puerperal fever. His life was one of unceasing struggle: a fight against the illness he wished to make an end of; a fight to secure the acceptance of his teaching, since he was firmly convinced of its soundness; and a fight against the numerous disappointments which life brought him.

Having studied medicine in Vienna and in Budapest, in 1846 he became assistant at the first Viennese Lying-in Hospital. In that same year, Skoda had been appointed professor, two years before Rokitansky. The new Viennese school stood at its climax. In the Lying-in Hospital, however, matters were at a bad pass. The mortality from puerperal fever was enormous, was terrifying. A remarkable feature of the case was that at the first Hospital, which was utilised for the instruction of medical students, the average mortality of women in childbed was 10 per cent. and in certain months was as high as 30 per cent., whereas at the second Hospital, where midwives were trained, the mortality was only 3 per cent. Doctors in those days had very vague ideas as to the nature of puerperal fever, regarding it as a peculiar form of epidemic disease. Naturally, in Vienna, there was much controversy as to what could be the cause of the differing mortality in the two hospitals. The authorities blamed all sorts of atmospheric, cosmic, and telluric influences; said that perhaps overcrowding was at fault; opined that the excessive mortality at the first Hospital must be due to the emotional strain to which the women in childbed there were subjected because they were examined by male students. In desperation, the foreign students were excluded from the first Hospital, on the ground that

354

they were rougher in their examinations than the Viennese.

Naturally enough, the first Hospital became notorious, and it is impossible, even after the lapse of years, to read Semmelweis' description without a sense of horror: "There were heart-rending scenes when patients knelt down, wringing their hands, to beg for a transfer to the second Hospital, having, by a mistake on their part, applied for admission to the first Hospital. . . . Women recently confined, with a pulse so frequent that it could not be counted, with abdomens enormously distended, with dry tongues—in a word, women suffering from severe puerperal fever—would insist, only a few hours before their death, that they were perfectly well, their object being to avoid medical treatment, since they knew that medical treatment was the immediate precursor of death." Several times a day a priest in full canonicals, preceded by a choir-boy tinkling a bell, would come to the hospital in order to give the last sacrament to the dying. We can readily imagine how distressing it must have been to a sensitive-minded physician to find himself helpless in face of such distresses. "It was a fresh shock to me every time I heard the bell as the priest passed my door, and once again I heaved a sigh for the victim who was to be destroyed by an unknown cause. The bell, in fact, became for me an exhortation to search with all my energies in order to elucidate the cause."

Illumination came. In the spring of 1847, Semmelweis made a trip to Venice, "hoping, through the sight of the art treasures in that city, to recover the equanimity which had been so greatly shaken by the events in the lying-in hospital." Immediately after his return to Vienna he was informed of the sudden death of his intimate friend Kolletschka, professor of medical jurisprudence, whose finger had been pricked by a maladroit student during a post-mortem examination and who had died of blood-poisoning. "I was instantly struck with the close resemblance of the malady from which Kolletschka had died to that from which I had seen countless numbers of women perish after childbirth." The symptoms were, in truth, identical.

The facts were plain. Just as the post-mortem knife which had caused Kolletschka's death had been infected with materials from a dead body, so, likewise, were infected the fingers of the examining physicians and students who, in Vienna where post-mortem examinations were so frequent, continually handled the viscera of the bodies of the dead. Semmelweis himself used to make post-mortem examinations every morning. Puerperal fever, then, was not due to any peculiar "epidemic constitution," but was a decomposition of the blood just like that caused by wound-infection. It became clear why the second Hospital was much less devastated by puerperal fever, seeing that the midwives had little opportunity of getting their fingers contaminated in this particular way. It was plain, too, why women who were delivered rapidly before an examination had taken place never sickened from puerperal fever, whereas those in whom labour was tedious and in whom numerous examinations were made were almost certain to die from the disease. It was comprehensible, moreover, why the mortality was much lower during the vacation, and also why puerperal fever was comparatively rare in country districts. Taking prompt action in the light of these considerations, Semmelweis insisted that in his clinic every doctor and student must disinfect the hands with chlorine water before making an examination—and immediately there was a great decline in mortality.

One might suppose that so epoch-making a discovery would speedily have achieved general recognition. This was far from being the case. Semmelweis declared: "It is owing to the doctors that there is so high a mortality in childbed." He himself frankly acknowledged: "As a logical outcome of my conviction I have to acknowledge that God only knows how many women I have prematurely brought down into the grave." Others were less frank. No doubt such men as Skoda and Hebra

were quick to appreciate the value of Semmelweis' work and
to proclaim the importance of his discovery. His fiercest
adversaries, however, were his own immediate colleagues, the
professors of midwifery, who regarded themselves as affronted.
There ensued a deplorable and long-lasting controversy
between Semmelweis and the most noted accoucheurs of
the day. On the one side there was a sincere conviction,
which often enough found expression in bitter phraseology;
and on the other side there was scorn and cold rejection.
"Murder must cease," wrote Semmelweis; "and I shall do
my utmost to ensure the cessation of murder, for everyone
who dares to disseminate dangerous fallacies concerning
puerperal fever will find in me an extremely active opponent.
I am firmly convinced that there is no other way of putting a
stop to these murders than the ruthless exposure of my
adversaries, and no one whose heart is in the right place will
blame me for the means I use."

Writing to Scanzoni, the famous Würzburg accoucheur,
he said: "If, Sir, without having refuted my doctrine, you
continue to teach the students and the midwives you train
that puerperal fever is an ordinary epidemic disease, I proclaim
you before God and the world to be an assassin, and the history
of puerperal fever would not do you an injustice were it, on
the grounds that you were the first to set yourself in opposition
to my life-saving discovery, to immortalise you as a medical
Nero."

It will readily be understood that such language as this did
not make Semmelweis popular. There was no chance of
promotion for him at the university of Vienna. His request
to be allowed to lecture there was at first bluntly rejected, and
was in the end granted only on the condition that he might
demonstrate operations upon the model exclusively. Naturally
he would not be content with this grudging concession. Five
days after his appointment as instructor, he shook the dust of
Vienna off his feet, and in 1851 returned to his native city

of Budapest, where he was able to work as honorary physician to the St. Rochus Hospital under the most unhygienic conditions imaginable. At length, after four years, he became ordinary professor of midwifery at the university of Budapest. He refused a call to Zurich, though made in gratifying terms, for he felt more at home in Buda.

His end was tragical. The joy of life, the exuberant cheerfulness, which, during the years when he was an assistant physician, had enabled him to divert himself many an evening in the Prater, and there to forget the troubles with which he was environed, had long since been damped by struggle and bitterness. His memory began to fail. His mind became clouded. At length he had to be put under restraint in an asylum. As a culmination of tragedy, he died when only forty-seven years of age of the very disease which had given him the hint needed for his discovery. He injured himself while performing an operation, and, like his friend Kolletschka long before, died of blood-poisoning.

Semmelweis wrote little, having no taste for it, as he himself declared. Apart from a few lectures and his notorious *Open Letters*, he published only one book of note, the *Aetiologie, Begriff und Prophylaxis des Kindbettfiebers*, which appeared in the year 1861. It is a small volume, simple and unadorned, but cogent through its presentation of hard facts and through its inexorable consistency—being a work which was intended to overcome the last resistance to his teaching. Semmelweis made his discovery empirically. He recognised that puerperal fever was a form of wound-infection. The post-partum uterus is like a huge wound, and can, like any other open wound, be readily contaminated by decomposing organic substances, with the result that a deadly form of blood-poisoning arises. He showed that certain chemicals could make these poisonous substances harmless. Thus he was a pioneer in the realisation of the modern notion of antisepsis. But he had no clear notion as to the nature of the virus. He was not aware that

358

living organisms were at work in producing wound-infection and puerperal fever. His doctrine lacked convincing force until these organisms had been discovered, but as soon as they had been discovered it became part of the general theory of infectious disorders. The actual discovery and demonstration of the contagia viva was the work of the men to whom we shall now turn.

CHAPTER FORTY-TWO

LOUIS PASTEUR
1822–1895

DOES Pasteur belong in this series of discoverers? Can we count him among the great doctors? He was a chemist, not a physician. History, however, is concerned, not with diplomas, but with achievements. Pasteur did far more for the prevention of illness, did far more in this respect on behalf of human welfare in general, than many "great doctors" who lived before and after him. Few men of science have become so widely known as he. Every child in France is familiar with his name and venerates him as a public benefactor.

Like Claude Bernard, Pasteur was a Burgundian. Born at Dôle in the year 1822, the son of a tanner, he was destined for the scholastic profession. Having been sent to Paris to study at the Ecole Normale, he showed from the outset noteworthy scientific talent. Becoming assistant to one of his teachers, Dumas the chemist, his first piece of original work was an important discovery. It was known that the chemical structure of tartaric acid and racemic acid was identical. But the two substances exhibited a noteworthy difference in their effect upon polarised light, tartaric acid being dextro-rotary, whereas racemic acid or paratartaric acid has no effect on the plane of polarised light, being optically neutral. Pasteur was able to prove that there are two kinds of tartaric acid which, though they have the same chemical formula, have the atoms arranged in inverse fashion, so that one of them, dextro-tartaric acid, rotates the place of polarised light to the right, whereas the other, laevo-tartaric acid, rotates it to the left. Racemic acid he showed to be a mixture of dextro-tartaric and laevo-tartaric acid in equal proportions. That is why it is optically neutral. This discovery laid the foundations of stereochemistry.

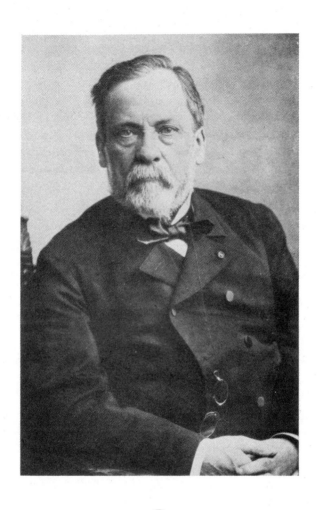

LOUIS PASTEUR, 1822–1897

After spending several years engaged in teaching activities at Dijon and Strasburg, Pasteur removed to Lille as dean of the newly founded faculty of natural science there. Lille being one of the chief centres of the manufacture of alcohol, the place gave him an opportunity of showing his inclination to attack practical problems and to solve them by scientific methods. Pasteur was not by temperament a man of the laboratory, although he spent the greater part of his life in laboratories. He was not a man of pure science, who studies science for its own sake from sheer joy in the process of scientific thought. He was, before all, practical. Life again and again confronted him with practical tasks, which he endeavoured to perform with the aid of science. Thus was it in Lille. The industry of the district being what it was, he naturally devoted special attention to fermentation. I have already related how Cagniard de la Tour and Schwann had recognised the part played by yeast in bringing about alcoholic fermentation. Pasteur retested their results, and was able to confirm them. He found it to be true that alcoholic fermentation was caused by the vital processes of small living creatures, the yeasts. What about other fermentations? Milk sours, butter turns rancid. What mechanisms are at work in such cases? Pasteur discovered that here, likewise, minute living organisms participated in the process. He found that lactose was converted into lactic acid and that butter fat was converted into butyric acid by the influence of microbes, but that there was a fundamental difference from the working of yeast, seeing that in lactic and butyric fermentations the change was caused by bacteria which throve only in the absence of free oxygen, by organisms which were anaerobic instead of aerobic—a discovery which was of fundamental importance to the understanding of the processes of putrefaction.

Coming as he did from a wine-growing district, Pasteur had often heard his compatriots complain that wine so readily "fell sick," just like living creatures. They did not know how to explain the process, and were therefore unable to ward it off and to avoid the losses it entailed. Now Pasteur's studies on fermentation showed him how wine was spoiled. Here, likewise, micro-organisms were at work, and if the organisms could be destroyed, or if contamination of the wine with them could be prevented, the undesirable change would not take place. He discovered that the microbes were killed by heat. If the wine were heated, it ought to keep perfectly. An experiment was made. A sailing vessel which was about to put to sea was supplied with two barrels of wine, the wine in one having been heated and that in the other not. After ten months, the wine that had been heated was unchanged and in good condition, whereas the unheated wine was scarcely fit to drink. A process for the preservation of wine had been discovered, and this was, after its discoverer, called "pasteurisation."

Next he had to tackle a far more thorny problem. The yeasts that were used to produce alcoholic fermentation were artificially added to the fermentable saccharine solution. But whence did the microbes come by which milk, wine, and beer were spoiled? Did they arise within the fermented substance, spontaneously, or were they introduced from without? The ticklish question of spontaneous generation had come up for solution once more. Pasteur, who had meanwhile become director of scientific studies at the Ecole Normale in Paris, devoted himself to the question, although many of his friends warned him that a number of noted investigators had burned their fingers in trying to handle this matter. Even at so late a date as the middle of the nineteenth century, spontaneous generation still had zealous defenders, one of whom was Pouchet, a fierce adversary of Pasteur. Whence could these millions of microbes derive if not from the decomposing substance itself? Pasteur, however, knowing that yeast was the cause and not the consequence of alcoholic fermentation, worked on the assumption that the micro-organisms in wine and in milk were causes and not consequences of the changes that occurred in those fluids. If, however, they were derived from without, whence could they come but from the environing atmosphere. For years Pasteur made experiments along these lines. Easily decomposable substances, such as urine above all, were sterilised by heating them in glass retorts—and remained unaltered so long as protected from the access of air. No germs appeared in them for in indefinite period, but they began to decompose as soon as air was admitted. These experiments proved beyond the shadow of a doubt that the germs of decomposition came from the air, from the environment at large, for in water too, in the earth, wherever human beings herd together, there are millions upon millions of bacteria, and they are more numerous the more closely people are packed upon the ground.

Now at length it was realised that in the entourage of human beings there are swarms of minute unicellular living creatures, bacteria and other microscopic fungi. It was known, furthermore, that these bacteria were not harmless, but that many of them were capable of bringing about extensive biological transformations. An obvious deduction was that certain microbes must constitute the contagium animatum.

Once more it was a practical problem which led Pasteur into a new field. In the year 1865 the silk-growing industry of southern France was faced by a catastrophe. The spotted disease of silkworms known as pébrine had broken out in epidemic form, and everywhere the caterpillars were dying. Whole districts were being impoverished. Pasteur was sent for to study the malady. He had never before had a silkworm in his hand. He went to the region, examined the question without prejudice, made experiments, and, after a few years, having had to cope with immense difficulties, he was able to elucidate the nature of the disease, to ascertain the method of infection, and to indicate a way of breeding healthy stock. The French silk industry was saved. Naturally the work done

363

upon this problem tended more and more to direct his attention to the infectious diseases in general.

He studied two epizootics, chicken cholera and splenic fever, which were causing enormous losses to stock-raisers. The latter deadly disease was also frequently transmitted to man (anthrax, malignant pustule, wool-sorters' disease, etc.). Earlier investigators had discovered a bacillus in the blood of animals that had died of splenic fever, and young Robert Koch had written an excellent little monograph upon the subject. A bacillus had also been found in cases of chicken cholera, had been artificially cultivated, and had then, inoculated into healthy birds, produced the fatal disease. Pasteur, one day, tried the effect of inoculating a culture several weeks old which had been overlooked in a corner of the laboratory, and found that, although the expected malady was produced, it did not, as was usually the case, prove fatal. The virulence of the bacteria had manifestly been weakened by storage. But when the birds which had just passed through a mild attack produced by the inoculation were reinoculated with fresh and fully virulent culture, they proved to be immune. The mild infection resulting from the mitigated virus protected them against further attacks of the disease.

The process was analogous to that of vaccination as an immuniser against smallpox, for here also a mitigated virus produced an active immunity. That which was possible in the case of smallpox was, then, possible in the case of other infectious disorders. What had to be done was to prepare a number of such mitigated viruses for different diseases, viruses which Pasteur termed "vaccines" by analogy with cowpox lymph. He was able to produce the vaccines requisite to cope with chicken cholera, splenic fever, and swine fever, thus saving stock-raisers from tremendous losses. Above all, however, Pasteur found a remedy for one of the illnesses which had long been a terror to mankind—hydrophobia. This was a peculiarly difficult task, and only after prolonged and laborious experiments was he able, by drying the spinal cord of animals infected with rabies, to produce a vaccine which, when injected into human beings who had been bitten by rabid dogs, was competent, during the lengthy incubation period, to produce immunity before the dreaded and invariably fatal attack of hydrophobia began. For practical purposes, this dreadful disease has been vanquished.

Like Claude Bernard, Pasteur did his early work under extremely primitive conditions. To-day in the Ecole Normale visitors are still shown a room so low-ceilinged that one cannot stand upright in it—the room where Pasteur performed the first of a series of experiments which showed spontaneous generation to be a chimera. Not until 1888, when he was already sixty-six years of age, were funds collected to establish the Pasteur Institute for the preventive treatment of hydrophobia and for far-reaching researches into the causes, prevention, and treatment of other infectious disorders.

Pasteur was a man of genius, impulsive, intuitive, full of fruitful ideas. Though he was a chemist, not a physician, medicine owes him much. His practical achievements and the knowledge he garnered were, in other hands, soon to produce even more important results.

CHAPTER FORTY-THREE

ROBERT KOCH
1843–1910

THE Franco-German war was over. When it broke out, Pasteur was above the age for military service. Nevertheless this war, this armed conflict between two great nations (and the two which throughout the nineteenth century had been most passionately devoted to the study of natural science), had been a profound shock to him. On the German side a young physician, Robert Koch, had taken part in the war as a volunteer. He was twenty years younger than Pasteur and sprang from a miner's family. From early youth he had shown a strong inclination towards scientific research. At Göttingen he studied mathematics and natural science, then entered himself as a medical student, and became one of Henle's pupils.

In 1872, when the war was over and done with, Robert Koch settled down as district medical officer at a little town named Bomst in Wollstein. The place had no more than four thousand inhabitants, but the new doctor soon secured a large practice, and his official duties made it necessary for him to travel extensively through the surrounding country. Already Koch was an ardent scientist. He established a primitive laboratory in his rooms, and he soon found himself faced with a great task. Again and again, in the region where he worked, epidemics of splenic fever occurred among the live-stock, and endangered the human population. What was the cause of this disease, and how was it transmitted? As far back as 1849, a veterinary surgeon, Pollender by name, had discovered rod-like organisms in the blood of animals that had died of the disease, specimens of a giant bacillus. Was this bacillus a cause or a consequence of the disease? The question was difficult to answer, for the organism was not constantly present

366

in the blood. Then, in 1863, Davaine, by the inoculation of blood containing these bacilli, was able to transmit the disease to healthy animals. This made it extremely probable that the bacillus was in actual fact the cause of splenic fever. Further investigations showed, however, that the malady could likewise be transmitted by the blood of infected animals when this blood was free from bacilli. Thus the whole question as to the exciting cause was rendered dubious once more.

Here was an extremely complicated problem for Koch to tackle. He kept a stock of mice infected with anthrax, examined their blood repeatedly under the microscope, and discovered that the anthrax bacilli grew into long threads, propagating themselves by transverse fission, and forming spores. Whereas the bacteria had comparatively slight powers of resistance, and soon perished outside the body of the infected animal, the spores retained their virulence for years. If they made their way, through the instrumentality of the food or of the air, into an animal body, they grew into bacteria, and gave rise to the disease. In this way the etiology of splenic fever was definitively elucidated. Koch went to Breslau to consult the botanist F. Cohn, at that time the most noted expert in the biology of the schizomycetes, and was able to satisfy Cohn of the accuracy of his observations. Not until this had been done did Koch publish his results, which appeared in Cohn's "Beiträge zur Biologie der Pflanzen," in the year 1876.

This work of Koch's was of fundamental importance. Not only did the paper, in its simplicity and lucidity, show itself to be the model of a scientific monograph; more momentous still, this was the first time when the causation of an infectious disorder had been demonstrated beyond the possibility of doubt. As regards splenic fever or anthrax it now became plain to everyone that miasma and contagium were not mysterious substances, were not vague ferments, but micro-organisms, schizomycetes, bacteria or their spores. The biology of one of these pathogenic bacilli was described in every detail, an account being given of its life-history both within and without the organism. Koch further showed how the investigator must work with such bacteria, how to obtain them from the infected animal, how to cultivate them artificially, and also how to destroy them, this being obviously the matter of primary significance. The destruction of the infective bacillus, the protection of the animal organism against the exciting cause of disease, was the main purpose of these researches. In the study of anthrax it was made perfectly clear that the exciting causes of infectious diseases are specific, this meaning that bacteria do not change haphazard into one another, and that a particular bacillus always causes a particular disease. It had already become plain to Koch that a bacterium could only be regarded as the exciting cause of a disease if its presence could invariably be demonstrated in this disease, if it could be artificially cultivated outside the organism, and if the injection of a pure culture into a healthy animal reproduced the original illness.

Now that the etiology of anthrax had thus been elucidated, there were adequate grounds for the assumption that every infectious disorder is caused by some specific organism. As early as 1873, three years before Koch's paper on anthrax was published, Obermeyer had discovered a spiral-shaped micro-organism, a spirochete, to be the exciting cause of relapsing fever. That same year Obermeyer died of cholera, so that his investigations were not followed up. In 1879, three years after the publication of Koch's paper, Neisser discovered the gonococcus as the exciting cause of gonorrhoea; in the following year, Eberth and Gaffky discovered the typhoid bacillus, Hansen discovered the exciting cause of leprosy, and Laveran discovered the exciting cause of malaria—this last not being one of the fission-fungi, but a minute animal organism, a protozoon. Thus rapidly did advances occur in this field.

Nor had Koch remained idle. Encouraged by the success of his first investigations, he devoted himself to the study of

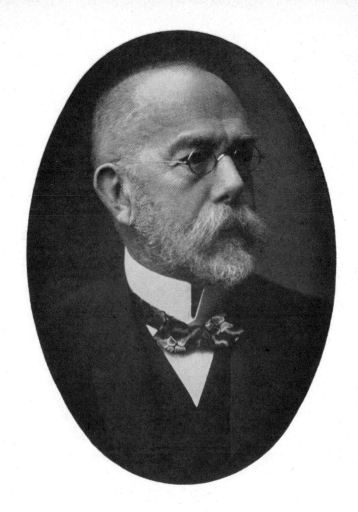

ROBERT KOCH

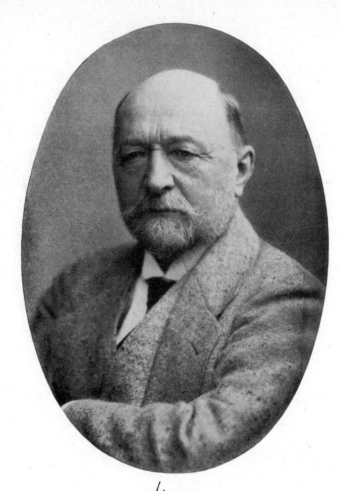

EMIL BEHRING, 1854–1917

wound-infections, and was able to demonstrate the existence of a number of specific bacteria giving rise to such maladies. He worked under very difficult conditions in his small private laboratory, and it speaks well for the intelligence of the German government that in 1880 Koch became a member of the Imperial Board of Health, and was thus afforded opportunities for continuing his labours under much more satisfactory auspices. The year before, vaccination had been made compulsory in the Empire and the Imperial Board of Health had been established to ensure the proper carrying-out of the Vaccination Act. This was in 1876, but ere long the Board was to become a central station for epidemiological research in general. It was in this institution that Koch elaborated the methods of bacteriological research which are still universally applied, and he developed above all the methodology of disinfection. Whereas hitherto the campaign against infective organisms had been mainly waged with chemical substances, and especially with acids of one sort or another, Koch showed that disinfection by steam was much more reliable, since this destroyed spores as well as the parent organisms.

On March 24, 1882, Koch informed the Berlin Physiological Society that he had discovered the tubercle bacillus, the exciting cause of tuberculosis. He had been able to prove that pulmonary consumption was not, as had been widely supposed, a chronic disorder of nutrition, but an infectious disorder that runs a chronic course. His work thus gave brilliant confirmation to the experiments of Villemin, who in 1865 had shown that tuberculosis could be transmitted from human beings to rabbits. Various other diseases, maladies of the skin, affections that had been classed as surgical, etc., were to disclose themselves as tubercular now that the exciting cause was known. In the bacillus, doctors had a trustworthy diagnostic sign, and they knew that destruction of the bacillus signified destruction of the infective material.

Koch now turned to new tasks. Cholera was on the march

once more. Setting out from India, it had reached Egypt and was threatening Europe. Koch travelled to meet it, and in 1883 discovered the exciting cause, the cholera vibrio, also known as the comma bacillus. He found that this exciting cause was mainly transmitted to human beings through the instrumentality of water.

Researches of the kind continued without pause. A whole generation of investigators devoted themselves to the campaign against pestilences. Each year brought fresh discoveries. In 1882, Löffler discovered the glanders bacillus; Bollinger and Harz discovered the actinomyces bovis, which is the cause of actinomycosis. Next year, Fehleisen discovered the exciting cause of erysipelas. The year 1884 was exceptionally fruitful, for in this came the discovery of the diphtheria bacillus by Löffler, of the tetanus bacillus by Nikolaier, and of the pneumonia bacillus by Fraenkel. In 1887, Weichselbaum discovered the exciting cause of epidemic cerebrospinal meningitis; in 1894, Kitasato and Yersin discovered the bacillus of bubonic plague; and in 1897, Kruse and Shiga discovered the exciting cause of dysentery. In 1901 came the discovery by Forde, Dutton, and Bruce of the exciting cause of sleeping-sickness; and 1905 was marked by Schaudinn's discovery of the spirochaete pallida, the exciting cause of syphilis.

Koch spent a considerable part of his life in travel. Many of the most destructive epidemics flourished mainly or exclusively in the tropics, and had to be studied in their homes. In South Africa, Koch made researches into the nature of rinderpest; and in Hindustan he supplemented the work which had been done by previous investigators upon bubonic plague, he and his collaborators being able to show that the malady is transmitted to human beings by the rat-flea. He also made expeditions to German East Africa for the study of diseases conveyed by the tse-tse fly; he examined the causation of another insect-borne disease, Texas fever; and he went to Java for researches upon malaria.

In the year 1885, Koch was appointed professor of hygiene and director of the Hygienic Institute at the university of Berlin. By temperament, however, he was wholly devoted to research, and his field of labour was the wide world. He could not hear of an epidemic anywhere without wanting to set forth and study it. It did not suit him to spend year after year teaching students the elements of hygiene. In 1891, therefore, he resigned his professorship and directorship to become chief of the Institute for Infectious Disorders brought into being for the conduct of his specialised researches and called by his name. He remained head of this until he retired in the year 1904.

One malady, above all, interested Koch throughout his life. Again and again he returned to the problem of tuberculosis. Far-reaching excitement was caused when, in 1890, at the Tenth International Medical Congress, sitting that year in Berlin, he announced that he had succeeded in isolating a substance which could "check the growth of tubercle bacilli, not only in a test-tube, but also in the animal body." Patients suffering from tuberculosis, inspired with fresh hope, flocked to Berlin from all over the world in order to try the new remedy which, as was subsequently disclosed, was a glycerine extract of a pure culture of tubercle bacilli and was known as tuberculin. But the new remedy failed to fulfil its discoverer's hopes. There was a reaction against its use. However, in subsequent years similar preparations, more or less modified, came into use. These are unquestionably of great value for diagnostic purposes, and some of them are perhaps of therapeutic value.

When, on May 21, 1910, an end came to Robert Koch's laborious life, it was possible to look back upon unexpected advances which were due to him, to Pasteur, and to their pupils. The infectious disorders had lost many of their terrors. They were better known than they had ever been known before. They could, as it were, be seen face to face. The struggle with them had become an open one. If we know our enemy, we have far less reason to dread his power. That is why cancer is so sinister, because it is an unknown adversary, one of whose nature we still know little or nothing, so that we cannot attack it at the root. Most of the infectious diseases, however, have now yielded up their secrets. By the time of Koch's retirement from active work, it was known, in the case of most of them, which was the best line, the best point, of attack. Many illnesses of the kind had been completely exterminated; others had been got largely under control; mortality was on the decline. Regions of the earth hitherto inaccessible for settlement by white men have now been made available, through mastery of the epidemic and endemic diseases that used to prevail there. Few pestilences, nowadays, are natural catastrophes which must be allowed to run their course unheeded and accepted as the decrees of fate, for most of the infectious disorders have become avoidable maladies, and society has devoted a large part of its energy to hindering the outbreak and spread of epidemics. I need hardly say that we are not yet at the end of the struggle. Countless thousands still die year after year of tuberculosis; and there are other infectious disorders against which we stand weaponless. Still, we have made close acquaintance with the methods by which we can hope to effect their conquest.

Within the lifetime of the elders among us, we have become more closely acquainted, not only with the biology of the exciting causes of disease, but also with the physiological mechanisms by which the organism protects itself against bacteria, and we have learned to turn these mechanisms purposively to account in our campaign against infectious disorders. It was above all to Emil Behring (1854–1917) that must be ascribed some of the most important advances in this field of knowledge. Behring was a pupil of Koch, and then his fellow-worker. After some preliminary years as army surgeon, Behring became assistant at the Berlin Institute of Hygiene, transferred with Koch to the new Institute for Infectious Diseases, became in 1894 professor of hygiene in Halle, and the following year professor in Marburg.

Bacteria which have become parasitic in an organism produce poison, toxins, chemical substances of an albuminous nature. For instance, it came to be recognised that the morbific agent of the diphtheria bacillus was the diphtheria toxin, which various observers had been able to detect in fluid cultures. Behring showed that the infected organism protects itself against such toxins by the formation of antitoxins, which combine with the toxins to form innocuous products. Thus in the blood serum of animals infected with diphtheria he found the diphtheria antitoxin, able in the animal body just as in a test-tube to combine with and thus neutralise the diphtheria toxin. Animals which have been immunised by the injection of this toxin in gradually increasing doses have large quantities of antitoxin in their blood. After extensive researches, Behring demonstrated that this diphtheria antitoxin, when injected into a human being, could not only bring about a transient immunity to diphtheritic infection, but could exert a remedial action in an individual in whom diphtheria had already begun. Thus by serotherapy, the diseased organism is helped to cope with its enemy. The means employed are those already being utilised by the organism. It creates antitoxins for itself, but cannot always create them fast enough or in sufficient quantities. We assist it, therefore, by artificially supplying it with antitoxin, with a larger supply of the defensive substance it needs to neutralise the toxin by entering into combination with it. We create a passive immunity.

The success of the serum treatment of diphtheria was amazing. Wherever the use of Behring's antitoxin was tried, there was an immediate and notable decline in mortality. In one of the Berlin hospitals, the death rate in cases of diphtheria fell from 48 per cent. to 13 per cent. In a hospital at Trieste, out of 236 patients injected with the antitoxic serum during a severe epidemic, 22 per cent. had died. Then the supply of serum ran short, and the lack could not be promptly supplied, whereupon the mortality instantly rose to 50 per cent. Even Virchow, who to begin with had been extremely sceptical about serology, had to admit: "Theoretical considerations must give way before the brute force of figures, which are so expressive as to defy contradiction."

Diphtheria, which used to be one of the most dreaded maladies of childhood, has lost much of its danger. In the year 1925, the total mortality from diphtheria in Germany was only 10 per cent. of that in the year 1877. Behring's services in this matter secured public recognition by the grant of the Nobel prize in the year 1901.

The principle of serotherapy and of artificial immunisation has been applied with great success to certain other diseases. One of the most notable of these is tetanus. If in every suspect wound the patient is given a dose of tetanus antitoxin, this dreaded disease will very rarely ensue. The Great War was, from that point of view, an experiment upon a vast scale to demonstrate the value of tetanus antitoxin.

CHAPTER FORTY-FOUR

JOSEPH LISTER
1827–1912

WE have traced the development of the anatomical concept
of disease step by step from the Renaissance onward. The
reader has been able to note how in the seventeenth century
physiology, in the eighteenth century pathology, and at the
opening of the nineteenth century clinical medicine and
diagnosis became dominated by anatomical outlooks. Obviously
this anatomical conception would in due course gain control
of the last important field of medicine, namely therapeutics. It
was the anatomical attitude which gave surgery its remarkable
fresh impetus during the latter half of the nineteenth
century. Surgery is, indeed, the most cogent expression of the
anatomical idea in therapeutics, inasmuch as surgical treatment
is primarily an anatomical correction.

There were two main hindrances to the free development of
surgery. Surgical intervention caused such intolerable pain that
the surgeon had to act swiftly and operations were necessarily
of brief duration. What was done had to be done in as few
minutes, and even in as few seconds, as possible. Furthermore,
the mortality among persons subjected to operations was
extraordinarily high. The surgeon was defenceless against
wound-infection, and in many cases the result of the best
planned and best performed operation would be completely
spoiled by subsequent infective processes. Every extensive
injury involved a terrible danger. An operation was something
that had to be regarded as a last resort, when all other methods
of treatment had been tried in vain.

During the nineteenth century, both these obstacles were
removed by purposive labour. In the 'forties came the
discovery of trustworthy methods of producing anaesthesia

375

by inhalation. Long before this there had been numerous attempts to secure a local numbing, and others to produce a generalised loss of sensation. Various methods had been tried, such as compression of the nerve trunks, electricity, the application of snow, and so on. The results, however, had been unsatisfactory. Then, within the space of a few years, three substances were discovered which could produce profound anaesthesia when inhaled. The first of these was nitrous oxide or "laughing gas," which an American dentist named Horace Wells was the first to use for an operation in the year 1844. Nitrous oxide was successful in this respect, that it caused complete anaesthesia, profound insensibility, but only of brief duration. Next came the discovery of ether as an anaesthetic, and once more it was an American dentist, William Morton, who was the first to induce ether anaesthesia. A year later, in 1847, Dr. Simpson, of Edinburgh, began to employ chloroform vapour as a means of producing anaesthesia, partial or complete, in certain surgical operations and painful diseases, as well as in ordinary obstetric practice.

Thus a great advance had been made. It was now possible to operate upon a patient kept perfectly insensible and with the body entirely relaxed. But even though this facilitated the task of undertaking prolonged and extensive operations, there always loomed in the background the spectre of wound-infection.

At length this obstacle likewise was removed, and Pasteur's researches led the way. The man who applied Pasteur's ideas to operative surgery was an Englishman, Joseph Lister.

Lister sprang from a Quaker family. His father was a wine-merchant, but also a man well versed in mathematics and physics, and one who devoted his leisure to microscopical studies. Having qualified in London, young Lister went to Scotland, where in 1854 he became Syme's house-surgeon at the Edinburgh Hospital. After distinguishing himself by various anatomical, physiological, and pathological researches, he was in 1861 appointed professor of surgery in Glasgow. It was there that his decisive life-work began. The general belief still was that contused wounds necessarily suppurated. Reflection upon this matter led Lister to ask himself the simple question why compound fractures always suppurated, whereas simple fractures, those in which the skin remained intact, never suppurated, however much the tissues had been contused. It seemed to him that the question answered itself. What is the difference between an open and a closed wound? Obviously this, that the air has access to the open wound, whereas the contused tissues of a simple fracture are secluded from the air. Pasteur had shown that the air was swarming with microbes, and that these minute living organisms were the causes of fermentation and putrefaction. If Pasteur was right, then the phenomena of putrefaction in an open wound must be caused by microbes which had entered it from the air. The surgeon must make it his business to destroy these microbes, or to protect the wound from their access. How could microbes be destroyed? Pasteur had taught that boiling was the best way, but the use of that method was impossible in the case of wounds. Another method must be sought: the micro-organisms must be killed by chemical substances. Lister made various experiments, first of all with chloride of zinc, then with sulphites, and finally with carbolic acid, which he found most successful. The air in the neighbourhood of the wound was purified by the use of a carbolic spray. The wound itself after the operation was dressed with gauze, eightfold-thick, drenched with carbolic acid, liquid resin, and paraffin; between the layers of gauze was a piece of mackintosh sheeting; and the whole was covered with a sheet of waxed taffeta as protective. Such was Lister's "occlusive dressing," which soon became famous all over the world. Beneath this dressing a scab formed, and the wound healed under the scab.

The results which Lister obtained by this method were amazing. During the first three years after the introduction of his new way of treating operative wounds, he had in his hospital only one case of wound erysipelas. Hospital gangrene, one of the most dreaded forms of wound infection, was rare in his wards, and occurred only in a comparatively mild form. Of 40 patients upon whom, during this period, he performed a major amputation, only 6 died, that is to say 15 per cent. In the two previous years before the introduction of the method, of 35 major amputation cases, 16 had died, a mortality of 45.7 per cent. From 1867 onward, Lister began to publish his results, but they secured little recognition, for his doctrine stood or fell with Pasteur's theories. One who differed from Pasteur, one who did not believe in the ubiquity of bacteria, was necessarily at odds with Lister; and Pasteur had powerful adversaries.

The Franco-German war gave an opportunity for the widespread application of the new method. "Listerism" was tried by many army surgeons, and with good results. After the war it was Volkmann, in especial, who in 1874 reported striking successes with Listerism at his surgical clinic in Halle. The work of Robert Koch a few years later concerning the exciting causes of wound infection clarified people's ideas. Antisepsis secured general approval, and the path was opened for a much freer use of operative surgery.

From antisepsis to asepsis was but a step, the step from chemical to physical methods of disinfection. Surgeons came to realise what Semmelweis had already observed, that a wound is much less threatened from the air than from the instruments used by the surgeon and the surgeon's own hands. Chemical disinfection persisted for the latter, since the surgeon's hands could not be boiled; but all the instruments and dressings that came into contact with the operation wound were sterilised in boiling water or in superheated steam. Bergmann in Berlin and his pupil Schimmelbusch were two of the surgeons who did most to elaborate the aseptic method which is to-day customary in every operating theatre.

In 1869, Lister succeeded his sometime teacher Syme as

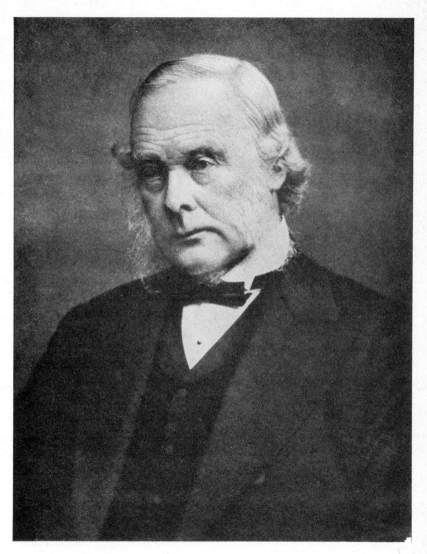

JOSEPH LISTER, 1827–1912

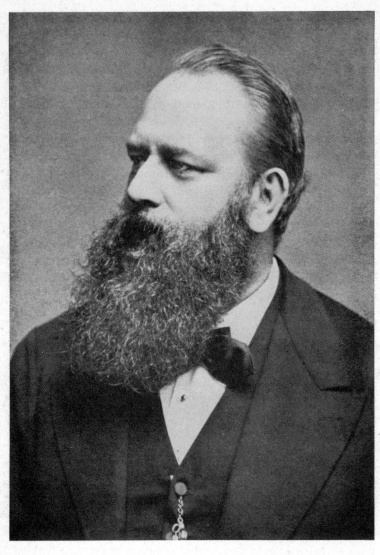

THEODOR BILLROTH, 1829–1894

professor of clinical surgery at Edinburgh. In 1877 he became professor at King's College, London, where he worked until his retirement in 1892. He laboured strenuously at the development of his method, and introduced the use of absorbable aseptic catgut for ligatures and sutures. He attained the great age of eighty-five, and was able to enjoy the satisfaction of seeing that his work had borne magnificent fruit.

CHAPTER FORTY-FIVE

THEODOR BILLROTH
1829–1894

THE barriers were down, and surgery could advance freely. One organ after another became accessible to the knife. The traditional boundaries between medicine and surgery faded away. Diseases which in former times had been regarded as purely "internal," such as gastric ulcer and cancer of the stomach, were made accessible to surgical treatment. The surgeon was no longer a mere handicraftsman. He was a physician, but a physician who used a particular therapeutic method. Remarkable successes were to increase the prestige of surgery year by year.

In all lands, surgery was advancing with giant strides. Almost every country in the world has contributed its part to this mighty impetus. From the plenitude of surgeons with impressive personalities, I will select for description one example, one of the most congenial characters known to the history of surgery—Theodor Billroth.

Billroth was a man of the intuitive type, an artist. The son of a pastor in the island of Rügen, he wanted to become a musician. Since his relatives dissuaded him from adopting this profession as one at which it would be hard to make a livelihood, he qualified as a doctor. All the same, he remained an artist, was an instrumentalist throughout his life, and was a close friend of Brahms and Hanslick. It is not by chance association that we find among the surgeons so many men of artistic temperament. Although surgery has become a science, the practice of surgery is still a skilled, an artistic handicraft.

Billroth studied at Greifswald and Göttingen, then in Berlin, while Schönlein still presided over the clinic in that city; he attended Traube's lectures; and he qualified in the year

1852. After post-graduate studies in Vienna and Paris, he took up his residence as a practitioner in Berlin. Things did not go well with him at first. For two months he waited in vain for a patient. Still, it would not do for him to spend all his time at music, since he had adopted medicine as his profession. When therefore he was offered an assistant post at the surgical clinic under Langenbeck, he accepted. Thus it was that he became a surgeon. Langenbeck was a man from whom he could learn much; not only how to operate, but also two of the other indispensable requisites of a good surgeon—fidelity and conscientiousness. As early as 1856 he became a member of the faculty as instructor in surgery and pathological anatomy. Most of the work he had done so far had been in the domain of pathological histology.

In 1860, Billroth accepted a call to Zurich. There he had a clinic of his own. The new hospital was considered one of the finest in Europe at that date, and Billroth speedily acquired a Europe-wide reputation. He remained seven years at Zurich, and during this period more than eight thousand surgical patients passed through his hands. Subsequently he published reports of his activities year by year, and these were characterised by a relentless sincerity and self-criticism. Surgical intervention was still far more often unsuccessful than successful, and much courage was needed to acknowledge the failures frankly. "Criticism," said Billroth on one occasion, "is the principal need of our day; and for this, knowledge, experience, and calm are requisite." Billroth began his criticism at home. An unsuccessful case is more instructive than ten successful ones, provided that no attempt is made to gloss over the mistake, and that the reasons for making it are thoroughly studied. Other surgical clinics followed Billroth's example in the publication of annual reports, and such reports, which did not consist merely of dry figures, but contained detailed descriptions of cases, contributed greatly to the advance of surgery.

The first important scientific task undertaken by Billroth was the study of wound infections, which were a burning problem of the day. The result of his numerous observations and experiments was published in 1862 under the title *Beobacht-ungsstudien über Wundfieber und accidentelle Wundkrankheiten.* One of the chief merits of this work was that it contained precise records of the observations which had been systemati-cally made upon the temperature of patients suffering from operative and other wounds. Just as for Wunderlich, in internal medicine, the temperature had become the main indication as to the course of the disease, so was it now for Billroth as regards surgical affections. He did not succeed, however, in discovering the true cause of wound infection. Bacteriology was still in its infancy, and the technique of making pure cultures outside the body had still to be worked out. Billroth, therefore, was not certain whether the exciting causes were in truth living organisms. If they were, he contended, their effect was not produced directly, but depended upon the chemical poisons which they formed in the blood and in the tissues.

It was while in Zurich, too, that Billroth published the finest of his books, *Die allgemeine chirurgische Pathologie und Therapie in fünfzig Vorlesungen,* one of the most splendid monuments in medical literature, a work of art in respect both of form and content, a book which ran through numerous editions and was translated into the chief languages of the world.

In 1867, he became professor of surgery at Vienna, and remained at work in the Austrian capital until shortly before his death at Abbazia in Istria on February 6, 1894. By degrees, antiseptic surgery was coming everywhere into use, so that it was possible to venture upon major abdominal operations, and it was Billroth who worked out the methods of gastro-intestinal surgery. Above all his name will remain associated with the history of the surgery of the stomach. He was the first, in the year 1881, to prove successful in the excision of the pylorus in a female patient who was suffering from cancer of that part of the gastro-intestinal tract. Before this he had

382

successfully extirpated a larynx, and these two operations of his attracted widespread attention. Billroth, however, did not aspire to create sensations, being an extremely cautious operator. He wrote: "We are only entitled to operate when there are reasonable chances of success. To use the knife when these chances are lacking is to prostitute the splendid art and science of surgery, and to render it suspect among the laity and among one's colleagues. We have to ask ourselves, then, by what standard we can measure the chances of success. We shall learn them through the indefatigable study of our science, through shrewd criticism of our own and others' observations, through careful consideration of individual cases, and through the meticulous appraisement of our results." He had no desire to establish "records," being far more concerned to elaborate sound ways of performing typical operations, to the end that operative surgery should not be solely effective in the hands of a small number of experts, but should be teachable to and learnable by the average operator.

Billroth was, in fact, mainly busied in teaching and in learning. He wrote a brilliant book upon these topics, pitilessly disclosing defects in the university curriculum—a work which brought him many enemies, but many friends as well. He was himself a great teacher. Many notable men were among his pupils, and were able to continue his work in responsible positions: Czerny, Gussenbauer, von Mikulicz, and von Eiselsberg, to name only a few of them. They all looked up to Billroth as their master, and remained faithful to his memory. Even in the pupils of these pupils, Billroth's spirit remains alive, for what he taught was something more than scientific principles, something more than operative methods; it was a medical ethos. At the close of his career he wrote: "What has given me the greatest joy in a diversified life has been the foundation of a school which is continuing the trend of my activities alike in scientific and in humanitarian directions, so that it seems destined to have a fair measure of durability."

383

CHAPTER FORTY-SIX

PAUL EHRLICH

1854–1915

BILLROTH and Ehrlich—how discordant an impression arises in our minds when we think of them together. Each name, considered singly, strikes a pure note; but altogether they are impossible. What could there be in common between Billroth the North-German and Ehrlich the Jew; between Billroth, who was an artist in every fibre of his being, and Ehrlich who was so thoroughly matter-of-fact. Ehrlich pursued his course purposively, as if obsessed, without ever glancing either to the right or to the left. He studied in Breslau, Strasburg, Freiburg, and Leipzig. He was mainly interested in histology and chemistry. Histology gave him an insight into the minutest formative elements of the organism. Chemistry provided him with the means of recognising the substance that lay beneath the form. It had long been known that each chemical substance has its own affiliations in, its own point of attack upon, the body. We see this most plainly when we stain sections of the organs or tissues. Certain parts of the cells are coloured by the stain, and other parts are not. This varying affinity for staining materials throws a great light upon structure. Towards the middle of the nineteenth century histological investigators began to stain thin slices or sections of the organs and tissues for microscopical examination, and it was this which first made histological investigation fruitful. At that time the number of available staining materials was still very small. Then, during Ehrlich's student days, a large number of aniline dyes were put upon the market.

The thesis with which Ehrlich took his degree was concerned with staining methods, with the theory and practice of histological examination as elucidated by the use of stains.

384

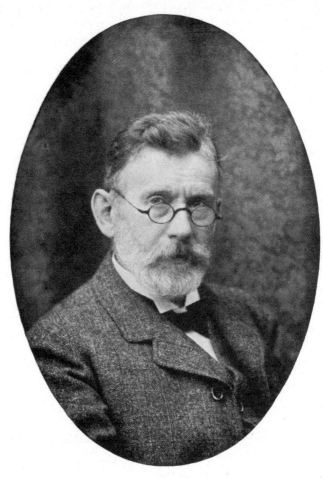

PAUL EHRLICH, 1854–1915

Frerichs summoned the young doctor as assistant at his clinic in Berlin. Recognising Ehrlich's talent, he allowed the junior to follow his own bent. Ehrlich applied his methods to the study of the blood. Of what does the blood consist? Of serum and blood corpuscles, the red corpuscles and the white, the erythrocytes and the leucocytes. But by this date it was already known that there were two kinds of "white" blood corpuscles, respectively termed lymphocytes and leucocytes. Virchow had come to that conclusion early in his career. Ehrlich made dry preparations of the blood upon cover-slips, and stained them by various methods. His researches disclosed that the morphology of the blood was far more complicated than had been previously assumed. There existed in the blood, certain cells which had affinities with alkaline dyes, others which had affinities with acid dyes, and yet others which had affinities with neutral dyes. The recognition of this was of the utmost importance to clinical medicine, inasmuch as the ratio of these various kinds of cells one to another varies in different diseases. Thus it became possible to learn vastly more about the diseases of the blood; and, over and above this, the microscopical examination of the blood developed into a diagnostic method which was of enormous value in diseases wherein the blood was not primarily disordered.

The blood which Ehrlich examined to begin with was dead; but he found that living tissues could also be stained. Methylene blue was a non-poisonous substance which could be absorbed by living tissues and could thus provide information where oxygen was being incorporated into the organism and where it was being given off. As the outcome of these investigations, in the year 1885 Ehrlich published his work entitled *Das Sauerstoffbedürfnis des Organismus* (the organism's need for oxygen). Ehrlich had devised a means for studying one of the functions of the living body while actually in progress. An additional outcome of these studies in the use of stains was what is known as the diazo-reaction. Ehrlich found that a certain chemical substance, diazo-benzene-sulphonic acid, combined with various substances in the urine to form a red colouring material. Thereby, once more, clinical medicine was enriched by a valuable diagnostic method.

Frerichs died. Gerhardt, his successor, had little interest in Ehrlich's investigations, and would not spare him any time for them. Consequently, in 1887, Ehrlich resigned his post at the Charité. Becoming affected with pulmonary tuberculosis, he had to stop work for a while. After a sojourn in Egypt, he returned to Berlin in good health, and set to work in a small private laboratory he established in his rooms. The problem to which he now devoted his attention was that of immunity. It was known that bacteria form toxins, and that the organism produces antitoxins to neutralise them. But there are other substances besides bacterial toxins which affect the organism in a similar way, for instance certain vegetable poisons, such as rizin. In the case of these intoxications, likewise, an immunity can be acquired. Ehrlich studied the laws of this immunity, and elaborated methods which proved extremely valuable for the promotion of immunity to infectious disorders. They enabled a precise gradation of the efficacy of antidiphtheritic serum to be effected. The fundamental notions of active and passive immunity were formulated by Ehrlich, and at length his studies culminated in a theory of immunity, known as the side-chain theory.

By now Robert Koch's attention had been directed towards Ehrlich. In 1890, Koch entrusted Ehrlich with the charge of an observation ward in the Moabit Hospital, for patients treated with tuberculin; and next year, when the Institute for Infectious Disorders was founded, Koch provided Ehrlich with more favourable opportunities of work. The remarkable success achieved by serum therapeutics led Althoff, the Prussian minister of State, to found a State institute for serum testing and serological research, of which Ehrlich was the chief. Three years later, the Royal Institute for Experimental

Therapeutics was founded at Frankfort-on-the-Main, and Ehrlich was put in charge. In 1906, the Georg Speyer Home for chemotherapeutics was affiliated to the foregoing.

At the Royal Institute, Ehrlich's studies took a new turn. He was still guided by the same idea, namely that the chemical substances in the organism had specific points of attack. It was by pursuing this notion and by applying staining materials to the study of histology that Ehrlich had done so much to further clinical diagnosis. The next step was to apply the same notion to therapeutics and to make it useful in that field. He wanted to find chemical substances which had very little affinity with the body cells and much affinity with bacteria; substances which would kill bacteria without harming the organism. The old Paracelsian ideal of specific remedies had re-emerged. Would it not be possible to discover a "therapia sterilisans magna"; a method of treatment thanks to which the injection of a syringe full of this sovereign remedy would destroy the bacteria which had invaded the organism? The "side-chain theory" was a guide to him in these investigations.

The first disease to which Ehrlich devoted his attention from this outlook was syphilis. He began with an arsenic compound, atoxyl, which had already given good results in the treatment of sleeping sickness. By systematic modifications of the molecules, he produced one arsenical combination after another in the hope of finding one which would comply with his theoretical demands. His experiments went on for years. The six-hundred-and-sixth preparation was salvarsan, or "606," which Ehrlich, with the collaboration of Bertheim and Benda, produced in the year 1910. The new remedy was tried with the utmost caution. Hata first demonstrated its efficacy in animals. To begin with, its use was found to be attended with danger, but, after a time, the investigators were able to obviate the noxious effects. Then an improved variant was manufactured, and was called neosalvarsan. A remedy of remarkable efficacy in the treatment of syphilis had been discovered.

These researches into the therapy of syphilis attracted attention throughout the world. Ehrlich was overwhelmed with honours. Even though salvarsan did not fulfil the desired end, and did not prove itself to be the therapia sterilisans magna as far as syphilis was concerned, it certainly did so in the case of another disease. A single injection of the drug effects a lasting cure of relapsing fever. Salvarsan has also been found extremely effective in certain other maladies. Framboesia or yaws, a contagious tropical disease, induced (like syphilis) by a spirillum, has been almost completely eradicated by salvarsan. The same drug has proved marvellously effective in a special form of angina, in Aleppo boil or oriental sore, and in a number of epizootics.

Thus once more had pure science, pursued for its own sake, produced remarkable practical results.

CHAPTER FORTY-SEVEN

MAX PETTENKOFER
1818–1901

WE learned in an earlier section that the current of the
hygienic movement which began to flow so mightily in the
eighteenth century became silted up in the opening years of
the nineteenth century. But the industrial revolution brought
in its train new dangers to public health, and compelled the
authorities to take action. Now that huge masses of human
beings were being concentrated in certain spots, thanks to the
speedy development of industry, and because they were living
under the most primitive hygienic conditions, grave dangers
to the public health ensued. Epidemic diseases were thus
provided with an appropriate soil. In 1830, Asiatic cholera
made its appearance in Europe, then and subsequently
devastating our continent for several years at a time. The
menace was grave.

The new hygienic movement began in England. It was in
Britain that industrialisation had made the greatest advances,
so naturally it was there that the first extensive attempts to
promote public hygiene were undertaken. In the year 1842,
a commission of inquiry was appointed. Statistical material
was accumulated. In 1848, the first Public Health Act was
passed. A centralised governmental authority was established
to control the efforts of local authorities on behalf of public
health. Widespread reforms were instituted. Waterworks for
town supply were established on the grand scale, the removal
of sewage was improved, the worst slums were demolished,
food-stuffs were subjected to public inspection.

But this great hygienic movement, valuable above all in that
it awakened a general sense of the importance of promoting
public health, remained for a long time purely empirical. There

were still lacking the scientific means requisite to ascertain whether a source of water supply was or was not free from danger. It was only when bacteriological research had advanced considerably that the necessary light was forthcoming. Insofar as bacteria had been recognised, the campaign of the hygienists was directed against them. These microscopic organisms must be kept away from human beings.

Throughout the nineteenth century the successive returns of cholera gave a shock to the hygienic conscience, and the reappearance of this disease was the touchstone of the value of the measures that had been adopted to further the public health. We have learned that in 1883 Robert Koch discovered the exciting cause of cholera, and further that he ascertained water to be the chief instrument of its distribution. For him, then, the road seemed clear. The comma bacillus polluted the soil or the water supply when these were contaminated with the evacuations of cholera patients, and thus the disease spread. Koch's views, however, were not universally accepted. Among those who opposed them strongly was the Munich hygienist Max Pettenkofer.

Pettenkofer had a totally different theory concerning the spread of cholera. Since 1854 he had been studying this epidemic disease in Bavaria. Like Koch, he was convinced that water had a great deal to do with its spread. Where he differed from Koch was in this, that he believed the subsoil water rather than drinking water to play the principal role. His opinion was that for the occurrence of a cholera epidemic a certain local and temporal disposition was essential. He held, in fact, that there were four requisites:

"1. An inhabited region in which the surface of the ground is permeable to water and air as far down as the level of the subsoil water.

"2. A temporary greater variation in the amount of moisture contained in this stratum—a variation which is most simply and plainly disclosed in alluvial soil by the varying level of the subsoil water, the phase of decline from an exceptionally high level being the time of exceptional danger.

"3. The presence of organic substances, especially those derived from excrements, in the receptive stratum of the soil.

"4. The specific germ, disseminable by human intercourse; the specific cause of cholera, derived for the main part from the intestinal evacuations of patients suffering from choleraic diarrhoea, but perhaps also from the evacuations of apparently healthy persons who have come from districts where cholera is endemic." [Such persons would to-day be called "carriers."]

The two theories were crassly opposed. On the one hand stood Koch and the contagionists, and on the other hand stood Pettenkofer and the localists. In conformity with their respective theories, the two parties advocated absolutely contrasted measures of defence. The contagionists held that the chief means of defence must be disinfection of the stools, the isolation of patients, the supervision of public intercourse, the supply of good drinking water. The localists, on the other hand, opined that isolation and disinfection were useless, inasmuch as the locality and not the patient was for them the originating factor of the disease. They held that the true line of defence was to be found in systematic sanation of the soil of predisposed localities. Of course the supply of good drinking water played a great part among the measures requisite for this sanation. Another indispensable measure was to flee from the cholera, to evacuate threatened settlements.

Koch held that the comma bacilli were the only causes of the disease. What could be easier than to demonstrate the truth or falsehood of this experimentally? On November 12, 1892, Pettenkofer swallowed one cubic centimetre of a fresh bouillon culture of cholera bacilli, enough to poison a regiment. "Even if I be mistaken, and this experiment that I am making imperils my life, I shall look death quietly in the face, for what I am doing is no frivolous or cowardly act of suicide, but I shall die in the service of science as a soldier perishes

391

on the field of honour. Health and life are doubtless worldly possessions of enormous value, but they are not the most valuable of human goods. Man, who wants to occupy a higher position than the beasts, must be ready to sacrifice even life and health on behalf of higher and more ideal goods." Pettenkofer had the luck to remain healthy. Obviously, then, the mere ingestion of the bacillus did not suffice to produce the disease. He was not predisposed, we say; his organism was equipped with natural defensive forces. Anyhow there can be no doubt that the contagionist doctrine which in subsequent years maintained the upper hand for a time, does not explain all the phenomena of an epidemic. No doubt there are plausible theories for explaining the rise and the decline of a pestilence, but they are little more than empty names, and it seems probable that the truth about the causation of cholera is to be found in some sort of combination of the rival theories.

Since 1865, Pettenkofer had been professor of hygiene at Munich. He had not originally intended to devote himself to public health, having reached it by a circuitous route. The son of a peasant, he was destined by the family to become an apothecary, like his uncle. For a time he was refractory, and went on the stage. Then he resumed his studies, becoming in 1843 a qualified apothecary, and at the same time taking his degree as doctor of medicine. In Würzburg, and in Giessen under Liebig, he made researches in physiological chemistry, discovering kreatinin, and what is still known as "Pettenkofer's test for the bile acids in the urine." In 1845 he became assistant at the Royal Mint in Munich, and two years later professor of medical chemistry at the university. Over and above his purely theoretical studies (which concerned, among other matters, the periodical system of the chemical elements), he was occupied in various domains of practical work, describing a method for obtaining illuminating gas from wood, and a plan for reviving the colours of old pictures. He gave lectures upon dietetic chemistry, and by this road advanced farther

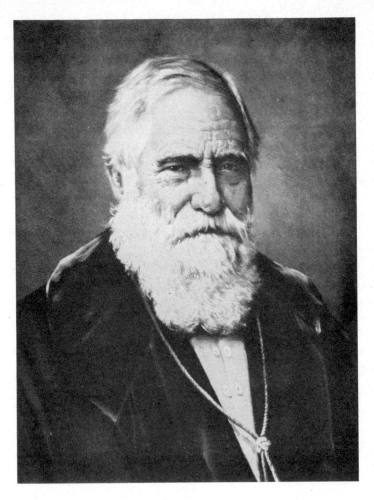

MAX PETTENKOFER, 1818–1901

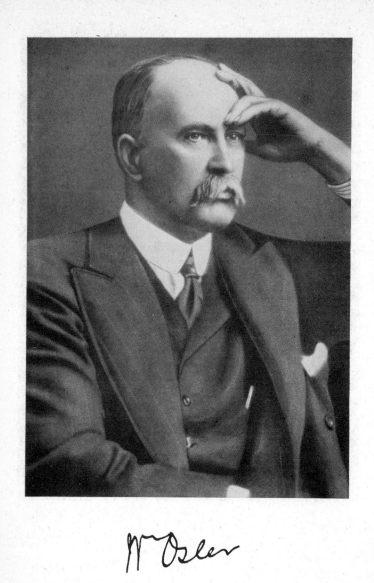

WILLIAM OSLER, 1849–1919

and farther into the domain of hygiene. In 1852 he was appointed ordinary professor, and was given scope for his specialised activities in the Physiological Institute.

Physiology studies the achievements and the apparatus of the organism under normal conditions. When are these conditions normal? At what point do they become abnormal, so that the reactions of the organism are no longer to be regarded as normal but as pathological? What are the best conditions under which to live, and how can these conditions be ensured? Such are the problems hygiene sets itself to solve, and the method for their solution resembles that of physiology, being primarily experimental. Hygiene, therefore, became an experimental science. Pettenkofer's chief service was that he founded this science of experimental hygiene. In the Physiological Institute, and after 1878 in his own Institute, he made researches into the effects of environment upon the life and health of human beings; he studied the atmosphere, clothing, dwelling houses and their ventilation, methods of heating and lighting, the soil, water, dietetics, the terminal products of metabolism and their excretion, the methods of disposing of the dead, etc. A science which had hitherto been purely empirical, was thenceforward placed upon a stable scientific and experimental foundation.

At the age of eighty-three, Pettenkofer, his health being broken, sought a voluntary death. His work was left as his monument. Hygiene had taken an outstanding place in the system of medicine. Since then it has continued to develop, achieving new conquests year by year. To it belongs the future.

CHAPTER FORTY-EIGHT

WILLIAM OSLER
1849–1919

THE New World, America, entered the medical stage!

It was a difficult entry, and all the phases of the history of medicine had to be traversed. At the outset, in the old colonial days, there were very few physicians, so that in this respect the story of New England opens in the period of priestly doctors. The clergy were the leaders of the people, were helpers in bodily distress as well as in spiritual matters. Moreover, just as in Europe the first medical document to be printed was not a textbook but a mere leaflet containing directions for bloodletting, so the medical incunabulum of America was a leaflet. Written by a minister whose name was Thomas Thatcher, it was printed at Boston in the year 1677, and contained advice as to behaviour in times when smallpox became epidemic. Life was hard in those early days, a perpetual struggle with the elements and with the hostile aborigines. The colonists were ravaged by one pestilence after another. Still, they kept their eyes open, following the progress of medical science in the homeland with close attention, so that inoculation with smallpox was introduced into Boston as early as 1721, long before it had obtained a footing upon the European continent.

Like the doctors of ancient Greece, the doctors of the North American colonists were handicraftsmen, who learned their profession as apprentices to a master physician. Moreover, even as a physician in Hellas sometimes took resident patients, housing them in the "iatreion," so did it happen here; and even as during the Middle Ages in Europe "xenodochia" came into being, rest-houses for the sick as well as for travellers (the precursors of our modern hospitals), so did it happen in America.

394

A good many doctors supplemented their apprenticeship by a period of study in foreign parts. In this respect, Edinburgh was the favourite university. The colonials took a medical degree there, recrossed the Atlantic, communicated what they had learned in the Old World, and engaged apprentices. Philadelphia was the busiest centre of intellectual life. It was there that Benjamin Franklin lived and worked; it was there that the first true hospital was established, in the year 1752; and it was there likewise that the first American medical faculty came into being, founded in 1765 by John Morgan, a young doctor who had been trained in Europe. Three years later, a medical school was started in New York, and in 1783 yet a third medical school was founded, this one being attached to Harvard University. A vigorous process had begun, and it closely resembled that which was taking place in Europe.

Then came the revolution, the war with England. On July 4, 1776, the thirteen colonies declared their independence and coalesced to form the United States of America. When the nineteenth century had opened, the great westward movement began, an epic conquest. In an endless succession, the pioneers marched forth into the West, clearing the primeval forest, cultivating the soil. When the forest belt had been traversed, they reached the prairie. This, too, they crossed; they climbed over the Rocky Mountains; until at length they reached the Pacific, where the coast had long ere this been occupied by the scattered Spanish missions. A vast area had been opened up, one fitted for the settlement of millions upon millions of human beings.

It need hardly be said that these developments imposed arduous tasks upon the medical science of the day. No one recognised this more clearly than Daniel Drake (1785–1852), a "hundred per cent. American," who never set foot upon European soil. He saw that the newly acquired territories must be scientifically studied in order to make them healthier, to make them more habitable for the settlers; and he wrote an epoch-making work, a *Treatise on the Principal Diseases of the Interior Valley of North America* (1850–1854). He was aware that the new country stood in great need of doctors, and he therefore founded several new medical schools. The movement caught on. Throughout the nineteenth century, these new schools came into being by the hundred, training doctors with the extremely inadequate means at their disposal. Obviously, in certain circumstances, the level of medical training could not fail to be a low one. When the Civil War broke out in 1861, imposing such severe stresses upon the Union, anarchical conditions prevailed in the medical art and science of America.

Yet even during this period of elementary expansion, the United States made important contributions to the healing art. In 1809, Ephraim McDowell, a doctor who lived in the highlands of Kentucky, was the first operator in the world who had the courage to remove an ovarian tumour. In 1833, another pioneer, a western army surgeon named William Beaumont, wrote (before Claude Bernard) a book upon the gastric juice and the physiology of digestion, the outcome of many years' observation and experiment upon a man suffering from a gastric fistula. The first to devise a successful method for operating upon vesico-vaginal fistulae was a South Carolina surgeon named James Marion Sims, who became the founder of operative gynecology, and who acquired a wide reputation on the eastern side of the Atlantic as well as in his native land. At Boston, in the year 1843, Oliver Wendell Holmes (poet, essayist, and novelist as well as physician) described, before Semmelweis, the infective nature and the contagious character of puerperal fever. Almost at the same date, and likewise from Boston, there came in 1846 the great boon of ether anaesthesia.

After the Civil War, the Americans began to become aware of the need for setting their medical house in order. The medical faculty of Johns Hopkins University at Baltimore played a notable part in this process of purification and reconstruction. The university, which took its name from the man of business who had been its founder, was opened in the year 1876. At first it consisted only of a philosophical faculty, affording instruction in letters and science to graduate students, and having attached to it a collegiate department for undergraduates; but in 1893 a medical school, opened by the Johns Hopkins Hospital, came to form part of the university. As far as the construction of the medical faculty was concerned, the scheme was worked out slowly and with the utmost care. Something entirely new for America was to be created, not a sort of elementary training school which should turn out doctors after two years' theoretical study, but a focus of medical research. Clinical instruction and laboratory work were to count for more than attendance at lectures. In fact, the Johns Hopkins medical school was to be a medical faculty in the European sense, and that was why the Hospital was built before the medical school was opened. Manifestly the fate of the institution would largely depend upon the choice of the medical and surgical staff. At this juncture, William Osler was called in to advise.

A Canadian of Celtic stock, the son of a minister of religion, he was originally intended to adopt his father's profession. Having grown up in a rural community, close to the primeval forest, he then went to study at Trinity College in Toronto. Having early begun to take an interest in natural science, he soon abandoned the idea of becoming a clergyman, and devoted himself to medicine. He studied the elements at the McGill University in Montreal, and took his degree there in 1872. Then he went abroad for post-graduate work. Whereas during the eighteenth century Edinburgh, and during the first half of the nineteenth century Paris, had been the Mecca of American medical students, these were now inclining more and more towards Germany and Austria. However, to begin with, Osler went to London, working there fifteen months at histology and physiology, and becoming an expert microscopist. Thereafter he proceeded to Berlin and to Vienna. Although German customs and ways of thought were so alien to his upbringing, he was quick to recognise the importance of German clinical medicine and of German laboratory research. He sat under Virchow, and attended the clinics of Frerichs and Traube at the Charité. In Vienna, Rokitansky and Skoda were still at work, but they were well up in years, and it was the Viennese specialists, above all, who were a lure to foreign students.

Returning to Canada in 1874, Osler soon became professor of medical institutions at McGill University. In 1884, he accepted a summons to become professor of clinical medicine in the University of Pennsylvania. Five years later, he removed to Baltimore.

Doctors who live on the continent of Europe find it hard to form a picture of Osler's influence. They know his name as that of a distinguished clinician; they know his scientific writings, and a good many of them are acquainted with his *Principles and Practice of Medicine*, which has been translated into various languages, including German. But as soon as a German physician enters English-speaking lands, he finds himself in a domain where Osler's spirit has universally made itself felt. As for the United States, from the Atlantic to the Pacific he will find a picture of Osler hanging on the wall in almost every doctor's house. Anecdotes regarding Osler are rife. A myth is beginning to accrete round his figure. We feel that in him a personality that radiated influence and induced profound conviction must have been at work, and that he has left deep traces in the history of medicine. In the endeavour to fathom the mystery of this influence, we turn to his writings. His textbook of medicine is unquestionably an admirable one, and even to-day, more than a dozen years after his death, it is still the most widely read work of the kind in England and the United States. But there have been many other excellent textbooks of medicine. Strümpell's probably had an even more remarkable success.

Osler did a great deal of original scientific work, not only in the domain of clinical medicine, but in a number of kindred fields. He was one of the first to describe the blood-platelets, and his name will remain associated with the clinical picture of a considerable number of diseases. But the period of his life activities was extraordinarily fruitful to medical science, and among his contemporaries there was an abundance of distinguished clinical investigators.

The explanation of Osler's fame is to be found elsewhere. His renown depends upon his personality as physician, as teacher, as man. We cannot but be struck by the parallel with Hermann Boerhaave. Boerhaave, too, made no outstanding discoveries. His books, valuable though they were, would never have accounted for his wide reputation. As we have learned in a previous chapter, what distinguished Boerhaave from his contemporaries was that he was the greatest clinical teacher in early eighteenth-century Europe, was a magnet continually attracting pupils to Leyden, was a man who taught juniors how to watch and how to think at the bedside of the sick, was one who inspired medical students with an enthusiasm for the healing art and filled them with the physician's ethos.

It was the same with Osler. But what made his influence so persistent was the fortunate circumstance that he came to the right place at the right moment. The Johns Hopkins Hospital was opened in 1889. Clinical work was begun there at once, though four years were to elapse before the medical faculty was completed. In the autumn of 1893, the medical school opened its doors. Here was now assembled a galaxy of talent unprecedented in America: William H. Welsh, the organiser of scientific medicine in America, a student under Ludwig and Cohnheim, was pathologist; Franklin Paine Mall, who had worked in Leipzig with His and Ludwig, was anatomist; John J. Abel, a pupil of Schmiedeberg, was pharmacologist; Halsted was surgeon; Kelly was gynecologist; and Osler was the leading clinician. Most of them had studied under German teachers, and they were fully aware of the importance of the task they had undertaken.

Those first years at Johns Hopkins were glorious years. Everything was new. There was no tradition to impose fetters upon growth. All the workers were young and enthusiastic, and Osler had scope for the full development of his personality. He worked with his pupils, lived with them, joked with them made doctors and investigators of them. His clinic was like a seething kettle of scientific life.

What gave the man so widespread an influence was that, in contradistinction to so many of the noted European clinicians of that day, he was no mere one-sided man of science. Although he did more than any one else to introduce precise laboratory methods and exact science into the field of American clinical medicine, he was a born humanist. He loved books, collected them, and read them by the score. But he was not one of those neo-humanists who believe that the world can be bettered in accordance with some fixed program. Scientific synthesis was for him something to be regarded as a matter of course, and was achieved in his character and in his work. In 1889, at the very opening of his activities at Johns Hopkins, he founded a society for the study of the history of medicine which is still an active nucleus of humanism.

In 1905, Osler left Baltimore. He was suffering from overwork, and therefore accepted a call to Oxford as professor of medicine—the highest distinction open to a British physician. But though he was absent in the flesh, in the spirit he remained active in America, for his ideas continued to bear fruit among his pupils and pupils' pupils. He had worked for twenty years in the United States, creating a ferment which will prove undying.

At Oxford, his hospitable home was always open to American

doctors. A heavy blow befell him in 1917 when his only son was killed at Ypres. Two years later, when William Osler was hard upon seventy, he also passed away. His library was sent back to America, to the McGill University in Montreal, where he had taken his medical degree.

The example of Johns Hopkins University exercised a lasting influence. The reorganisation of American medicine was greatly accelerated. In 1901, the Rockefeller Institute for Medical Research was opened. The less creditable medical faculties were closed, and new, admirably designed institutions took their places. The United States, in these matters, had the advantage of being able to study the millenniary experience of Europe. But the pioneer spirit played its part as well. Where, only three centuries ago, medicine-men still practised their unsavoury art, the methods of research and the methods of treatment are among the most advanced in the world. America is now coming to play a more and more important part in the concert of universal medicine.

POSTFACE

I HAVE reached the end of my story of the great doctors. But history continues its unceasing march. Acting and creating, each of us in his place, we form part of its progress. The tempo of evolution has slackened a little as compared with that of a few decades back. The stage, on the other hand, has widened, for now the United States of America, Russia, and Japan form parts of it, each of these countries being actively engaged in our common struggle against illness. The last few years have brought new and important discoveries, those, for instance, which have given doctors fresh powers of coping with such diseases as diabetes and pernicious anaemia. Wider and ever wider strata of the population receive medical care. The idea of prophylaxis perpetually gains ground. The average duration of life is continually increasing, so that one who is born to-day has an expectation of life which is nearly sixty years, whereas half a century ago the expectation was only thirty-five years.

Strange and multifarious figures have passed before our gaze, men of the most diversified kind, simple practitioners, persons exclusively devoted to surgery, adventurers, philosophers, and above all students of natural science—those who, with the scalpel, the microscope, and the test-tube, did their utmost to wrest her secrets from nature in order to win control over nature, in order to burst the fetters that hamper us, so that man may become free to fulfil his mission. Epic figures many of them have been, heroes who were unwearied in cutting off the heads of the hydra of disease wherever these might show themselves.

Many years of study have made me acquainted with the lives and works of the great doctors. Their lives have, in a sense, become part of my own, and I have tried to hand on my experience to others. The reader must decide how far I have succeeded. I have invented nothing. All that I have related in the foregoing book, down to the minutest detail, is vouched for by the writings of the doctors concerned or by contemporary sources. Still, what I have chiefly tried to do is to make the sources intelligible to the minds of my contemporaries. The reader must take my word for it that I have chapter and verse for every statement. I did not wish to swell my book by the needless citation of authorities, which would have interrupted the thread of my discourse. The expert knows the sources, and for the non-expert their mention would have been superfluous.

The illustrations are not added for merely ornamental purposes. A man's countenance, when we know how to look at it, will often tell us more than many words. Even his signature may be a guide to us, for it is certainly part of his personality.

To the private persons and public authorities whose kindness has enabled me to enrich my book in this way, I tender my sincerest thanks.

It is with regret that I bid farewell to the great doctors with whom this year I have been living day in and day out. They make their bow and bid you farewell. My hope is that they will have convinced you of the grandeur of the struggle which, in this domain, the human mind has carried on and is still carrying on against nature untamed.

HENRY E. SIGERIST

LEIPZIG, *September* 1931

BIBLIOGRAPHY

THE author has not aimed at compiling a full bibliography, having been content to mention a few of the more important and especially the most recent works relating to the subjects of the various chapters. He hopes that enough has been done to guide the reader who needs additional information regarding the great doctors whose lives and works are discussed in this book.

I. GENERAL TREATISES ON THE HISTORY OF MEDICINE AND KINDRED TOPICS

Sudhoff, Karl, *Kurzes Handbuch der Geschichte der Medizin* (third and fourth editions of J. L. Pagel's Einführung in die Geschichte der Medizin, Berlin, 1922).

Meyer-Steineg, T., and Sudhoff, Karl, *Geschichte der Medizin im Ueberblick mit Abbildungen*, third edition, Jena, 1928.

Neuburger, Max, *Geschichte der Medizin*, two vols., Stuttgart, 1906–1911.

Neuburger, Max, and Pagel, Julius, *Handbuch der Geschichte der Medizin*, originated by T. Puschmann, three vols., Jena, 1902–1905.

Diepgen, Paul, *Geschichte der Medizin* (Goeschen Collection), five vols., Berlin and Leipzig, 1914–1928.

Castiglioni, Arturo, *Storia della medicina*, Milan, 1927.

Garrison, Fielding H., *An Introduction to the History of Medicine*, fourth edition, Philadelphia and London, 1929.

Sigerist, Henry E., *Einführung in die Medizin*, Leipzig, 1931.— English translation by Margaret Boise, *Man and Medicine*, George Allen and Unwin, Ltd., London, 1932.

II. SPECIAL WORKS ON GREAT DOCTORS

ASCLEPIADES OF PRUSA.

Vilas, Hans von, *Der Arzt und Philosoph Asklepiades von Bithynien*, Vienna and Leipzig, 1903.

Wellmann, Max, *Asklepiades aus Bithynien von einem herrschenden Vorurteil befreit*, "Neue Jahrb. f. d. klass. Altertum, Geschichte u. deutsche Literatur," vol. xxi, Leipzig, 1909.

AESCULAPIUS.

Wilamowitz-Moellendorf, M. von, *Isyllos von Epidauros*, Berlin, 1886.

Jayne, Walter Addison, *The Healing Gods of Ancient Civilisation*, New Haven, 1925.

Herzog, Rudolf, *Die Wunderheilungen von Epidauros*, Leipzig, 1931.

Defrasse, A., and Lechat, H., *Epidaure*, Paris, 1895.

Besnier, Maurice, *L'île tiberine dans l'antiquité*, Paris, 1902.

Sigerist, H. E., *Sebastian-Apollo*, "Arch. f. Geschichte d. Med.," vol. xix, 1927, pp. 301–317.

AUENBRUGGER, LEOPOLD.

Neuburger, Max, *Leopold Auenbruggers Inventum Novum*, a facsimile of the first edition, with Corvisart's French translation, Forbes' English translation, Ungar's German translation, and a biographical sketch, Vienna and Leipzig, 1922.

Fossel, V., a translation of the *Inventum Novum*, "Klassiker der Medizin," Leipzig, 1912.

Clar, *Leopold Auenbrugger, der Erfinder der Perkussion des Brustkorbs u. s. Inventum Novum*, Graz, 1867.

AVICENNA.

Wüstenfeld, F., *Geschichte der arabischen Aerzte und Naturforscher*, Göttingen, 1840.

Leclerc, L., *Histoire de la médecine arabe*, Paris, 1876.

Browne, E. G., *Arabian Medicine*, Cambridge, 1921.

Carra de Vaux, *Avicenna*, Paris, 1900.

BAGLIVI, GIORGIO.

Salomon, Max, *Giorgio Baglivi und seine Zeit*, Berlin, 1889.

Fabre, Paul, *Un médecin italien de la fin du XVII*e *siècle, Georges Baglivi, rectifications biographiques*, Paris, 1896.

Castiglioni, Arturo, *Di un illustre medico raguseo del secolo decimosetto (Giorgio Baglivi)*, "Riv. di Storia crit. delle Scienze mediche e naturali," vol. iv, 1921, pp. 1–11.

BERNARD, CLAUDE.

L'oeuvre de Claude Bernard (Bibliography, with essays by E. Renan, Paul Bert, Armand Moreau), Paris, 1881.

Faure, Jean Louis, *Claude Bernard*, Paris, 1925.

BICHAT, XAVIER.

Corvisart, *Notice sur X. Bichat*, Paris, 1802.

Roux, *Boyer et Bichat*, Paris, 1851.

BILLROTH, THEODOR.

Briefe von Theodor Billroth, eighth edition, Hanover and Leipzig, 1910.

Fischer, I., *Theodor Billroth und seine Zeitgenossen, in Briefen an Billroth*, Berlin and Vienna, 1929.

BIBLIOGRAPHY

Huber, Arnold, *Theodor Billroth in Zürich*, 1860–1867, Zurich, 1924.

Gersuny, R., *Theodor Billroth*, Vienna, 1922.

BOERHAAVE, HERMANN.

Hirzel, Ludwig (as editor) *Albrecht Hallers Tagebücher seiner Reisen nach Deutschland, Holland und England*, 1723–1727, Leipzig, 1883.

Articles by van Leersum, Zeeman, Neuburger, Cohen, Kroon, Hunger, de Lint, and Martin, in "Janus, Archives internationales pour l'Histoire de la Médecine et la Géographie Médicale," vol. xxiii, 1918.

BROUSSAIS, F. J. V.

Reis, Paul, *Etude sur Broussais et sur son oeuvre*, Paris, 1869.

CONSTANTINE OF AFRICA.

Creutz, Rudolf, *Der Arzt Constantinus Africanus von Montekassino*, "Stud. u. Mitt. z. Gesch. d. Benedictinerordens," vol. xlvii, 1929, pp. 1–44.

Creutz, Rudolf, *Die Ehrenrettung Konstantins von Afrika*, ibid., vol. xlix, 1931, pp. 25–44.

Sudhoff, Karl, *Konstantin der Afrikaner und die Medizinschule von Salerno*, "Arch. f. Gesch. d. Med.," vol. xxiii, 1930, pp. 293–298.

CORVISART, JEAN NICOLAS.

Héchemann, Louis, *Corvisart et la percussion*, Paris, 1906.

Lassus, J. M., *Corvisart et la cardiologie*, Paris, 1927.

Busquet, Paul, *Aphorismes de médecine clinique par le baron Corvisart*, Paris, 1929.

DE HAEN, ANTON.

See the entries under van Swieten. Also:

Lebert, H., *Ueber den Einfluss der Wiener Schule des vorigen Jahrhunderts auf den positiven Fortschritt in der Medizin*, Berlin, 1865.

Petersen, J., *Hauptmomente in der älteren Geschichte der med. Klinik*, Copenhagen, 1890.

Neuburger, M., *Anton de Haen als Experimentalforscher*, "Wiener Med. Presse," 1898, no. 42.

DIOCLES OF CARYSTUS.

Wellman, M. (as editor), *Die Fragmente der sikelischen Aerzte Akron, Philistion und des Diokles von Karystos*, Berlin, 1901.

EHRLICH, PAUL.

Festschrift zu Ehrlichs 60. Geburtstag, Jena, 1914.

Lazarus, *Paul Ehrlich*, 1922.

Marquardt, Martha, *Paul Ehrlich als Mensch und Arbeiter*, Berlin and Leipzig, 1924.

ERASISTRATUS.

Fuchs, Robert, *Erasistratea quae in librorum memoria latent, congesta enarrantur*, a dissertation, Berlin, 1892.

FRACASTORO, GIROLAMO.

Biography, in the introduction to *Opera omnia*, Venice, 1555.

Barberini, E., *Girolamo Fracastoro e le sue opere*, Venice, 1891.

Rossi, G., *Girolamo Fracastoro in relazione all' Aristotelismo e alle scienze nel rinascimento*, Pisa, 1893.

Massalongo, R., *Girolamo Fracastoro e la rinascenza della medicina in Italia*, Venice, 1915.

FRANK, JOHANN PETER.

Autobiography, Vienna, 1802.

Doll, K., *Dr. J. P. Frank*, Carlsruhe, 1909.

Schmitz, K. E. F., *Die Bedeutung Johann Peter Franks für die Entwicklung der sozialen Hygiene*, Berlin, 1917.

Neuburger, Max, *Das alte medizinische Wien in zeitgenössischen Schilderungen*, Vienna and Leipzig, 1921.

GALEN.

Galeni opera omnia, edited by C. G. Kühn, Leipzig, 1821–1833.

Oeuvres anatomiques, physiologiques et médicales de Galien, translated by Charles Daremberg, two vols., Paris, 1854–1856.

Ilberg, J., *Ueber die Schriftstellerei des Klaudios Galenos*, "Rheinisches Museum," vols. xliv, xlvii, li, and lii, 1889–1897.

Ilberg, J., *Aus Galens Praxis, ein Kulturbild aus der römischen Kaiserzeit*, Leipzig, 1905.

HAEN, ANTON DE, see De Haen.

HALLER, ALBRECHT VON.

Irsay, S. d', *Albrecht von Haller, eine Studie zur Geistesgeschichte der Aufklärung*, "Arbeiten des Instituts für Geschichte der Medizin an der Universität Leipzig," vol. i, Leipzig, 1930 (contains additional bibliographical material).

Zimmermann, Johann Georg, *Das Leben des Herrn von Haller*, Zurich, 1755.

Hirzel, Ludwig, *Albrecht von Hallers Gedichte*, vol. i, *Hallers Leben und Dichtungen*, Frauenfeld and Leipzig, 1917.

Sigerist, H. E. (as editor), *Albrecht von Hallers Briefe an Johannes Gesner* (1728–1777), "Abhandl. d. Kgl. Gesell. d. Wiss. zu Göttingen," New Series, vol. xi, Berlin, 1923.

BIBLIOGRAPHY

HARVEY, WILLIAM.

Sigerist, H. E. (as editor), *Exercitatio anatomica de motu cordis et sanguinis in animalibus*, a facsimile, in "Monumenta Medica," vol. v, Florence, 1928.

Die Bewegung des Herzens und des Blutes, a translation by R. von Töply, "Klassiker der Medizin," vol. i, Leipzig, 1910.

Willis, R., *William Harvey*, London, 1878.

Singer, Charles, *The Discovery of the Circulation of the Blood*, London, 1922.

Sigerist, H. E., *William Harveys Stellung in der europäischen Geistesgeschichte*, "Arch. f. Kulturgesch," vol. xix, 1928, pp. 158–168.

HELMHOLTZ, HERMANN.

Königsberger, Leo, *Hermann von Helmholtz*, three vols., Brunswick, 1903.

HELMONT, see Van Helmont.

HENLE, JAKOB.

The section on Miasmata and Contagia, *Pathologische Untersuchungen*, in "Klassiker der Medizin," vol. iii, Leipzig, 1910.

Merkel, F., *Jakob Henle, ein deutsches Gelehrtenleben*, Brunswick, 1891.

HERACLIDES OF TARENTUM.

Deichgräber, Karl, *Die griechische Empirikerschule, Sammlung der Fragmente und Darstellung der Lehre*, Berlin, 1930.

HEROPHILUS OF CHALCEDON.

Marx, K. F. H., *Herophilos, ein Beitrag zur Geschichte der Medizin*, Carlsruhe and Baden, 1838.

De Herophili celeberrimi medici vita scriptis atque in medicina meritis, Göttingen, 1842.

HIPPOCRATES.

Oeuvres complètes d'Hippocrate, new translation with the Greek text facing the French version, by E. Littré, ten vols., Paris, 1839–1861.

Editions of parts of the Hippocratic writings: by Ilberg and Kühlewein, Leipzig, 1894–1902; by W. H. S. Jones, with English translation, Loeb Classical Library, London, 1923; by Heiberg, in Corpus Medicorum Graecorum, Berlin and Leipzig, 1927.

Hippokrates sämmtliche Werke, a translation by R. Fuchs, three vols., Munich, 1895–1900.

Hirschberg, Julius, *Vorlesungen über hippokratische Heilkunde*, Leipzig, 1922.

Sudhoff, Karl, *Kos und Knidos*, Munich, 1927.

Edelstein, Ludwig, *Peri aëron und die Sammlung der hippokratischen Schriften*, Berlin, 1931.

HUNTER, JOHN.
Paget, Stephen, *John Hunter, Man of Science and Surgeon* (1728–1793), London, 1897.

IMHOTEP.
Sethe, Kurt, *Imhotep, der Asklepios der Aegypter, ein vergötteter Mensch aus der Zeit des Königs Doser*, Leipzig, 1902.
Hurry, Jamieson B., *Imhotep the Vizier and Physician of King Zoser and afterwards the Egyptian God of Medicine*, Oxford, 1928.

JENNER, EDWARD.
A facsimile of the Inquiry was published at Milan in 1923, and a German translation appeared in "Klassiker der Medizin," vol. x, Leipzig, 1911.
Baron, John, *The Life of Edward Jenner*, London, 1827.
Creighton, Charles, *Jenner and Vaccination*, London, 1889.

KOCH, ROBERT.
Writings on Anthrax and Tuberculosis in "Klassiker der Medizin," vols. ix and xix, Leipzig, 1910 and 1912.
Becher, W., *Robert Koch*, Berlin (undated).
Wezel, Karl, *Robert Koch*, Berlin, 1912.
Kirchner, Martin, *Robert Koch*, Vienna and Berlin, 1924.

LAENNEC, R. T. H.
Saintignon, H., *Laennec, sa vie et son oeuvre*, Paris, 1904.
Rouxeau, Alfred, *Laennec avant* 1806; *Laennec après* 1806; Paris, 1912, 1920.

LISTER, JOSEPH.
First publications regarding the antiseptic treatment of wounds, "Klassiker der Medizin," vol. xvii, Leipzig, 1912.
Wrench, G. T., *Lord Lister, his Life and Work*, London, 1913.
Godlee, Rickman John, *Six Papers by Lord Lister, with a Short Biography and Explanatory Notes*, London, 1921.
Cheyne, W. Watson, *Lister and his Achievement*, New York, 1925.

MALPIGHI, MARCELLO.
Möbius, M. (as editor and translator), *Marcellus Malpighi's Die Anatomie der Pflanzen*, Ostwald's "Klassiker," no. 120, Leipzig, 1901.
Atti, Gaetano, *Notizie edite ed inedite della vita e delle opere di Marcello Malpighi e di Lorenzo Bellini*, Bologna, 1847.

BIBLIOGRAPHY

Cardini, M., *La vita e l'opera di Marcello Malpighi*, Rome, 1927.

Franchini, F., *Marcello Malpighi*, Bologna, 1930.

MORGAGNI, GIOVANNI BATTISTA.

Virchow, R., *Morgagni und der anatomische Gedanke*, Berlin, 1894.

Falk, F., *Die pathologische Anatomie und Physiologie der Joh. Bapt. Morgagni*, Berlin, 1887.

Carteggio inedito di Giambattista Morgagni con Giovanni Bianchi, with introduction and notes by G. Bilancioni and A. Bignami, Bari, 1914.

Bilancioni, Guglielmo, *Giambattista Morgagni*, Rome, 1922.

MÜLLER, JOHANNES.

Virchow, R., *Johannes Müller, ein Gedächtnisrede*, Berlin, 1888.

Bois-Reymond, Emil du, *Gedächtnisrede auf Johannes Müller*, Berlin, 1860.

Haberling, Wilhelm, *Johannes Müller, das Leben des rheinischen Naturforschers*, Leipzig, 1924.

Müller, Martin, *Ueber die philosophischen Anschauungen des Naturforschers Johannes Müller*, Leipzig, 1927.

OSLER, WILLIAM.

Cushing, Harvey, *The Life of Sir William Osler*, two vols., Oxford, 1925.

Reid, Edith Gittings, *The Great Physician, a Short Life of Sir William Osler*, London, New York, and Toronto, 1931.

"Bulletin of the International Association of Medical Museums and Journal of Technical Methods," Sir William Osler Memorial Number, Appreciations and Reminiscences, Montreal, 1926.

PARACELSUS.

Theophrast von Hohenheim gen. Paracelsus, *Sämtliche Werke*, I. Abt. *Medizinische naturwissenschaftliche und philosophische Schriften*, edited by Karl Sudhoff, Munich, 1922 and foll.

Paracelsus, *Sämtliche Werke*, translated into modern German by Berhard Aschner, Jena, 1926 and foll.

Paracelsus, *Volumen Paramirum* (Of Disease and a Healthy Life), edited and annotated by Joh. Daniel Achelis, Jena, 1928.

Theophrastus Paracelsus, *Das Buch Paragranum*, edited by Franz Strunz, Leipzig, 1903.

Theophrast von Hohenheim (Paracelsus), *Sieben Defensiones und Labyrinthus medicorum errantium*, edited by Karl Sudhoff, Leipzig, 1916.

Theophrastus Paracelsus, *Labyrinthus medicorum* (Doctors' Blunders), Insel-Bücherei, no. 366, Leipzig (undated).

Schriften, *Theophrasts von Hohenheim gen. Paracelsus,* selections by H. Kayser, Leipzig, 1921.

Netzhammer, Pater Raymund, O.S.B., *Theophrastus Paracelsus,* Einsiedeln, Waldshut, and Cologne, 1901.

Strunz, Franz, *Theophrastus Paracelsus, sein Leben und seine Persön-lichkeit,* Leipzig, 1903.

Gundolf, Friedrich, *Paracelsus,* Berlin, 1927.

PARÉ, AMBROISE.

Malgaigne, J. F., *Oeuvres complètes d'Ambroise Paré,* three vols., Paris, 1840.

Sigerist, H. E. (as editor and translator), *Ambroise Paré, Die Behandlung der Schusswunden,* Leipzig, 1923.

Le Paulmier, *Ambroise Paré,* Paris, 1884.

Paget, Stephen, *Ambroise Paré and his Times,* London, 1897.

Packard, Francis R., *Life and Times of Ambroise Paré,* New York, 1921.

Mirabaud, Robert, *Une grande âme: Ambroise Paré,* Paris, 1928.

Escheviennes, Carlos d', *La vie d'Ambroise Paré,* Paris, 1930.

PASTEUR, LOUIS E.

Duclaux, E., *Pasteur,* Paris, 1896.

Vallery-Radot, René, *La vie de Pasteur,* 1903.

PETTENKOFER, MAX.

Voit, Carl von, *Max von Pettenkofer zum Gedächtnis,* Munich, 1902.

Erismann, F., *Max von Pettenkofer,* Leipzig, 1901.

PIETRO D'ABANO.

Ferrari, S., *I tempi, la vita, la dottrine di Pietro d'Abano,* Genoa, 1900.

Norpoth, Leo, *Zur Bio- Bibliographie und Wissenschaftslehre des Pietro d'Abano,* "Kyklos," vol. iii, 1930, pp. 292–353.

PINEL, PHILIPPE.

Semelaigne, R., *Aliénistes et philanthropes, Les Pinels et les Tukes,* Paris, 1912.

RHAZES.

Consult the literature under Avicenna. Also:

Ruska, *Al-Biruni als Quelle für das Leben und die Schriften al-Razis,* "Isis," vol. v, 1923, pp. 26–50.

ROKITANSKY, KARL.

Wunderlich, C. A., *Wien und Paris,* Stuttgart, 1841.

Müller, Martin, *Rokitanskys Krasenlehre,* "Arch. f. Gesch. d. Med.," vol. xxiii, 1930, pp. 10–39.

SANTORIO, SANTORIO.

Castiglioni, Arturo, *La vita e l'opera di Santorio Santorio Capodi-striano,* Bologna and Trieste, 1920.

BIBLIOGRAPHY

SCHÖNLEIN, JOHANN LUKAS.
  Virchow, R., *Gedächtnisrede auf Joh. Lukas Schönlein*, Berlin, 1865.
SCHOOL OF SALERNO.
  Renzi, S. de, *Collectio Salernitana*, five vols., Naples, 1852–1859.
  Renzi, S. de, *Storia documentata della Scuola di Salerno*, Naples, 1857.
  Giacosa, Piero, *Magistri Salernitani nondum editi*, Turin, 1901.
  Capparoni, Pietro, *Magistri Salernitani nondum cogniti*, London, 1923.
  Hartmann, F., *Die Literatur von Früh- und Hochsalerno*, a dissertation, Leipzig, 1919.
SEMMELWEIS, IGNAZ PHILIPP.
  Semmelweis, I. P., *Gesammelte Werke*, edited by T. von Györy, 1905.
  Semmelweis, I. P., *Aetiologie, Begriff und Prophylaxis des Kindbettfiebers*, "Klassiker der Medizin," vol. xviii, Leipzig, 1912.
  Hegar, A., *I. P. Semmelweis, sein Leben und seine Lehre*, Freiburg, 1882.
  Holmes, Oliver Wendell, "The Contagiousness of Puerperal Fever," in *Medical Essays*, Boston and New York, 1861.
  Schürer von Waldheim, Felix, *I. P. Semmelweis, sein Leben und Wirken*, Vienna, 1905.
  Malade, Theo, *Semmelweis, der Retter der Mütter, der Roman eines ärztlichen Lebens*, Munich, 1924.
SKODA, JOSEPH.
  Wunderlich, C. A., *Wien und Paris*, Stuttgart, 1841.
  Sternberg, Maximilian, *Josef Skoda*, Vienna, 1924.
SORANUS OF EPHESUS.
  Sorani Gynaeciorum libri IV, de signis fracturarum, de fasciis, vita Hippocratis secundum Soranum, ed. J. Ilberg, Leipzig and Berlin, 1927.
  Die Gynaekologie des Soranus von Ephesus, translated into German by H. Lüneberg, Munich, 1894.
  Meyer-Steineg, T., *Das medizinische System der Methodiker*, Jena, 1916.
  Buchheim, Ernst, *Die geburtshilflichen Operationen und zugehörigen Instrumente des Klassischen Altertums*, Jena, 1916.
STAHL, GEORG ERNST.
  Koch, Richard, *War Georg Ernst Stahl ein selbständiger Denker?* "Arch. f. Gesch. d. Med.," vol. xviii, 1926, pp. 20–50.
  Metzger, Hélène, *Newton, Stahl, Boerhaave et la doctrine chimique*, Paris, 1930.
  Lemoine, Albert, *Stahl et l'animisme*, Paris, 1858.
  Lemoine, Albert, *Le vitalisme et l'animisme de Stahl*, Paris, 1864.
SWIETEN, see Van Swieten.

SYDENHAM, THOMAS.
Sydenham, *Tractatus de Podagra et Hydrope*, reprinted in German translation in "Klassiker der Medizin," vol. vi, Leipzig, 1910.
Comrie, John D., *Selected Works of Thomas Sydenham*, London, 1922.
Picard, Frédéric, *Sydenham, sa vie, ses oeuvres*, Paris and London, 1889.
Payne, Joseph Frank, *Thomas Sydenham*, London, 1900.
Andrae, Heinrich, *Ueber die Medizin Thomas Sydenhams*, Leipzig, 1900.
Riesman, David, *Thomas Sydenham, Clinician*, New York, 1926.
Temkin, O., *Die Krankheitsauffassung von Hippokrates und Sydenham in ihren "Epidemien,"* "Arch. f. Gesch. d. Med.," vol. xx, 1928, pp. 327–352.
SYLVIUS, FRANZ DE LE BOË.
See under Part I of this Bibliography, General Treatises, etc.

VAN HELMONT, JAN BAPTISTA VON.
Pagel, Walter, *Joh. Bapt. van Helmont, Einführung in die philosophische Medizin des Barock*, Berlin, 1930.
Pagel, Walter, *Helmont, Leibnitz, Stahl*, "Arch. f. Gesch. d. Med.," vol. xxiv, 1931, pp. 19–59.
Strunz, Franz, *Johann Baptist van Helmont, ein Beitrag zur Geschichte der Naturwissenschaften*, Leipzig and Vienna, 1907.
VAN SWIETEN, GERHARD.
Müller, W., *Gerhard van Swieten. Biographischer Beitrag zur Geschichte der Aufklärung in Oesterreich*, Vienna, 1883.
Puschmann, T., *Die Medizin in Wien während der letzten 100 Jahre*, Vienna, 1889.
Neuburger, M., *Entwicklung der Medizin in Oesterreich*, Vienna and Leipzig, 1918.
VERSALIUS, ANDREAS.
Holl, M., and Sudhoff, Karl (as editors), *Des Andreas Vesalius sechs anatomische Tafeln vom Jahre* 1538, Leipzig, 1920.
Roth, M., *Andreas Vesalius Bruxellensis*, Berlin, 1892.
Sudhoff, Karl, *Andreas Vesalius zu Ehren*, "Arch. f. Gesch. d. Med.," vol. xxi, 1929, pp. 131–155.
Spielmann, M. H., *The Iconography of Andreas Vesalius*, London, 1925.
VIRCHOW, RUDOLF.
Virchow, Rudolf, *Briefe an seine Eltern, 1839–1864*, Leipzig, 1906.
Sudhoff, Karl, *Rudolf Virchow und die Deutschen Naturforscherversammlungen*, Leipzig, 1922.
Becher, W., *Rudolf Virchow, eine Biographische Studie*, Berlin, 1894.

BIBLIOGRAPHY

Marchand, F., *Rudolf Virchow als Pathologe*, Munich, 1902.
Waldeyer, W., *Gedächtnisrede auf Rudolf Virchow*, Berlin, 1903.
Pagel, J., *Rudolf Virchow*, Berlin, 1906.
Posner, C., *Rudolf Virchow*, Vienna, 1921.
Hirschfeld, E., *Virchow*, "Kyklos," vol. ii, 1929, pp. 106–116.
Pagel, Walter, *Rudolf Virchow*, Jena, 1932.

WUNDERLICH, CARL AUGUST.
Heubner, O., *C. A. Wunderlich*, Leipzig, 1878.

INDEX

INDEX

INDEX

421

INDEX

INDEX

428

INDEX

INDEX

435

A CATALOGUE OF SELECTED DOVER BOOKS
IN ALL FIELDS OF INTEREST

A CATALOGUE OF SELECTED DOVER BOOKS
IN ALL FIELDS OF INTEREST

AMERICA'S OLD MASTERS, James T. Flexner. Four men emerged unexpectedly from provincial 18th century America to leadership in European art: Benjamin West, J. S. Copley, C. R. Peale, Gilbert Stuart. Brilliant coverage of lives and contributions. Revised, 1967 edition. 69 plates. 365pp. of text.
21806-6 Paperbound $3.00

FIRST FLOWERS OF OUR WILDERNESS: AMERICAN PAINTING, THE COLONIAL PERIOD, James T. Flexner. Painters, and regional painting traditions from earliest Colonial times up to the emergence of Copley, West and Peale Sr., Foster, Gustavus Hesselius, Feke, John Smibert and many anonymous painters in the primitive manner. Engaging presentation, with 162 illustrations. xxii + 368pp.
22180-6 Paperbound $3.50

THE LIGHT OF DISTANT SKIES: AMERICAN PAINTING, 1760-1835, James T. Flexner. The great generation of early American painters goes to Europe to learn and to teach: West, Copley, Gilbert Stuart and others. Allston, Trumbull, Morse; also contemporary American painters—primitives, derivatives, academics—who remained in America. 102 illustrations. xiii + 306pp.
22179-2 Paperbound $3.00

A HISTORY OF THE RISE AND PROGRESS OF THE ARTS OF DESIGN IN THE UNITED STATES, William Dunlap. Much the richest mine of information on early American painters, sculptors, architects, engravers, miniaturists, etc. The only source of information for scores of artists, the major primary source for many others. Unabridged reprint of rare original 1834 edition, with new introduction by James T. Flexner, and 394 new illustrations. Edited by Rita Weiss. 6⅝ x 9⅝.
21695-0, 21696-9, 21697-7 Three volumes, Paperbound $13.50

EPOCHS OF CHINESE AND JAPANESE ART, Ernest F. Fenollosa. From primitive Chinese art to the 20th century, thorough history, explanation of every important art period and form, including Japanese woodcuts; main stress on China and Japan, but Tibet, Korea also included. Still unexcelled for its detailed, rich coverage of cultural background, aesthetic elements, diffusion studies, particularly of the historical period. 2nd, 1913 edition. 242 illustrations. lii + 439pp. of text.
20364-6, 20365-4 Two volumes, Paperbound $6.00

THE GENTLE ART OF MAKING ENEMIES, James A. M. Whistler. Greatest wit of his day deflates Oscar Wilde, Ruskin, Swinburne; strikes back at inane critics, exhibitions, art journalism; aesthetics of impressionist revolution in most striking form. Highly readable classic by great painter. Reproduction of edition designed by Whistler. Introduction by Alfred Werner. xxxvi + 334pp.
21875-9 Paperbound $2.50

VISUAL ILLUSIONS: THEIR CAUSES, CHARACTERISTICS, AND APPLICATIONS, Matthew Luckiesh. Thorough description and discussion of optical illusion, geometric and perspective, particularly; size and shape distortions, illusions of color, of motion; natural illusions; use of illusion in art and magic, industry, etc. Most useful today with op art, also for classical art. Scores of effects illustrated. Introduction by William H. Ittleson. 100 illustrations. xxi + 252pp.

21530-X Paperbound $2.00

A HANDBOOK OF ANATOMY FOR ART STUDENTS, Arthur Thomson. Thorough, virtually exhaustive coverage of skeletal structure, musculature, etc. Full text, supplemented by anatomical diagrams and drawings and by photographs of undraped figures. Unique in its comparison of male and female forms, pointing out differences of contour, texture, form. 211 figures, 40 drawings, 86 photographs. xx + 459pp. 5⅜ x 8⅜.

21163-0 Paperbound $3.50

150 MASTERPIECES OF DRAWING, Selected by Anthony Toney. Full page reproductions of drawings from the early 16th to the end of the 18th century, all beautifully reproduced: Rembrandt, Michelangelo, Dürer, Fragonard, Urs, Graf, Wouwerman, many others. First-rate browsing book, model book for artists. xviii + 150pp. 8⅜ x 11¼.

21032-4 Paperbound $2.50

THE LATER WORK OF AUBREY BEARDSLEY, Aubrey Beardsley. Exotic, erotic, ironic masterpieces in full maturity: Comedy Ballet, Venus and Tannhauser, Pierrot, Lysistrata, Rape of the Lock, Savoy material, Ali Baba, Volpone, etc. This material revolutionized the art world, and is still powerful, fresh, brilliant. With *The Early Work,* all Beardsley's finest work. 174 plates, 2 in color. xiv + 176pp. 8⅛ x 11.

21817-1 Paperbound $3.00

DRAWINGS OF REMBRANDT, Rembrandt van Rijn. Complete reproduction of fabulously rare edition by Lippmann and Hofstede de Groot, completely reedited, updated, improved by Prof. Seymour Slive, Fogg Museum. Portraits, Biblical sketches, landscapes, Oriental types, nudes, episodes from classical mythology—All Rembrandt's fertile genius. Also selection of drawings by his pupils and followers. "Stunning volumes," *Saturday Review.* 550 illustrations. lxxviii + 552pp. 9⅛ x 12¼.

21485-0, 21486-9 Two volumes, Paperbound $7.00

THE DISASTERS OF WAR, Francisco Goya. One of the masterpieces of Western civilization—83 etchings that record Goya's shattering, bitter reaction to the Napoleonic war that swept through Spain after the insurrection of 1808 and to war in general. Reprint of the first edition, with three additional plates from Boston's Museum of Fine Arts. All plates facsimile size. Introduction by Philip Hofer, Fogg Museum. v + 97pp. 9⅜ x 8¼.

21872-4 Paperbound $2.00

GRAPHIC WORKS OF ODILON REDON. Largest collection of Redon's graphic works ever assembled: 172 lithographs, 28 etchings and engravings, 9 drawings. These include some of his most famous works. All the plates from *Odilon Redon: oeuvre graphique complet,* plus additional plates. New introduction and caption translations by Alfred Werner. 209 illustrations. xxvii + 209pp. 9⅛ x 12¼.

21966-8 Paperbound $4.00

DESIGN BY ACCIDENT; A BOOK OF "ACCIDENTAL EFFECTS" FOR ARTISTS AND DESIGNERS, James F. O'Brien. Create your own unique, striking, imaginative effects by "controlled accident" interaction of materials: paints and lacquers, oil and water based paints, splatter, crackling materials, shatter, similar items. Everything you do will be different; first book on this limitless art, so useful to both fine artist and commercial artist. Full instructions. 192 plates showing "accidents," 8 in color. viii + 215pp. 8⅜ x 11¼.   21942-9 Paperbound $3.50

THE BOOK OF SIGNS, Rudolf Koch. Famed German type designer draws 493 beautiful symbols: religious, mystical, alchemical, imperial, property marks, runes, etc. Remarkable fusion of traditional and modern. Good for suggestions of timelessness, smartness, modernity. Text. vi + 104pp. 6⅛ x 9¼.
                    20162-7 Paperbound $1.25

HISTORY OF INDIAN AND INDONESIAN ART, Ananda K. Coomaraswamy. An unabridged republication of one of the finest books by a great scholar in Eastern art. Rich in descriptive material, history, social backgrounds; Sunga reliefs, Rajput paintings, Gupta temples, Burmese frescoes, textiles, jewelry, sculpture, etc. 400 photos. viii + 423pp. 6⅜ x 9¾.   21436-2 Paperbound $4.00

PRIMITIVE ART, Franz Boas. America's foremost anthropologist surveys textiles, ceramics, woodcarving, basketry, metalwork, etc.; patterns, technology, creation of symbols, style origins. All areas of world, but very full on Northwest Coast Indians. More than 350 illustrations of baskets, boxes, totem poles, weapons, etc. 378 pp.
                    20025-6 Paperbound $3.00

THE GENTLEMAN AND CABINET MAKER'S DIRECTOR, Thomas Chippendale. Full reprint (third edition, 1762) of most influential furniture book of all time, by master cabinetmaker. 200 plates, illustrating chairs, sofas, mirrors, tables, cabinets, plus 24 photographs of surviving pieces. Biographical introduction by N. Bienenstock. vi + 249pp. 9⅞ x 12¾.   21601-2 Paperbound $4.00

AMERICAN ANTIQUE FURNITURE, Edgar G. Miller, Jr. The basic coverage of all American furniture before 1840. Individual chapters cover type of furniture— clocks, tables, sideboards, etc.—chronologically, with inexhaustible wealth of data. More than 2100 photographs, all identified, commented on. Essential to all early American collectors. Introduction by H. E. Keyes. vi + 1106pp. 7⅞ x 10¾.
                    21599-7, 21600-4 Two volumes, Paperbound $11.00

PENNSYLVANIA DUTCH AMERICAN FOLK ART, Henry J. Kauffman. 279 photos, 28 drawings of tulipware, Fraktur script, painted tinware, toys, flowered furniture, quilts, samplers, hex signs, house interiors, etc. Full descriptive text. Excellent for tourist, rewarding for designer, collector. Map. 146pp. 7⅞ x 10¾.
                    21205-X Paperbound $2.50

EARLY NEW ENGLAND GRAVESTONE RUBBINGS, Edmund V. Gillon, Jr. 43 photographs, 226 carefully reproduced rubbings show heavily symbolic, sometimes macabre early gravestones, up to early 19th century. Remarkable early American primitive art, occasionally strikingly beautiful; always powerful. Text. xxvi + 207pp. 8⅜ x 11¼.   21380-3 Paperbound $3.50

ALPHABETS AND ORNAMENTS, Ernst Lehner. Well-known pictorial source for decorative alphabets, script examples, cartouches, frames, decorative title pages, calligraphic initials, borders, similar material. 14th to 19th century, mostly European. Useful in almost any graphic arts designing, varied styles. 750 illustrations. 256pp. 7 x 10.   21905-4 Paperbound $4.00

PAINTING: A CREATIVE APPROACH, Norman Colquhoun. For the beginner simple guide provides an instructive approach to painting: major stumbling blocks for beginner; overcoming them, technical points; paints and pigments; oil painting; watercolor and other media and color. New section on "plastic" paints. Glossary. Formerly *Paint Your Own Pictures*. 221pp.   22000-1 Paperbound $1.75

THE ENJOYMENT AND USE OF COLOR, Walter Sargent. Explanation of the relations between colors themselves and between colors in nature and art, including hundreds of little-known facts about color values, intensities, effects of high and low illumination, complementary colors. Many practical hints for painters, references to great masters. 7 color plates, 29 illustrations. x + 274pp.
20944-X Paperbound $2.75

THE NOTEBOOKS OF LEONARDO DA VINCI, compiled and edited by Jean Paul Richter. 1566 extracts from original manuscripts reveal the full range of Leonardo's versatile genius: all his writings on painting, sculpture, architecture, anatomy, astronomy, geography, topography, physiology, mining, music, etc., in both Italian and English, with 186 plates of manuscript pages and more than 500 additional drawings. Includes studies for the Last Supper, the lost Sforza monument, and other works. Total of xlvii + 866pp. 7⅞ x 10¾.
22572-0, 22573-9 Two volumes, Paperbound $10.00

MONTGOMERY WARD CATALOGUE OF 1895. Tea gowns, yards of flannel and pillow-case lace, stereoscopes, books of gospel hymns, the New Improved Singer Sewing Machine, side saddles, milk skimmers, straight-edged razors, high-button shoes, spittoons, and on and on . . . listing some 25,000 items, practically all illustrated. Essential to the shoppers of the 1890's, it is our truest record of the spirit of the period. Unaltered reprint of Issue No. 57, Spring and Summer 1895. Introduction by Boris Emmet. Innumerable illustrations. xiii + 624pp. 8½ x 11⅝.
22377-9 Paperbound $6.95

THE CRYSTAL PALACE EXHIBITION ILLUSTRATED CATALOGUE (LONDON, 1851). One of the wonders of the modern world—the Crystal Palace Exhibition in which all the nations of the civilized world exhibited their achievements in the arts and sciences—presented in an equally important illustrated catalogue. More than 1700 items pictured with accompanying text—ceramics, textiles, cast-iron work, carpets, pianos, sleds, razors, wall-papers, billiard tables, beehives, silverware and hundreds of other artifacts—represent the focal point of Victorian culture in the Western World. Probably the largest collection of Victorian decorative art ever assembled—indispensable for antiquarians and designers. Unabridged republication of the Art-Journal Catalogue of the Great Exhibition of 1851, with all terminal essays. New introduction by John Gloag, F.S.A. xxxiv + 426pp. 9 x 12.
22503-8 Paperbound $4.50

A History of Costume, Carl Köhler. Definitive history, based on surviving pieces of clothing primarily, and paintings, statues, etc. secondarily. Highly readable text, supplemented by 594 illustrations of costumes of the ancient Mediterranean peoples, Greece and Rome, the Teutonic prehistoric period; costumes of the Middle Ages, Renaissance, Baroque, 18th and 19th centuries. Clear, measured patterns are provided for many clothing articles. Approach is practical throughout. Enlarged by Emma von Sichart. 464pp.   21030-8 Paperbound $3.50

Oriental Rugs, Antique and Modern, Walter A. Hawley. A complete and authoritative treatise on the Oriental rug—where they are made, by whom and how, designs and symbols, characteristics in detail of the six major groups, how to distinguish them and how to buy them. Detailed technical data is provided on periods, weaves, warps, wefts, textures, sides, ends and knots, although no technical background is required for an understanding. 11 color plates, 80 halftones, 4 maps. vi + 320pp. 6⅛ x 9⅛.   22366-3 Paperbound $5.00

Ten Books on Architecture, Vitruvius. By any standards the most important book on architecture ever written. Early Roman discussion of aesthetics of building, construction methods, orders, sites, and every other aspect of architecture has inspired, instructed architecture for about 2,000 years. Stands behind Palladio, Michelangelo, Bramante, Wren, countless others. Definitive Morris H. Morgan translation. 68 illustrations. xii + 331pp.   20645-9 Paperbound $2.50

The Four Books of Architecture, Andrea Palladio. Translated into every major Western European language in the two centuries following its publication in 1570, this has been one of the most influential books in the history of architecture. Complete reprint of the 1738 Isaac Ware edition. New introduction by Adolf Placzek, Columbia Univ. 216 plates. xxii + 110pp. of text. 9½ x 12¾.
21308-0 Clothbound $10.00

Sticks and Stones: A Study of American Architecture and Civilization, Lewis Mumford.One of the great classics of American cultural history. American architecture from the medieval-inspired earliest forms to the early 20th century; evolution of structure and style, and reciprocal influences on environment. 21 photographic illustrations. 238pp.   20202-X Paperbound $2.00

The American Builder's Companion, Asher Benjamin. The most widely used early 19th century architectural style and source book, for colonial up into Greek Revival periods. Extensive development of geometry of carpentering, construction of sashes, frames, doors, stairs; plans and elevations of domestic and other buildings. Hundreds of thousands of houses were built according to this book, now invaluable to historians, architects, restorers, etc. 1827 edition. 59 plates. 114pp. 7⅞ x 10¾.
22236-5 Paperbound $3.00

Dutch Houses in the Hudson Valley Before 1776, Helen Wilkinson Reynolds. The standard survey of the Dutch colonial house and outbuildings, with constructional features, decoration, and local history associated with individual homesteads. Introduction by Franklin D. Roosevelt. Map. 150 illustrations. 469pp. 6⅝ x 9¼.   21469-9 Paperbound $4.00

THE ARCHITECTURE OF COUNTRY HOUSES, Andrew J. Downing. Together with Vaux's *Villas and Cottages* this is the basic book for Hudson River Gothic architecture of the middle Victorian period. Full, sound discussions of general aspects of housing, architecture, style, decoration, furnishing, together with scores of detailed house plans, illustrations of specific buildings, accompanied by full text. Perhaps the most influential single American architectural book. 1850 edition. Introduction by J. Stewart Johnson. 321 figures, 34 architectural designs. xvi + 560pp.
22003-6 Paperbound $4.00

LOST EXAMPLES OF COLONIAL ARCHITECTURE, John Mead Howells. Full-page photographs of buildings that have disappeared or been so altered as to be denatured, including many designed by major early American architects. 245 plates. xvii + 248pp. 7⅞ x 10¾.
21143-6 Paperbound $3.50

DOMESTIC ARCHITECTURE OF THE AMERICAN COLONIES AND OF THE EARLY REPUBLIC, Fiske Kimball. Foremost architect and restorer of Williamsburg and Monticello covers nearly 200 homes between 1620-1825. Architectural details, construction, style features, special fixtures, floor plans, etc. Generally considered finest work in its area. 219 illustrations of houses, doorways, windows, capital mantels. xx + 314pp. 7⅞ x 10¾.
21743-4 Paperbound $4.00

EARLY AMERICAN ROOMS: 1650-1858, edited by Russell Hawes Kettell. Tour of 12 rooms, each representative of a different era in American history and each furnished, decorated, designed and occupied in the style of the era. 72 plans and elevations, 8-page color section, etc., show fabrics, wall papers, arrangements, etc. Full descriptive text. xvii + 200pp. of text. 8⅜ x 11¼.
21633-0 Paperbound $5.00

THE FITZWILLIAM VIRGINAL BOOK, edited by J. Fuller Maitland and W. B. Squire. Full modern printing of famous early 17th-century ms. volume of 300 works by Morley, Byrd, Bull, Gibbons, etc. For piano or other modern keyboard instrument; easy to read format. xxxvi + 938pp. 8⅜ x 11.
21068-5, 21069-3 Two volumes, Paperbound $10.00

KEYBOARD MUSIC, Johann Sebastian Bach. Bach Gesellschaft edition. A rich selection of Bach's masterpieces for the harpsichord: the six English Suites, six French Suites, the six Partitas (Clavierübung part I), the Goldberg Variations (Clavierübung part IV), the fifteen Two-Part Inventions and the fifteen Three-Part Sinfonias. Clearly reproduced on large sheets with ample margins; eminently playable. vi + 312pp. 8⅛ x 11.
22360-4 Paperbound $5.00

THE MUSIC OF BACH: AN INTRODUCTION, Charles Sanford Terry. A fine, nontechnical introduction to Bach's music, both instrumental and vocal. Covers organ music, chamber music, passion music, other types. Analyzes themes, developments, innovations. x + 114pp.
21075-8 Paperbound $1.25

BEETHOVEN AND HIS NINE SYMPHONIES, Sir George Grove. Noted British musicologist provides best history, analysis, commentary on symphonies. Very thorough, rigorously accurate; necessary to both advanced student and amateur music lover. 436 musical passages. vii + 407 pp.
20334-4 Paperbound $2.75

JOHANN SEBASTIAN BACH, Philipp Spitta. One of the great classics of musicology, this definitive analysis of Bach's music (and life) has never been surpassed. Lucid, nontechnical analyses of hundreds of pieces (30 pages devoted to St. Matthew Passion, 26 to B Minor Mass). Also includes major analysis of 18th-century music. 450 musical examples. 40-page musical supplement. Total of xx + 1799pp.
(EUK) 22278-0, 22279-9 Two volumes, Clothbound $17.50

MOZART AND HIS PIANO CONCERTOS, Cuthbert Girdlestone. The only full-length study of an important area of Mozart's creativity. Provides detailed analyses of all 23 concertos, traces inspirational sources. 417 musical examples. Second edition. 509pp. (USO) 21271-8 Paperbound $3.50

THE PERFECT WAGNERITE: A COMMENTARY ON THE NIBLUNG'S RING, George Bernard Shaw. Brilliant and still relevant criticism in remarkable essays on Wagner's Ring cycle, Shaw's ideas on political and social ideology behind the plots, role of Leitmotifs, vocal requisites, etc. Prefaces. xxi + 136pp.
21707-8 Paperbound $1.50

DON GIOVANNI, W. A. Mozart. Complete libretto, modern English translation; biographies of composer and librettist; accounts of early performances and critical reaction. Lavishly illustrated. All the material you need to understand and appreciate this great work. Dover Opera Guide and Libretto Series; translated and introduced by Ellen Bleiler. 92 illustrations. 209pp.
21134-7 Paperbound $1.50

HIGH FIDELITY SYSTEMS: A LAYMAN'S GUIDE, Roy F. Allison. All the basic information you need for setting up your own audio system: high fidelity and stereo record players, tape records, F.M. Connections, adjusting tone arm, cartridge, checking needle alignment, positioning speakers, phasing speakers, adjusting hums, trouble-shooting, maintenance, and similar topics. Enlarged 1965 edition. More than 50 charts, diagrams, photos. iv + 91pp. 21514-8 Paperbound $1.25

REPRODUCTION OF SOUND, Edgar Villchur. Thorough coverage for laymen of high fidelity systems, reproducing systems in general, needles, amplifiers, preamps, loudspeakers, feedback, explaining physical background. "A rare talent for making technicalities vividly comprehensible," R. Darrell, High Fidelity. 69 figures. iv + 92pp. 21515-6 Paperbound $1.25

HEAR ME TALKIN' TO YA: THE STORY OF JAZZ AS TOLD BY THE MEN WHO MADE IT, Nat Shapiro and Nat Hentoff. Louis Armstrong, Fats Waller, Jo Jones, Clarence Williams, Billy Holiday, Duke Ellington, Jelly Roll Morton and dozens of other jazz greats tell how it was in Chicago's South Side, New Orleans, depression Harlem and the modern West Coast as jazz was born and grew. xvi + 429pp.
21726-4 Paperbound $2.50

FABLES OF AESOP, translated by Sir Roger L'Estrange. A reproduction of the very rare 1931 Paris edition; a selection of the most interesting fables, together with 50 imaginative drawings by Alexander Calder. v + 128pp. 6½x9¼.
21780-9 Paperbound $1.50

AGAINST THE GRAIN (A REBOURS), Joris K. Huysmans. Filled with weird images, evidences of a bizarre imagination, exotic experiments with hallucinatory drugs, rich tastes and smells and the diversions of its sybarite hero Duc Jean des Esseintes, this classic novel pushed 19th-century literary decadence to its limits. Full unabridged edition. Do not confuse this with abridged editions generally sold. Introduction by Havelock Ellis. xlix + 206pp.   22190-3 Paperbound $2.00

VARIORUM SHAKESPEARE: HAMLET. Edited by Horace H. Furness; a landmark of American scholarship. Exhaustive footnotes and appendices treat all doubtful words and phrases, as well as suggested critical emendations throughout the play's history. First volume contains editor's own text, collated with all Quartos and Folios. Second volume contains full first Quarto, translations of Shakespeare's sources (Belleforest, and Saxo Grammaticus), Der Bestrafte Brudermord, and many essays on critical and historical points of interest by major authorities of past and present. Includes details of staging and costuming over the years. By far the best edition available for serious students of Shakespeare. Total of xx + 905pp.
21004-9, 21005-7, 2 volumes, Paperbound $7.00

A LIFE OF WILLIAM SHAKESPEARE, Sir Sidney Lee. This is the standard life of Shakespeare, summarizing everything known about Shakespeare and his plays. Incredibly rich in material, broad in coverage, clear and judicious, it has served thousands as the best introduction to Shakespeare. 1931 edition. 9 plates. xxix + 792pp.   (USO) 21967-4 Paperbound $3.75

MASTERS OF THE DRAMA, John Gassner. Most comprehensive history of the drama in print, covering every tradition from Greeks to modern Europe and America, including India, Far East, etc. Covers more than 800 dramatists, 2000 plays, with biographical material, plot summaries, theatre history, criticism, etc. "Best of its kind in English," New Republic. 77 illustrations. xxii + 890pp.
20100-7 Clothbound $8.50

THE EVOLUTION OF THE ENGLISH LANGUAGE, George McKnight. The growth of English, from the 14th century to the present. Unusual, non-technical account presents basic information in very interesting form: sound shifts, change in grammar and syntax, vocabulary growth, similar topics. Abundantly illustrated with quotations. Formerly Modern English in the Making. xii + 590pp.
21932-1 Paperbound $3.50

AN ETYMOLOGICAL DICTIONARY OF MODERN ENGLISH, Ernest Weekley. Fullest, richest work of its sort, by foremost British lexicographer. Detailed word histories, including many colloquial and archaic words; extensive quotations. Do not confuse this with the Concise Etymological Dictionary, which is much abridged. Total of xxvii + 830pp. 6½ x 9¼.
21873-2, 21874-0 Two volumes, Paperbound $6.00

FLATLAND: A ROMANCE OF MANY DIMENSIONS, E. A. Abbott. Classic of science-fiction explores ramifications of life in a two-dimensional world, and what happens when a three-dimensional being intrudes. Amusing reading, but also useful as introduction to thought about hyperspace. Introduction by Banesh Hoffmann. 16 illustrations. xx + 103pp.   20001-9 Paperbound $1.00

POEMS OF ANNE BRADSTREET, edited with an introduction by Robert Hutchinson. A new selection of poems by America's first poet and perhaps the first significant woman poet in the English language. 48 poems display her development in works of considerable variety—love poems, domestic poems, religious meditations, formal elegies, "quaternions," etc. Notes, bibliography. viii + 222pp.

22160-1 Paperbound $2.00

THREE GOTHIC NOVELS: THE CASTLE OF OTRANTO BY HORACE WALPOLE; VATHEK BY WILLIAM BECKFORD; THE VAMPYRE BY JOHN POLIDORI, WITH FRAGMENT OF A NOVEL BY LORD BYRON, edited by E. F. Bleiler. The first Gothic novel, by Walpole; the finest Oriental tale in English, by Beckford; powerful Romantic supernatural story in versions by Polidori and Byron. All extremely important in history of literature; all still exciting, packed with supernatural thrills, ghosts, haunted castles, magic, etc. xl + 291pp.

21232-7 Paperbound $2.00

THE BEST TALES OF HOFFMANN, E. T. A. Hoffmann. 10 of Hoffmann's most important stories, in modern re-editings of standard translations: Nutcracker and the King of Mice, Signor Formica, Automata, The Sandman, Rath Krespel, The Golden Flowerpot, Master Martin the Cooper, The Mines of Falun, The King's Betrothed, A New Year's Eve Adventure. 7 illustrations by Hoffmann. Edited by E. F. Bleiler. xxxix + 419pp. 21793-0 Paperbound $2.50

GHOST AND HORROR STORIES OF AMBROSE BIERCE, Ambrose Bierce. 23 strikingly modern stories of the horrors latent in the human mind: The Eyes of the Panther, The Damned Thing, An Occurrence at Owl Creek Bridge, An Inhabitant of Carcosa, etc., plus the dream-essay, Visions of the Night. Edited by E. F. Bleiler. xxii + 199pp. 20767-6 Paperbound $1.50

BEST GHOST STORIES OF J. S. LEFANU, J. Sheridan LeFanu. Finest stories by Victorian master often considered greatest supernatural writer of all. Carmilla, Green Tea, The Haunted Baronet, The Familiar, and 12 others. Most never before available in the U. S. A. Edited by E. F. Bleiler. 8 illustrations from Victorian publications. xvii + 467pp. 20415-4 Paperbound $3.00

THE TIME STREAM, THE GREATEST ADVENTURE, AND THE PURPLE SAPPHIRE— THREE SCIENCE FICTION NOVELS, John Taine (Eric Temple Bell). Great American mathematician was also foremost science fiction novelist of the 1920's. *The Time Stream,* one of all-time classics, uses concepts of circular time; *The Greatest Adventure,* incredibly ancient biological experiments from Antarctica threaten to escape; The *Purple Sapphire,* superscience, lost races in Central Tibet, survivors of the Great Race. 4 illustrations by Frank R. Paul. v + 532pp.

21180-0 Paperbound $3.00

SEVEN SCIENCE FICTION NOVELS, H. G. Wells. The standard collection of the great novels. Complete, unabridged. *First Men in the Moon, Island of Dr. Moreau, War of the Worlds, Food of the Gods, Invisible Man, Time Machine, In the Days of the Comet.* Not only science fiction fans, but every educated person owes it to himself to read these novels. 1015pp. 20264-X Clothbound $5.00

LAST AND FIRST MEN AND STAR MAKER, TWO SCIENCE FICTION NOVELS, Olaf Stapledon. Greatest future histories in science fiction. In the first, human intelligence is the "hero," through strange paths of evolution, interplanetary invasions, incredible technologies, near extinctions and reemergences. Star Maker describes the quest of a band of star rovers for intelligence itself, through time and space: weird inhuman civilizations, crustacean minds, symbiotic worlds, etc. Complete, unabridged. v + 438pp. 21962-3 Paperbound $2.50

THREE PROPHETIC NOVELS, H. G. WELLS. Stages of a consistently planned future for mankind. *When the Sleeper Wakes,* and *A Story of the Days to Come,* anticipate *Brave New World* and *1984,* in the 21st Century; *The Time Machine,* only complete version in print, shows farther future and the end of mankind. All show Wells's greatest gifts as storyteller and novelist. Edited by E. F. Bleiler. x + 335pp. (USO) 20605-X Paperbound $2.25

THE DEVIL'S DICTIONARY, Ambrose Bierce. America's own Oscar Wilde—Ambrose Bierce—offers his barbed iconoclastic wisdom in over 1,000 definitions hailed by H. L. Mencken as "some of the most gorgeous witticisms in the English language." 145pp. 20487-1 Paperbound $1.25

MAX AND MORITZ, Wilhelm Busch. Great children's classic, father of comic strip, of two bad boys, Max and Moritz. Also Ker and Plunk (Plisch und Plumm), Cat and Mouse, Deceitful Henry, Ice-Peter, The Boy and the Pipe, and five other pieces. Original German, with English translation. Edited by H. Arthur Klein; translations by various hands and H. Arthur Klein. vi + 216pp.
20181-3 Paperbound $2.00

PIGS IS PIGS AND OTHER FAVORITES, Ellis Parker Butler. The title story is one of the best humor short stories, as Mike Flannery obfuscates biology and English. Also included, That Pup of Murchison's, The Great American Pie Company, and Perkins of Portland. 14 illustrations. v + 109pp. 21532-6 Paperbound $1.00

THE PETERKIN PAPERS, Lucretia P. Hale. It takes genius to be as stupidly mad as the Peterkins, as they decide to become wise, celebrate the "Fourth," keep a cow, and otherwise strain the resources of the Lady from Philadelphia. Basic book of American humor. 153 illustrations. 219pp. 20794-3 Paperbound $1.50

PERRAULT'S FAIRY TALES, translated by A. E. Johnson and S. R. Littlewood, with 34 full-page illustrations by Gustave Doré. All the original Perrault stories—Cinderella, Sleeping Beauty, Bluebeard, Little Red Riding Hood, Puss in Boots, Tom Thumb, etc.—with their witty verse morals and the magnificent illustrations of Doré. One of the five or six great books of European fairy tales. viii + 117pp. 8⅛ x 11. 22311-6 Paperbound $2.00

OLD HUNGARIAN FAIRY TALES, Baroness Orczy. Favorites translated and adapted by author of the *Scarlet Pimpernel.* Eight fairy tales include "The Suitors of Princess Fire-Fly," "The Twin Hunchbacks," "Mr. Cuttlefish's Love Story," and "The Enchanted Cat." This little volume of magic and adventure will captivate children as it has for generations. 90 drawings by Montagu Barstow. 96pp.
(USO) 22293-4 Paperbound $1.95

THE RED FAIRY BOOK, Andrew Lang. Lang's color fairy books have long been children's favorites. This volume includes Rapunzel, Jack and the Bean-stalk and 35 other stories, familiar and unfamiliar. 4 plates, 93 illustrations x + 367pp.
21673-X Paperbound $2.50

THE BLUE FAIRY BOOK, Andrew Lang. Lang's tales come from all countries and all times. Here are 37 tales from Grimm, the Arabian Nights, Greek Mythology, and other fascinating sources. 8 plates, 130 illustrations. xi + 390pp.
21437-0 Paperbound $2.50

HOUSEHOLD STORIES BY THE BROTHERS GRIMM. Classic English-language edition of the well-known tales — Rumpelstiltskin, Snow White, Hansel and Gretel, The Twelve Brothers, Faithful John, Rapunzel, Tom Thumb (52 stories in all). Translated into simple, straightforward English by Lucy Crane. Ornamented with headpieces, vignettes, elaborate decorative initials and a dozen full-page illustrations by Walter Crane. x + 269pp.
21080-4 Paperbound $2.50

THE MERRY ADVENTURES OF ROBIN HOOD, Howard Pyle. The finest modern versions of the traditional ballads and tales about the great English outlaw. Howard Pyle's complete prose version, with every word, every illustration of the first edition. Do not confuse this facsimile of the original (1883) with modern editions that change text or illustrations. 23 plates plus many page decorations. xxii + 296pp.
22043-5 Paperbound $2.50

THE STORY OF KING ARTHUR AND HIS KNIGHTS, Howard Pyle. The finest children's version of the life of King Arthur; brilliantly retold by Pyle, with 48 of his most imaginative illustrations. xviii + 313pp. 6⅛ x 9¼.
21445-1 Paperbound $2.50

THE WONDERFUL WIZARD OF OZ, L. Frank Baum. America's finest children's book in facsimile of first edition with all Denslow illustrations in full color. The edition a child should have. Introduction by Martin Gardner. 23 color plates, scores of drawings. iv + 267pp.
20691-2 Paperbound $2.25

THE MARVELOUS LAND OF OZ, L. Frank Baum. The second Oz book, every bit as imaginative as the Wizard. The hero is a boy named Tip, but the Scarecrow and the Tin Woodman are back, as is the Oz magic. 16 color plates, 120 drawings by John R. Neill. 287pp.
20692-0 Paperbound $2.50

THE MAGICAL MONARCH OF MO, L. Frank Baum. Remarkable adventures in a land even stranger than Oz. The best of Baum's books not in the Oz series. 15 color plates and dozens of drawings by Frank Verbeck. xviii + 237pp.
21892-9 Paperbound $2.00

THE BAD CHILD'S BOOK OF BEASTS, MORE BEASTS FOR WORSE CHILDREN, A MORAL ALPHABET, Hilaire Belloc. Three complete humor classics in one volume. Be kind to the frog, and do not call him names . . . and 28 other whimsical animals. Familiar favorites and some not so well known. Illustrated by Basil Blackwell. 156pp.
(USO) 20749-8 Paperbound $1.25

EAST O' THE SUN AND WEST O' THE MOON, George W. Dasent. Considered the best of all translations of these Norwegian folk tales, this collection has been enjoyed by generations of children (and folklorists too). Includes True and Untrue, Why the Sea is Salt, East O' the Sun and West O' the Moon, Why the Bear is Stumpy-Tailed, Boots and the Troll, The Cock and the Hen, Rich Peter the Pedlar, and 52 more. The only edition with all 59 tales. 77 illustrations by Erik Werenskiold and Theodor Kittelsen. xv + 418pp. 22521-6 Paperbound $3.00

GOOPS AND HOW TO BE THEM, Gelett Burgess. Classic of tongue-in-cheek humor, masquerading as etiquette book. 87 verses, twice as many cartoons, show mischievous Goops as they demonstrate to children virtues of table manners, neatness, courtesy, etc. Favorite for generations. viii + 88pp. 6½ x 9¼. 22233-0 Paperbound $1.25

ALICE'S ADVENTURES UNDER GROUND, Lewis Carroll. The first version, quite different from the final Alice in Wonderland, printed out by Carroll himself with his own illustrations. Complete facsimile of the "million dollar" manuscript Carroll gave to Alice Liddell in 1864. Introduction by Martin Gardner. viii + 96pp. Title and dedication pages in color. 21482-6 Paperbound $1.25

THE BROWNIES, THEIR BOOK, Palmer Cox. Small as mice, cunning as foxes, exuberant and full of mischief, the Brownies go to the zoo, toy shop, seashore, circus, etc., in 24 verse adventures and 266 illustrations. Long a favorite, since their first appearance in St. Nicholas Magazine. xi + 144pp. 6⅝ x 9¼. 21265-3 Paperbound $1.75

SONGS OF CHILDHOOD, Walter De La Mare. Published (under the pseudonym Walter Ramal) when De La Mare was only 29, this charming collection has long been a favorite children's book. A facsimile of the first edition in paper, the 47 poems capture the simplicity of the nursery rhyme and the ballad, including such lyrics as I Met Eve, Tartary, The Silver Penny. vii + 106pp. 21972-0 Paperbound $1.25

THE COMPLETE NONSENSE OF EDWARD LEAR, Edward Lear. The finest 19th-century humorist-cartoonist in full: all nonsense limericks, zany alphabets, Owl and Pussycat, songs, nonsense botany, and more than 500 illustrations by Lear himself. Edited by Holbrook Jackson. xxix + 287pp. (USO) 20167-8 Paperbound $2.00

BILLY WHISKERS: THE AUTOBIOGRAPHY OF A GOAT, Frances Trego Montgomery. A favorite of children since the early 20th century, here are the escapades of that rambunctious, irresistible and mischievous goat—Billy Whiskers. Much in the spirit of Peck's Bad Boy, this is a book that children never tire of reading or hearing. All the original familiar illustrations by W. H. Fry are included: 6 color plates, 18 black and white drawings. 159pp. 22345-0 Paperbound $2.00

MOTHER GOOSE MELODIES. Faithful republication of the fabulously rare Munroe and Francis "copyright 1833" Boston edition—the most important Mother Goose collection, usually referred to as the "original." Familiar rhymes plus many rare ones, with wonderful old woodcut illustrations. Edited by E. F. Bleiler. 128pp. 4½ x 6⅜. 22577-1 Paperbound $1.25

TWO LITTLE SAVAGES; BEING THE ADVENTURES OF TWO BOYS WHO LIVED AS INDIANS AND WHAT THEY LEARNED, Ernest Thompson Seton. Great classic of nature and boyhood provides a vast range of woodlore in most palatable form, a genuinely entertaining story. Two farm boys build a teepee in woods and live in it for a month, working out Indian solutions to living problems, star lore, birds and animals, plants, etc. 293 illustrations. vii + 286pp.

20985-7 Paperbound $2.50

PETER PIPER'S PRACTICAL PRINCIPLES OF PLAIN & PERFECT PRONUNCIATION. Alliterative jingles and tongue-twisters of surprising charm, that made their first appearance in America about 1830. Republished in full with the spirited woodcut illustrations from this earliest American edition. 32pp. 4½ x 6⅜.

22560-7 Paperbound $1.00

SCIENCE EXPERIMENTS AND AMUSEMENTS FOR CHILDREN, Charles Vivian. 73 easy experiments, requiring only materials found at home or easily available, such as candles, coins, steel wool, etc.; illustrate basic phenomena like vacuum, simple chemical reaction, etc. All safe. Modern, well-planned. Formerly *Science Games for Children*. 102 photos, numerous drawings. 96pp. 6⅛ x 9¼.

21856-2 Paperbound $1.25

AN INTRODUCTION TO CHESS MOVES AND TACTICS SIMPLY EXPLAINED, Leonard Barden. Informal intermediate introduction, quite strong in explaining reasons for moves. Covers basic material, tactics, important openings, traps, positional play in middle game, end game. Attempts to isolate patterns and recurrent configurations. Formerly *Chess*. 58 figures. 102pp. (USO) 21210-6 Paperbound $1.25

LASKER'S MANUAL OF CHESS, Dr. Emanuel Lasker. Lasker was not only one of the five great World Champions, he was also one of the ablest expositors, theorists, and analysts. In many ways, his Manual, permeated with his philosophy of battle, filled with keen insights, is one of the greatest works ever written on chess. Filled with analyzed games by the great players. A single-volume library that will profit almost any chess player, beginner or master. 308 diagrams. xli x 349pp.

20640-8 Paperbound $2.75

THE MASTER BOOK OF MATHEMATICAL RECREATIONS, Fred Schuh. In opinion of many the finest work ever prepared on mathematical puzzles, stunts, recreations; exhaustively thorough explanations of mathematics involved, analysis of effects, citation of puzzles and games. Mathematics involved is elementary. Translated by F. Göbel. 194 figures. xxiv + 430pp. 22134-2 Paperbound $3.00

MATHEMATICS, MAGIC AND MYSTERY, Martin Gardner. Puzzle editor for Scientific American explains mathematics behind various mystifying tricks: card tricks, stage "mind reading," coin and match tricks, counting out games, geometric dissections, etc. Probability sets, theory of numbers clearly explained. Also provides more than 400 tricks, guaranteed to work, that you can do. 135 illustrations. xii + 176pp.

20338-2 Paperbound $1.50

MATHEMATICAL PUZZLES FOR BEGINNERS AND ENTHUSIASTS, Geoffrey Mott-Smith. 189 puzzles from easy to difficult—involving arithmetic, logic, algebra, properties of digits, probability, etc.—for enjoyment and mental stimulus. Explanation of mathematical principles behind the puzzles. 135 illustrations. viii + 248pp.
20198-8 Paperbound $1.75

PAPER FOLDING FOR BEGINNERS, William D. Murray and Francis J. Rigney. Easiest book on the market, clearest instructions on making interesting, beautiful origami. Sail boats, cups, roosters, frogs that move legs, bonbon boxes, standing birds, etc. 40 projects; more than 275 diagrams and photographs. 94pp.
20713-7 Paperbound $1.00

TRICKS AND GAMES ON THE POOL TABLE, Fred Herrmann. 79 tricks and games— some solitaires, some for two or more players, some competitive games—to entertain you between formal games. Mystifying shots and throws, unusual caroms, tricks involving such props as cork, coins, a hat, etc. Formerly *Fun on the Pool Table*. 77 figures. 95pp.
21814-7 Paperbound $1.00

HAND SHADOWS TO BE THROWN UPON THE WALL: A SERIES OF NOVEL AND AMUSING FIGURES FORMED BY THE HAND, Henry Bursill. Delightful picturebook from great-grandfather's day shows how to make 18 different hand shadows: a bird that flies, duck that quacks, dog that wags his tail, camel, goose, deer, boy, turtle, etc. Only book of its sort. vi + 33pp. 6½ x 9¼.   21779-5 Paperbound $1.00

WHITTLING AND WOODCARVING, E. J. Tangerman. 18th printing of best book on market. "If you can cut a potato you can carve" toys and puzzles, chains, chessmen, caricatures, masks, frames, woodcut blocks, surface patterns, much more. Information on tools, woods, techniques. Also goes into serious wood sculpture from Middle Ages to present, East and West. 464 photos, figures. x + 293pp.
20965-2 Paperbound $2.00

HISTORY OF PHILOSOPHY, Julián Marias. Possibly the clearest, most easily followed, best planned, most useful one-volume history of philosophy on the market; neither skimpy nor overfull. Full details on system of every major philosopher and dozens of less important thinkers from pre-Socratics up to Existentialism and later. Strong on many European figures usually omitted. Has gone through dozens of editions in Europe. 1966 edition, translated by Stanley Appelbaum and Clarence Strowbridge. xviii + 505pp.
21739-6 Paperbound $3.00

YOGA: A SCIENTIFIC EVALUATION, Kovoor T. Behanan. Scientific but non-technical study of physiological results of yoga exercises; done under auspices of Yale U. Relations to Indian thought, to psychoanalysis, etc. 16 photos. xxiii + 270pp.
20505-3 Paperbound $2.50

Prices subject to change without notice.
Available at your book dealer or write for free catalogue to Dept. GI, Dover Publications, Inc., 180 Varick St., N. Y., N. Y. 10014. Dover publishes more than 150 books each year on science, elementary and advanced mathematics, biology, music, art, literary history, social sciences and other areas.